*Presented as an
Educational Service*

by

Lederle Laboratories

 *Committed to Pediatric Medicine*

Otitis Media in Infants and Children

Charles D. Bluestone, M.D.

Professor of Otolaryngology
University of Pittsburgh School of Medicine
Director
Department of Pediatric Otolaryngology
Children's Hospital of Pittsburgh
Pittsburgh, PA

Jerome O. Klein, M.D.

Professor of Pediatrics
Boston University School of Medicine
Director
Division of Pediatric Infectious Diseases
Maxwell Finland Laboratory for Infectious Diseases
Associate Director
Department of Pediatrics
Boston City Hospital
Boston, MA

W.B. SAUNDERS COMPANY
Harcourt Brace Jovanovich, Inc.

Philadelphia London Toronto Montreal Sydney Tokyo

W. B. SAUNDERS COMPANY
Harcourt Brace Jovanovich, Inc.

The Curtis Center
Independence Square West
Philadelphia, PA 19106

Library of Congress Cataloging-in-Publication Data

Bluestone, Charles D., 1932–

Otitis media in infants and children.

(Major problems in clinical pediatrics; v. 31)

1. Otitis media in children. I. Klein, Jerome O.,
  1931–   . II. Title. III. Series. [DNLM:
  1. Otitis Media—in infancy and childhood.
  W1 MA492M v.31 / WV 232 B6580]

RF225.B57 1988   618.92′09784   87–4561

ISBN 0–7216–1759–X

Editor: Darlene Cooke
Designer: Karen Giacomucci
Production Manager: Carolyn Naylor
Manuscript Editor: Linda Mills
Illustration Coordinator: Lisa Lambert
Indexer: Ellen Murray

OTITIS MEDIA IN INFANTS AND CHILDREN   ISBN 0–7216–1759–X

Last digit is the print number: 9   8   7   6   5   4   3

To our wives
Patricia and Linda
and to our children
Mark and James
Andrea, Bennett, Adam, Zachary
and grandchildren
Alexander and Evan
for their love, support, and understanding

IN MEMORIAM

The authors dedicate this monograph to the memory of Ben H. Senturia, M.D. (1910–1982), our constant source of inspiration and our colleague and friend, who contributed to our understanding of otitis media. Dr. Senturia was Emeritus Professor of Otolaryngology, Washington University, St. Louis, and Editor of the *Annals of Otology, Rhinology, and Laryngology* for over a decade.

Foreword

To the practicing pediatrician, the problems of acute otitis media and otitis media with effusion are so frequent that in terms of numbers of children involved, this monograph by Charles D. Bluestone and Jerome O. Klein constitutes a very significant publication in this area.

Charles D. Bluestone is an eminent pediatric otolaryngologist, one who has had total immersion in the problems of otitis media. I have elsewhere referred to him as the "Emperor of Otitis Media with Effusion!" Dr. Bluestone received his undergraduate and medical degrees from the University of Pittsburgh. In 1975, he turned his back on Boston, where he had been Professor of Otolaryngology at Tufts University School of Medicine and Director of the Department of Otolaryngology at the Boston City Hospital, to return to Pittsburgh as Professor of Otolaryngology at the University of Pittsburgh School of Medicine and Director of the Department of Otolaryngology at the Children's Hospital of Pittsburgh. (I have yet to forgive him for leaving us.) He has received the Certificate of Award of the American Academy of Otolaryngology—Head and Neck Surgery and has been a member of national and international otolaryngology boards and commissions too numerous to list.

Jerome O. Klein received his undergraduate degree from Union College and his M.D. from Yale University. I have known him since the day when I had the remarkable good sense to appoint him as a pediatric resident at the Boston City Hospital. Following his pediatric training and a fellowship in infectious diseases, he received a Career Development Award from the National Institutes of Health and has been a major contributor to the field of infectious diseases ever since. He became Associate Professor of Pediatrics at the Harvard Medical School and subsequently was appointed Professor of Pediatrics at Boston University School of Medicine and Director of Pediatric Infectious Diseases at Boston City Hospital. He was Editor of the *Red Book* (Report of the Committee on Infectious Diseases, American Academy of Pediatrics, 19th edition, 1982). Dr. Klein has exhibited the same energy and determination as Dr. Bluestone in pursuing the causes and management of acute otitis media and otitis media with effusion in children.

With two such distinguished investigators combining their knowledge and skills, this monograph represents a landmark in pediatrics. One might say of the collaboration of these two individuals that theirs is a medical marriage that had to be made in heaven, if not in the Boston City Hospital.

Drs. Bluestone and Klein have taken on the task of answering or trying to answer the host of questions raised by pediatricians dealing with infants and children who have repeated bouts of acute otitis media or otitis media with effusion. Do the many children who have persistent otitis media with effusion following acute otitis media represent a change in the course of acute otitis media? Did as many children or more have otitis media with effusion in the preantibiotic era? Did antibiotics bring an end to children with chronic draining ears and mastoiditis but set the stage for a low-grade inflammatory process leading to otitis media with effusion? There seems to be no way to compare the two eras, owing to the fact that the diagnosis of middle ear effusion depends so frequently on pneumotoscopy and tympanometry, techniques that were not available in the preantibiotic era. Did the much more commonly used paracentesis or the unaltered course of the infection in the preantibiotic era lessen the likelihood of persistence of otitis media with effusion? With the present widespread use of antibiotics, are viral infections more significant in the etiology of acute otitis media and otitis media with effusion? Is our present-day antimicrobial treatment of acute otitis media too long or too short? After effusion has been present for over three months, is paracentesis as successful as placement of tubes in the termination of effusion? How important is an underlying atopic state in the etiology of acute or recurrent otitis media or otitis media with effusion?

Although the authors do not have all the answers to these and many more questions, their continued collaboration and investigation will reduce the number of questions. In the meantime, let us be grateful for their interest and involvement in these common but important disorders of childhood.

SYDNEY S. GELLIS, M.D.
Professor of Pediatrics
Chairman Emeritus, Department of Pediatrics
Tufts University School of Medicine
Boston, Massachusetts

Preface

Otitis media is one of the most common diseases of childhood, but only in recent years have a growing number of clinicians and scientists concentrated their efforts on studying the epidemiology, etiology, pathogenesis, microbiology, immunology, diagnosis, and management of the disease. We have combined our respective backgrounds in otolaryngology, pediatrics, and infectious disease with our interest in otitis media to present in this monograph the state of knowledge about the inflammatory conditions of the middle ear in infants and children. The text is organized and the information presented in a way that is meant to convey to the reader that otitis media and its related conditions, complications, and sequelae frequently represent a continuum of disease, especially in certain high-risk children and populations. The chapters have not been divided into the classic divisions employed in the past. Terms such as "acute suppurative otitis media" and "chronic serous otitis media" are no longer appropriate or relevant and therefore are not used. The transition from the acute to the chronic stage is only a temporal one, and the etiology and pathogenesis are more than likely the same. The clinician may examine the child at various intervals during this continuum, thus receiving and giving a false impression of the disease. The purpose of the organization and method of presenting the material in this text is to make the clinician aware that even though otitis media may have various causes, the clinical appearance may be similar despite the cause, and conversely, the clinical appearance may be different at different stages of the disease, but the etiology and pathogenesis are likely to be the same.

In addition, information derived from the past literature is difficult to interpret, since most investigators failed to or could not specifically define the disease being studied. For example, an investigation of acute otitis media in children would describe the event, but it was not known whether or not the child had pre-existing chronic disease and the episode being studied represented only a sudden onset of signs and symptoms of an acute process superimposed on the chronic disease. Likewise, past studies of the chronic forms of the disease have only cut across one stage in the disease process without consideration of the antecedent events that might have occurred months or years before.

Much of the information presented in this monograph appeared first in chapters on otitis media written by the same authors in the textbook *Pediatric Otolaryngology* (Bluestone, C. D., and Stool, S. E., eds., W. B. Saunders Co., Philadelphia, Pa., 1983), which was written primarily for the otolaryngologist. This book focuses on material of specific interest to otolaryngologists, physicians responsible for the care of infants and children, audiologists, specialists in speech and language, and psychologists. It includes more recent material based on investigations by the authors and a review of the literature to April, 1987.

We sincerely hope that after reading this monograph, a new concept of otitis media will be evident to the clinician that will aid in the management and prevention of this disease in infants and children.

CHARLES D. BLUESTONE
JEROME O. KLEIN

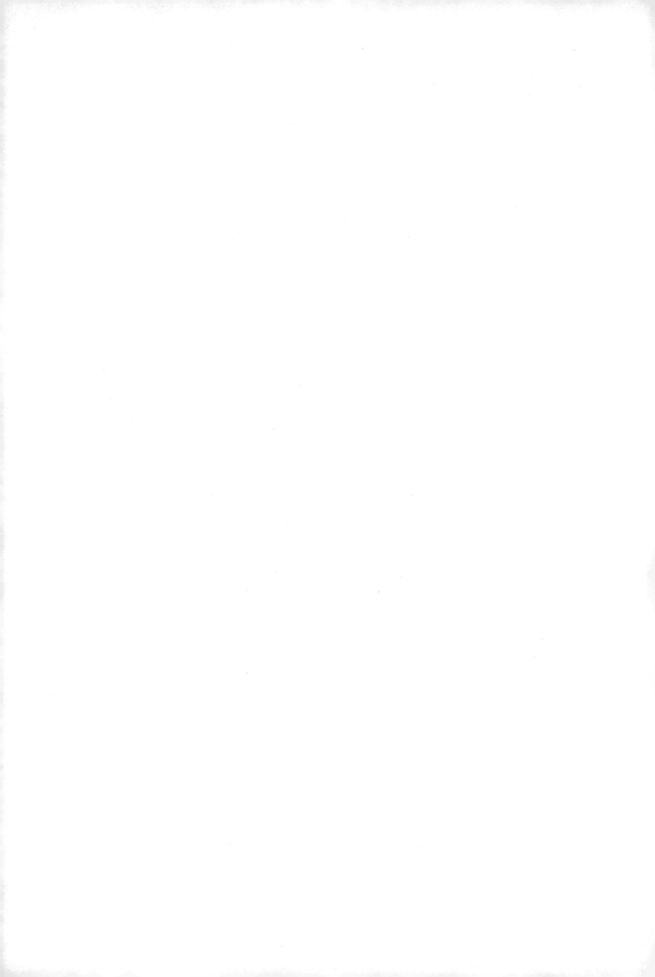

Acknowledgment

The authors are indebted to Sandra K. Arjona, M.L.S., and Mary D. Scheetz, M.L.S., for their editorial assistance in the preparation of this monograph, Mrs. Minnie Johnson for her secretarial assistance, Jon Coulter for his excellent artwork, Robert Coulter and Norman Rabinowitz for their photographic contributions, and William J. Doyle, Ph.D., for assistance in writing the chapter on anatomy.

Contents

1

Definitions, Terminology, and Classification

During the past century, a multitude of terms has emerged to describe the inflammatory conditions of the middle ear. This has resulted in confusion and misunderstanding among clinicians who provide health care to infants and children with ear disease. This confusion impedes appropriate evaluation of studies reported in the literature, since interpretation of results of these investigations depends upon precise definition of the disease studied. In an effort to eliminate ambiguity as much as possible, we have used terminology that meets current understanding of the disease process and have organized the information in a manner that we believe will aid the clinician's understanding of otitis media (Bluestone, 1984).

TERMINOLOGY AND DEFINITIONS

Otitis media is an inflammation of the middle ear, without reference to etiology or pathogenesis.

Middle ear effusion is the liquid resulting from otitis media. The effusion may be either *serous*—thin, watery liquid; *mucoid*—thick, viscid, mucus-like liquid; or *purulent*—pus-like liquid.

Otorrhea is a discharge from the ear.

CLASSIFICATION

The classification presented here is derived from our present knowledge of the disease,

but it is often difficult to determine by history and visual inspection of the tympanic membrane the specific type and stage of otitis media. The physician usually arrives at a presumptive diagnosis of the variety of otitis media present in the patient from limited data, but a more definitive diagnosis could be determined by: (1) Knowledge of the condition of the middle ear prior to onset of the present illness. Such information would differentiate acute, subacute, and chronic forms. A child may have classic signs and symptoms of acute otitis media, but whether or not the middle ear was effusion-free prior to onset of this episode may not be known. (2) Tympanocentesis to determine the characteristics of the middle ear effusion (i.e., serous, mucoid, or purulent). Appropriate cultures of the effusion would define the microbiological features. (3) Biopsy of the middle ear mucosa. Although rarely necessary in the clinical setting, examination of the tissue would define the pathological condition of the middle ear (Senturia et al., 1980).

Otitis Media without Effusion

In certain cases, inflammation of the middle ear mucous membrane and tympanic membrane will be present only, without any evidence of a middle ear effusion. The appearance of the tympanic membrane by pneumatic otoscopy will reveal only *myringitis*,

1

in which there is usually erythema and opacification of the eardrum but relatively normal mobility to applied positive and negative pressure. Blebs or bullae may be present when the disease is acute. Otitis media without effusion is usually present in the early stages of acute otitis media but may also be found in the stage of resolution of acute otitis media or may even be chronic. Evidence for the existence of this type of otitis media has been provided by the examination of histopathological specimens of temporal bone. The absence of a middle ear effusion when a myringotomy is performed in the presence of otitis media has provided clinical proof that this condition exists in certain cases.

Acute Otitis Media

The rapid and short onset of signs and symptoms of inflammation in the middle ear is termed acute otitis media. Synonyms such as acute *suppurative* or *purulent* otitis media are acceptable. One or more local or systemic signs are present: otalgia (or pulling of the ear in the young infant), otorrhea, fever, recent onset of irritability, anorexia, vomiting, or diarrhea. The tympanic membrane is full or bulging, opaque, and has limited or no mobility to pneumatic otoscopy—indicative of a middle ear effusion. Erythema of the eardrum is an inconsistent finding. The acute onset of ear pain, fever, and a purulent discharge (otorrhea) through a perforation of the tympanic membrane (or tympanotomy tube) would also be evidence of acute otitis media. Following an episode of acute otitis media, a middle ear effusion that persists for longer than three months is termed chronic otitis media with effusion.

Otitis Media with Effusion

The presence of a relatively asymptomatic middle ear effusion has many synonyms, such as *secretory*, *nonsuppurative*, or *serous* otitis media, but the most acceptable term is *otitis media with effusion*. Since the effusion may be serous (transudate), the term *secretory* may not be correct in all cases. Likewise, the term *nonsuppurative* may not be correct, since asymptomatic middle ear effusion may contain bacteria and may even be purulent. The term *serous otitis media* is appropriate if an amber or bluish effusion can be visualized

through a translucent tympanic membrane; however, the most frequent otoscopic finding is opacification of the tympanic membrane, which makes assessment of the type of effusion (i.e., serous, mucoid, or purulent) not possible. Pneumatic otoscopy will frequently reveal either a retracted or convex tympanic membrane in which the mobility is impaired. However, fullness or even bulging may be visualized. In addition, an air-fluid level or bubbles, or both, may be observed through a translucent tympanic membrane. The duration (not the severity) of the effusion can be *acute* (less than three weeks), *subacute* (three weeks to two to three months), or *chronic* (greater than two to three months). The most important distinction between this type of disease and acute otitis media (acute "suppurative" otitis media) is that the signs and symptoms of acute infection are lacking in otitis media with effusion (e.g., otalgia, fever), but hearing loss may be present in both conditions.

Atelectasis of the Tympanic Membrane–Middle Ear

Atelectasis of the tympanic membrane, which may or may not be associated with otitis media, is defined as either collapse or retraction of the tympanic membrane. Collapse implies passivity, whereas retraction implies active pulling inward of the tympanic membrane, usually from negative middle ear pressure. A *retraction pocket* is a localized area of atelectasis of the tympanic membrane. Atelectasis of the tympanic membrane is not strictly a type of otitis media but is a related condition. It may be present prior to, concurrent with, or after an episode of otitis media with effusion. It also may be present in some patients without evidence of otitis media, and if persistent and progressive, it can lead to complications or sequelae commonly attributed to otitis media, such as hearing loss, ossicular chain discontinuity, and cholesteatomas.

COMPLICATIONS AND SEQUELAE

The complications and sequelae of otitis media are divided into those that occur within the middle ear and temporal bone and those that occur within the intracranial cavity. It should be noted that these conditions are listed as complications and sequelae of otitis media, but they also may develop from causes other than otitis media. For example, ossicular chain discontinuity may occur, among other possible means, as the result of trauma to the middle ear. On the other hand, several of these conditions listed may be complications or sequelae not of otitis media but of a related condition. An example of this situation would be the presence of atelectasis of the tympanic membrane without otitis media in which a discontinuity of the ossicular chain occurs or an acquired cholesteatoma develops (Bluestone et al., 1977, 1978). The term *chronic suppurative otitis media* is included in the classification but has been specifically defined since there has been some confusion concerning this disease entity. For example, an acquired cholesteatoma may have a purulent discharge secondary to inflammation within the confines of the sac-like structure but the middle ear is not inflamed; therefore, the term *chronic suppurative otitis media* would be inaccurate. On the other hand, a cholesteatoma that is present in association with in- flammation of the middle ear would be defined as chronic suppurative otitis media with cholesteatoma (see Chapter Nine, Complications and Sequelae: Intratemporal).

References

Bluestone, C. D.: State of the art: Definitions and classifications. *In* Lim, D. J., Bluestone, C. D., Klein, J. O., and Nelson, J. D.: *Recent Advances in Otitis Media with Effusion.* Toronto, B. C. Decker, 1984, pp. 1–4.

Bluestone, C. D., Cantekin, E. I., Beery, Q. C., Douglas, G. S., Stool, S. E., and Doyle, W. J.: Functional eustachian tube obstruction in acquired cholesteatoma and related conditions. *In* McCabe, B. F., Sade, J., and Abramson, M. (Eds.): *Cholesteatoma, First International Conference.* Birmingham, Aesculapius Publishing Co., 1977, pp. 325–335.

Bluestone, C. D., Cantekin, E. I., Beery, Q. C., and Stool, S. E.: Function of the eustachian tube related to surgical management of acquired aural cholesteatoma in children. Laryngoscope 88:1155–1163, 1978.

Senturia, B. S., Bluestone, C. D., Klein, J. O., Lim, D., and Paradise, J. L.: Report of the ad hoc committee on definition and classification of otitis media with effusion. Ann. Otol. Rhinol. Laryngol. 89(68):3–4, 1980.

2

Anatomy

The middle ear is part of a system of contiguous organs including the nose, nasopharynx, eustachian tube, middle ear, and mastoid. Respiratory mucosa is continuous through the system. Thus, signs and effects of inflammation, infection, or obstruction in one area are likely to be reflected in other areas (Fig. 2–1).

NASOPHARYNX

The nasopharynx lies behind the nasal cavities and above the soft palate. Unlike the oral cavity, it is continually patent, communicating with the nasal cavities anteriorly via the paired choanae. The communication with the oral cavity is by means of the velopharyngeal port, which may be closed by elevation

of the soft palate (its inferior boundary) and inward movement of the constrictor muscles of the oropharynx. On the lateral wall is a prominence, the torus tubarius, which protrudes into the nasopharynx. This prominence is formed by the abundant soft tissue overlying the cartilage of the eustachian tube. Anterior to this is the triangularly shaped nasopharyngeal orifice of the tube. From the torus a raised ridge of mucous membrane, the salpingopharyngeal fold, descends vertically. On the posterior wall lie the adenoids, or pharyngeal tonsil, composed of abundant lymphoid tissue. Above the tonsil is a variable depression within the mucous membrane called the pharyngeal bursa. Behind the torus lies a deep pocket, extending the nasopharynx posteriorly along the medial border of the eustachian tube. This pocket, the fossa of

Figure 2–1. Nasopharynx–eustachian tube–middle ear–mastoid system.

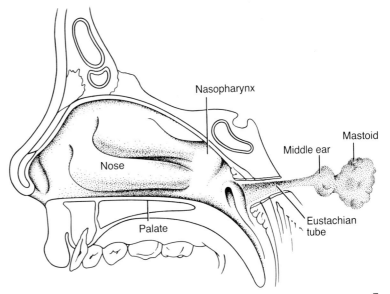

Rosenmüller (Fig. 2–2), varies in height from 8 to 10 mm and in depth from 3 to 10 mm (Proctor, 1967). Adenoid tissue usually extends into this pocket, giving soft tissue support to the tube.

EUSTACHIAN TUBE

In adults the tube lies at an angle of 45° in relation to the horizontal plane, whereas in infants this inclination is only 10° (Proctor, 1967) (Fig. 2–3). The tube is longer in the adult than in the infant and young child, and its length varies with race; it has been reported to be as short as 30 mm (Speilberg, 1927) and as long as 40 mm (Bacher, 1912), but the usual range of length reported in the literature is 31 to 38 mm (Anson, 1967; Anson and Donaldson, 1967; Doyle, 1977; Goss, 1967; Macbeth, 1960; Proctor, 1967). It is generally accepted that the posterior

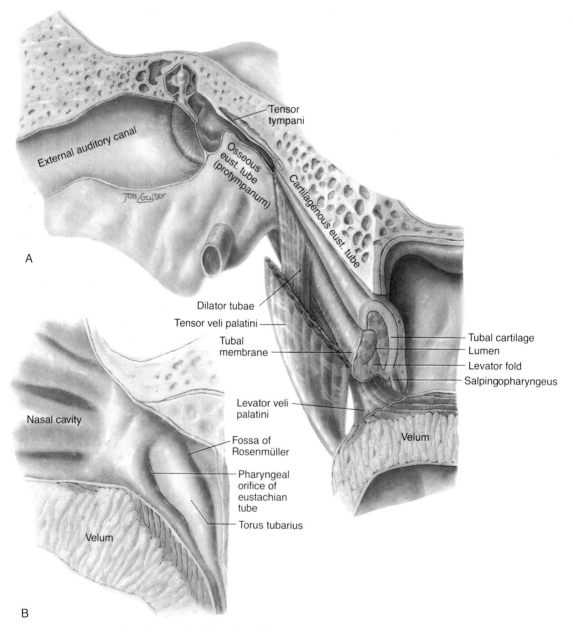

Figure 2–2. *A*, Illustration of a complete dissection of the eustachian tube and middle ear. Especially evident are the relations of the eustachian tube, paratubal muscles, and cranial base, as well as the positioning of the juncture between the osseous portion of the eustachian tube and the middle ear. *B*, Appearance of the nasopharyngeal orifice of the eustachian tube. Note the large torus tubarius and its inferior continuation at the salpingopharyngeal fold.

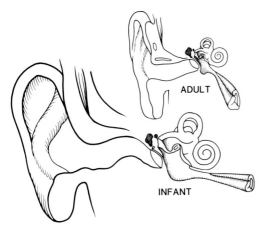

Figure 2–3. Illustration showing difference in angles of eustachian tubes in infants and adults.

third (11 to 14 mm) of the adult tube is osseous and the anterior two thirds (20 to 25 mm) is composed of membrane and cartilage (Graves and Edwards, 1944; Proctor, 1967).

The morphology of the eustachian tube and relation to other structures are presented in Figure 2–2A. The osseous eustachian tube (protympanum) lies completely within the petrous portion of the temporal bone and is directly continuous with the anterior wall of the superior portion of the middle ear. The juncture of the osseous tube and the epitympanum lies 4 mm above the floor of the tympanic cavity (Graves and Edwards, 1944). This relationship, although valid, is misrepresented in the more popular descriptions and depictions of the tubal–middle ear juncture and is of some importance in the functional clearance of middle ear fluids. As depicted in Figure 2–4, the course of the osseous tube is linear anteromedially, following the petrous apex and deviating little from the horizontal plane. The lumen is roughly triangular, measuring 2 to 3 mm vertically and 3 to 4 mm along the horizontal base. The healthy osseous portion is open at all times, in contrast to the fibrocartilaginous portion, which is closed at rest and opens during swallowing or when forced open, such as during the Valsalva maneuver. The osseous and cartilaginous portions of the eustachian tube meet at an irregular bony surface and form an angle of about 160° with each other.

The cartilaginous tube then courses anteromedially and inferiorly, angled in most cases 30° to 40° to the transverse plane and 45° to the sagittal plane (Graves and Edwards, 1944). The tube is closely applied to the basal

aspect of the skull and is fitted to a sulcus tubae between the greater wing of the sphenoid bone and the petrous portion of the temporal bone. The cartilaginous tube is firmly attached at its posterior end to the osseous orifice by fibrous bands and usually extends some distance (3 mm) into the osseous portion of the tube. At its inferomedial end it is attached to a tubercle on the posterior edge of the medial pterygoid lamina (Anson and Donaldson, 1967; Bryant, 1907; Doyle, 1977; Graves and Edwards, 1944; Proctor, 1967; Rood and Doyle, 1982).

The cartilaginous tube has a crook-shaped mediolateral superior wall (see Fig. 2–2). It is completed laterally and inferiorly by a veiled membrane (Terracol et al., 1949; Anson, 1967; Proctor, 1967), which serves as the site for the attachment of the fibers of the dilator tubae, or tensor veli palatini muscle (Bryant, 1907; Rood and Doyle, 1978). The tubal lumen is shaped like two cones joined at their apices. The juncture of the cones is the narrowest point of the lumen and has been called the "isthmus," and its position is usually described as at or near the juncture of the osseous and cartilaginous portions of the tube. The lumen at this point is approximately 2 mm high and 1 mm wide (Proctor, 1967). From the isthmus, the lumen expands to approximately 8 to 10 mm in height and 1 to 2 mm in diameter at the pharyngeal orifice (Rees-Jones and McGibbon, 1941). Tubal cartilage increases in mass from birth to puberty, and this development has physiological implications (see Chapter Three, Physiology, Pathophysiology, and Pathogenesis).

The cartilaginous eustachian tube does not follow a straight course in the adult but extends along a curve from the junction of the osseous and cartilaginous portions to the medial pterygoid plate, approximating the cranial base for the greater part of its course. The eustachian tube crosses the superior border of the superior constrictor muscle immediately posterior to its terminus within the nasopharynx. The thickened anterior fibrous investment of the medial cartilage of the tube presses against the pharyngeal wall to form a prominent fold, the torus tubarius, which measures 10 to 15 mm in thickness (Proctor, 1967). The torus is the site of origin of the salpingopalatine muscle (Simkins, 1943) and is the point of origin of the salpingopharyngeal muscle, which lies within the inferoposteriorly directed salpingopharyngeal fold (see Fig. 2–2B) (Rosen, 1970).

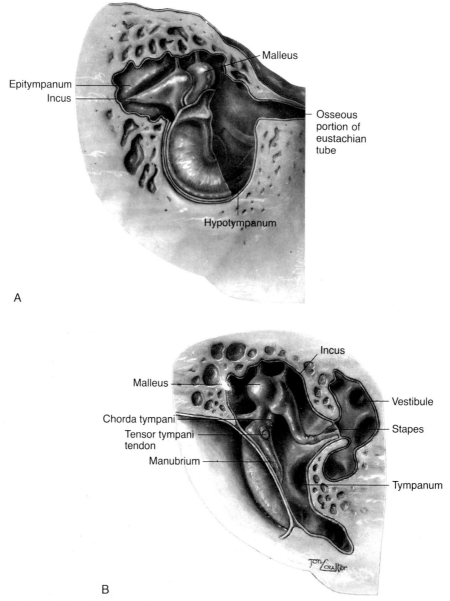

Figure 2–4. *A*, View of the middle ear and osseous portion of eustachian tube, drawn from dissection and illustrating the positioning of the middle ear ossicles and middle ear protympanic juncture in a coronally rotated sagittal plane. *B*, Sagittally rotated coronal view of the middle ear, its ossicles, and its relation to the inner ear.

The mucosal lining of the eustachian tube is continuous with that of the nasopharynx and middle ear and is characterized as respiratory epithelium. Structural differentiation of this mucosal lining is evident; mucous glands predominate at the nasopharyngeal orifice, and there is graded change to a mixture of goblet, columnar, and ciliated cells near the tympanum (Tos, 1984).

Muscles Associated with the Eustachian Tube

Traditionally there are four muscles that are commonly cited as being associated with the eustachian tube: the tensor veli palatini, levator veli palatini, salpingopharyngeus, and tensor tympani. Each has at one time or another been directly or indirectly implicated in tubal function (Anson, 1967; Brash, 1951; Bryant, 1907; Goss, 1967; Rood, 1973; Thomsen, 1957; Van Dishoeck, 1947).

Usually the eustachian tube is closed; it opens during such actions as swallowing, yawning, or sneezing and thereby permits the equalization of middle ear and atmospheric pressures. Although controversy still exists as to the mechanism of tubal dilation, most anatomical and physiological evidence supports active dilation induced solely by the tensor veli palatini muscle (Cantekin et al., 1979; Rich, 1920). Closure of the tube has been attributed to passive reapproximation of tubal walls by extrinsic forces exerted either by the surrounding deformed tissues, by the recoil of elastic fibers within the tubal wall, or by both mechanisms. More recent experimental and clinical data suggest that, at least for certain abnormal populations, the closely applied internal pterygoid muscle may assist tubal closure by an increase in its mass within the pterygoid fossa; this increase applies medial pressure to the tensor veli palatini muscle and consequently to the lateral membranous wall of the eustachian tube (Cantekin et al., 1979; Doyle et al., 1980; Ross, 1971).

The tensor veli palatini is composed of two fairly distinct bundles of muscle fibers divided by a layer of fibroelastic tissue. The bundles lie mediolateral to the tube. The more lateral bundle (the tensor veli palatini proper) is of an inverted triangular design, taking its origin from the scaphoid fossa and entire lateral osseous ridge of the sulcus tubae for the course of the eustachian tube, as depicted in Figure 2–2A. The bundles

descend anteriorly, laterally, and inferiorly to converge in a tendon that rounds the hamular process of the medial pterygoid lamina about an interposed bursa (Fig. 2–5). This fiber group then inserts into the posterior border of the horizontal process of the palatine bone and into the palatine aponeurosis of the anterior portion of the velum (Fig. 2–6). The more posteroinferior muscle fibers lack an osseous origin, extending instead into the semicanal of the tensor tympani muscle. Here, the latter group of muscle fibers receive a second muscle slip, which originates from the tubal cartilages and sphenoid bone. These muscle masses converge to a tendon that rounds the cochleariform process and inserts into the manubrium of the malleus. This arrangement imposes a bipennate form to the tensor tympani muscle (Lupin, 1969; Rood and Doyle, 1978). The tensor tympani does not appear to be involved in the function of the eustachian tube (Honjo et al., 1983).

The medial bundle of the tensor veli palatini muscle lies immediately adjacent to the lateral membranous wall of the eustachian tube and is called the dilator tubae muscle (Goss, 1967; Rood and Doyle, 1978). It takes its superior origin from the posterior third of the lateral membranous wall of the eusta-

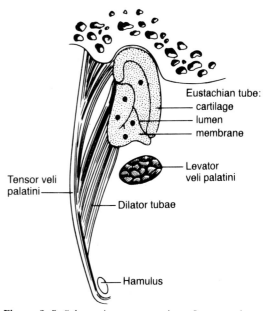

Figure 2–5. Schematic representation of a coronal section through the eustachian tube and its related musculature. Note that this section is from the posterior third of the cartilaginous portion of the eustachian tube and that the position of the hamulus is highly schematized to illustrate its relation to the tensor veli palatini tendon.

chian tube. The fibers descend sharply to enter and blend with the fibers of the lateral bundle of the tensor veli palatini muscle. It is this inner bundle that is responsible for active dilation of the tube by inferolateral displacement of the membranous wall (Rood, 1973; Rood and Doyle, 1978; Ross, 1971).

The levator veli palatini muscle arises from the inferior aspect of the petrous apex and from the lower border of the medial lamina of the tubal cartilage. The fibers pass inferomedially, paralleling the tubal cartilage and lying within the vault of the tubal floor (see Fig. 2–2A). They fan out and blend with the dorsal surface of the soft palate (Bryant, 1907; Graves and Edwards, 1944; Rood, 1973). Most investigators deny a tubal origin for this muscle and believe that in fact it is related to the tube only by loose connective tissue (McMyn, 1940; Simkins, 1943). The levator is not an active opener of the tube but probably adds support (Cantekin et al., 1983).

The salpingopharyngeal muscle arises from the medial and inferior borders of the tubal cartilage via slips of muscular and tendinous fibers (see Fig. 2–2A). The muscle then courses inferoposteriorly to blend with the mass of the palatopharyngeal muscle (Graves and Edwards, 1944; McMyn, 1940). Rosen (1970) examined 10 hemisected human heads and identified the muscle in nine specimens. However, in all cases the muscle fibers were few in number and appeared to lack any ability to perform physiologically.

Infant Eustachian Tube

The eustachian tube in the infant is about half as long as that in the adult; it averages about 18 mm. The cartilaginous tube represents somewhat less than two thirds of this distance, whereas the osseous portion is relatively longer and wider in diameter than it is in the adult. The height of the pharyngeal orifice of the infant eustachian tube is about one half that of the adult, but the width is similar. The ostium of the tube is more exposed in the infant than it is in the adult, since it lies lower in the shallower nasopharyngeal vault. The direction of the tube varies, from horizontal to an angle of about 10° to the horizontal, and the tube is not angulated at the isthmus but merely narrows (Fig. 2–3) (Graves and Edwards, 1944). Holborow (1975) demonstrated that in infants the medial cartilaginous lamina is relatively shorter since there is less tubal mass and stiffness in the infant tube than there is in that of the older child and adult. The tensor veli palatini muscle is less efficient in the infant.

MIDDLE EAR

The middle ear is an irregular, laterally compressed, air-filled space lying within the petrous portion of the temporal bone between the external auditory canal and the inner ear (Fig. 2–7). This cavity can be considered to be divided into three parts superoinferiorly in relation to the tympanic membrane. The epitympanum, or attic, refers to that space lying above the superior border of the tympanic membrane. The mesotympanum lies opposite the membrane, and the hypotympanum lies below the membrane. At birth, the cavity and associated structures are of adult size. The vertical and anteroposterior diameters measure about 15 mm,

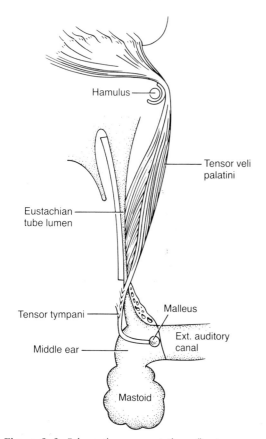

Figure 2–6. Schematic representation of a transverse section through the eustachian tube and its musculature, emphasizing the relation of the tripartite muscle bundle (tensor tympani–dilator tubae–tensor tympani) to the tube (see text).

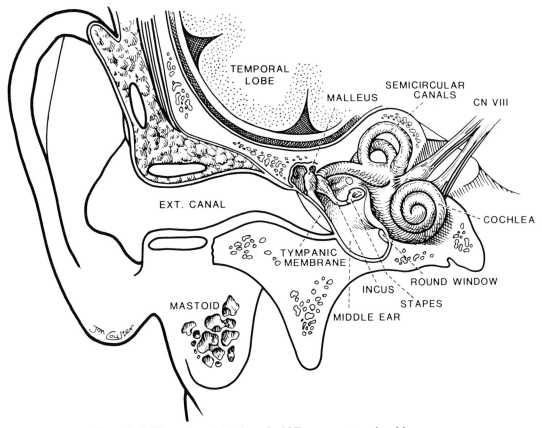

Figure 2–7. Illustration of relation of middle ear to external and inner ears.

whereas the transverse diameter measures 4 mm at the epitympanum, 2 mm at the mesotympanum, and 6 mm at the hypotympanum (Goss, 1967). Because of these dimensions, the middle ear has been termed a cleft or a narrow box.

Walls of the Middle Ear and the Contiguous Structures

The middle ear and its contents are depicted in Figure 2–8. Superiorly, the cavity is bounded by a thin plate of bone, the tegmen tympani, which extends forward to cover the semicanal of the tensor tympani muscle and posteriorly to cover the attic, thereby isolating the middle ear from the middle cranial fossa. The floor of the cavity consists of a bony plate that separates the cavity anteriorly from the jugular fossa and the posterior wall of the ascending portion of the carotid canal. Dehiscences are common in these bony structures occupying the floor of the middle ear.

Anteriorly, the floor of the middle ear cavity is raised to become continuous with

that of the bony portion of the eustachian tube. Superiorly and beneath the tegmen tympani lies the cylindrical semicanal for the tensor tympani muscle, which is separated from the eustachian tube by an upwardly concave thin bony septum, the cochleariform process. This process enters the middle ear along its superomedial margin to end just above the oval window, at which point it flares laterally. This termination of the cochleariform process serves as a pulley about which the tendon of the tensor tympani muscle makes a right-angled turn to proceed laterally to its insertion on the muscular process of the malleus.

The middle ear is bounded medially by the lateral surface of the bone covering the labyrinth of the inner ear. The bone is twice interrupted by areas of middle ear–inner ear communication—the oval window and the round window. The oval window is an opening leading from the middle ear into the vestibule of the inner ear. It is located at about the level of the superior border of the tympanic membrane. The raised facial prominence demarcating the position of the bony canal of the facial nerve is immediately su-

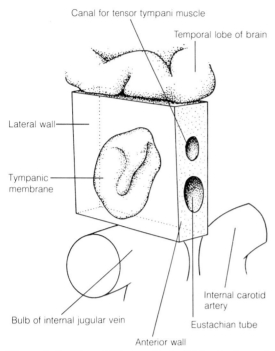

Figure 2–8. The middle ear. From Klein, J. O., and Daum, R. S.: The Diagnosis and Management of the Patient with Otitis Media. Copyright © Biomedical Information Corporation, New York, 1985.

perior to the oval window and curves vertically downward along its posterior border. The footplate of the stapes occupies the window and is tightly tied to the margin by an annular ligament. The round window is situated below and behind the oval window and is located within a funneled depression, the round window niche. The window is closed by the secondary tympanic membrane, which consists of three layers: a lateral mucosal layer derived from the middle ear lining, an internal layer derived from the lining of the cochlea, and an intermediate fibrous layer. The membrane is drawn into the cochlea, giving it a concave appearance from the middle ear. A bulbous, hollowed prominence formed by the outward projection of the basal turn of the cochlea occupies the position between the oval and round windows. This structure, the promontory, is crosshatched by the various branches of the tympanic plexus of nerves.

The lateral wall is formed by the tympanic membrane (eardrum), the tympanic ring, and a portion of the squamous temporal bone called the septum. The tympanic ring is superiorly incomplete, thereby forming the notch of Rivinus.

The posterior border of the middle ear is

demarcated by the anterior wall of the mastoid cavity, pyramidal prominence, and mastoid antrum. The pyramidal prominence is a hollow, forward-projecting bony pyramid located behind the round window and anterior to the vertical portion of the facial nerve. It contains the stapedius muscle, whose tendon exits through a small hole in the apex of the pyramid. A small branch of the facial nerve pierces the pyramid to innervate the stapedius muscle. In the posterior part of the epitympanum is a small depression that lodges the short process of the incus.

Mucosa

The mucous membrane of the middle ear and mastoid is continuous with that of the nasopharynx via the eustachian tube. This membrane covers all structures within the middle ear, including the ossicles, vessels, and nerves. Examination of cells of the mucous membrane within the tympanic cavity reveals a gradual change from tall, columnar cells with interspersed goblet cells to shorter cuboidal cells at the posterior portion of the promontory and aditus ad antrum (Fig. 2–9).

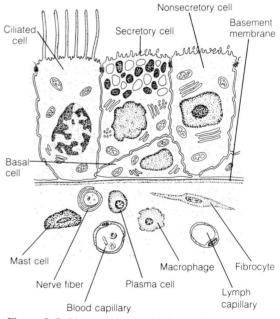

Figure 2–9. Mucosa of the middle ear. From Klein, J. O., and Daum, R. S.: The Diagnosis and Management of the Patient with Otitis Media. Copyright © Biomedical Information Corporation, New York, 1985.

Nerve Supply

The tympanic cavity and contained structures are innervated by branches of the tympanic plexus of nerves. Jacobson's nerve, a branch of the glossopharyngeal nerve, enters the cavity through its floor, divides, and ramifies about the promontory to contribute to the plexus. Sympathetic innervation to the plexus is provided by the superior and interior caroticotympanic nerves and parasympathetic fibers by the smaller superficial petrosal nerve.

Also contained within the middle ear cavity is the chorda tympani nerve, which arises from the sensory part of the descending facial nerve. It enters the cavity through the iter chordae posterior, transverses the cavity by crossing the manubrium of the malleus and the long process of the incus, and exits via the iter chordae anterius.

Tympanic Membrane

The eardrum is a thin, semitransparent membrane that separates the middle ear from the external ear canal. It measures about 8 to 10 mm in diameter and is positioned downward and inward. The outer margin is thickened and forms a fibrocartilaginous ring, the tympanic annulus, which is fitted into a sulcus in the bony tympanic ring. Superiorly, where the ring is deficient, the eardrum is lax and thin. This triangular region of the eardrum is called the pars flaccida, or flaccid part, and communication between the external and middle ears may occur in this area. The remaining eight ninths of the eardrum is called the pars tensa. The most depressed part of this concavity is called the umbo. The tympanic membrane has three layers. The most lateral layer is derived from the skin of the external ear canal. The medial layer is derived from the mucous membrane of the middle ear. The intermediate fibrous layer consists of two sublayers: a radial layer with fibers diverging out from the manubrium like the spokes on a bicycle tire, and a circumferential layer with abundant fibers near the circumference and few fibers near the center.

The Ossicles

Tiny bones, or ossicles, bridge the middle ear cavity and provide a mechanical trans-

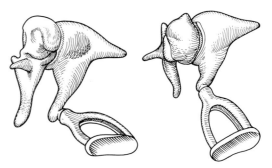

Figure 2–10. Middle ear ossicles viewed from medial to lateral *(left)* and from above *(right)*.

mission of vibrations from the eardrum to the oval window and inner ear (Fig. 2–10). The most lateral of these is the malleus. The malleus has a superior rounded head containing a posteriorly facing facet for articulation with the incus, a neck from which various processes are extended, and a manubrium, or handle, which is connected to the tympanic membrane on its internal surface. These ligaments attach to the processes arising from the neck, and they support the malleus within the cavity. The tendon of the tensor tympani muscle is inserted on a posteriorly directed muscular process. The middle ossicle is called the incus and has a body and two crura, or legs, which project at right angles to each other. The body is compressed transversely and presents a concavoconvex facet on its anterior surface for articulation with the head of the malleus. The short crus projects backward and gives rise to a ligament that connects the incus to the fossa incudis of the epitympanic recess. The long crus descends vertically and bends medially to end in a small lens-shaped structure, the lenticular process, which provides an articulating surface for the stapes. The most medial ossicle is the stapes, which has a head, a neck, two crura, and a footplate. The small head presents a concavity at its termination for articulation with the lenticular process of the incus. Below the head, the stapes narrows to its neck, which provides insertion for the stapedius muscle tendon. From the neck the two crura diverge and are connected at their end to the flattened oval footplate. The footplate fills the oval window, to which it is affixed by an annular ligament.

MASTOID AIR SPACE

Directly posterior to the epitympanum is a large air space called the mastoid antrum (see

Fig. 2–1). The antrum serves as a patent communication between the middle ear and the mastoid air cells. The mastoid refers to that portion of the petrous temporal bone that lies posterior to the middle ear cavity. In the adult, the mastoid is extended exteriorly and interiorly to form a process to which the sternocleidomastoid muscle is attached superficially. The mastoid cavity is partitioned by numerous air cells of variable size that intercommunicate in varying ways.

In the young infant, the mastoid process is small and the degree of pneumatization low. By between five and 10 years of age, the process of pneumatization is for the most part complete. Incomplete development of the air cell system has been associated with frequent bouts of otitis media in infancy and childhood.

References

Anson, B. (Ed.): *Morris' Human Anatomy.* McGraw-Hill Co., New York, 1967, pp. 1195–1196.

Anson, B., and Donaldson, J.: *The Surgical Anatomy of the Temporal Bone and Ear.* Philadelphia, W. B. Saunders Co., 1967, pp. 29–30.

Bacher, J. A.: The applied anatomy of the eustachian tube. Laryngoscope 22:21–37, 1912.

Brash, J. (Ed.): *Cunningham's Textbook of Anatomy.* 9th ed. London, Oxford Press, 1951.

Bryant, W. S.: The eustachian tube: Its anatomy and its movement: With a description of the cartilages, muscles, fasciae, and the fossa of Rosenmuller. Med. Rec. 71:931–934, 1907.

Cantekin, E. I., Doyle, W. J., Reichert, T. J., Phillips, D. C., and Bluestone, C. D.: Dilation of the eustachian tube by electrical stimulation of the trigeminal nerve. Ann. Otol. Rhinol. Laryngol. 88:40–51, 1979.

Cantekin, E. I., Doyle, W. J., and Bluestone, C. D.: Effect of levator veli palatini muscle excision of eustachian tube function. Arch. Otolaryngol. 109:281–284, 1983.

Doyle, W. J.: A functiono-anatomic description of eustachian tube vector relations in four ethnic populations—an osteologic study. Ph.D. Dissertation, University of Pittsburgh, 1977.

Doyle, W. J., Cantekin, E. I., Bluestone, C. D., Phillips, D. C., Kimes, K. K., and Siegel, M. I.: A nonhuman primate model of cleft palate and its implications for middle ear pathology. Ann. Otol. Rhinol. Laryngol. 89(68):41–46, 1980.

Goss, C. (Ed.): *Gray's Anatomy of the Human Body.* Philadelphia, Lea & Febiger, 1967, p. 1087.

Graves, G. O., and Edwards, L. F.: The eustachian tube: Review of its descriptive, microscopic, topographic, and clinical anatomy. Arch. Otolaryngol. 39:359–397, 1944.

Holborow, C.: Eustachian tube function: Changes throughout childhood and neuro-muscular control. J. Laryngol. Otol. 89:47–55, 1975.

Honjo, I., Ushiro, K., Hajo, T., Nozoe, T., and Matsui, H.: Role of tensor tympani muscle in eustachian tube function. Acta Otolaryngol. (Stockh.) 95:329–332, 1983.

Lupin, A. J.: The relationship of the tensor tympani and tensor palati muscles. Ann. Otol. Rhinol. Laryngol. 78:792–796, 1969.

Macbeth, R.: Some thoughts on the eustachian tube. Proc. R. Soc. Med. 53:151–161, 1960.

McMyn, J. K.: The anatomy of the salpingopharyngeus muscle. J. Laryngol. Otol. 55:1–22, 1940.

Proctor, B.: Embryology and anatomy of the eustachian tube. Arch. Otolaryngol. 86:503–526, 1967.

Rees-Jones, G. F., and McGibbon, J. E.: Radiological visualization of the eustachian tube. Lancet 241:660–662, 1941.

Rich, A. R.: The innervation of the tensor veli palatini and levator veli palatini muscles. Bull. J. Hopkins Hosp. 31:305–310, 1920.

Rood, S. R.: Morphology of m. tensor veli palatini in the five-month human fetus. Am. J. Anat. 138:191–196, 1973.

Rood, S. R., and Doyle, W. J.: The morphology of the tensor veli palatini, tensor tympani, and dilator tubae muscles. Ann. Otol. Rhinol. Laryngol. 87(2):202–211, 1978.

Rood, S. R., and Doyle, W. J.: The nasopharyngeal orifice of the auditory tube: Implications for tubal dynamics anatomy. Cleft Pal. J. 19:119–128, 1982.

Rosen, L. M.: The morphology of the salpingopharyngeus muscle. Unpublished Master's Thesis, University of Pittsburgh, 1970.

Ross, M.: Functional anatomy of the tensor palati—its relevance in cleft palate surgery. Arch. Otolaryngol. 93:1–8, 1971.

Simkins, C.: Functional anatomy of the eustachian tube. Arch. Otolaryngol. 38:476, 1943.

Speilberg, W.: Visualization of the eustachian tube by roentgen ray. Arch. Otolaryngol. 5:334–340, 1927.

Terracol, A., Corone, A., and Guerrier, G.: *La Trompe D'Eustache.* Paris, Masson, 1949.

Thomsen, K. A.: Studies on the function of the eustachian tube in a series of normal individuals. Acta Otolaryngol. (Stockh.) 48:516–529, 1957.

Tos, M.: Anatomy and histology of the middle ear. Clin. Rev. Aller. 2:267–284, 1984.

Van Dishoeck, H. A. E.: Resistance measuring of the eustachian tube and the ostium and isthmus valve mechanisms. Acta Otolaryngol. (Stockh.) 35:317–326, 1947.

3

Physiology, Pathophysiology, and Pathogenesis

The pathogenesis of acute otitis media is likely to follow the following pattern in most children: the patient has an antecedent event (due to allergy or infection) that results in congestion of the respiratory mucosa throughout the respiratory tract, including the nasopharynx, eustachian tube, and middle ear; congestion of the mucosa in the eustachian tube results in obstruction of the narrowest portion of the tube, the isthmus; secretions of the mucosa of the middle ear have no egress and accumulate in the middle ear; microbial pathogens (bacteria in most cases) may be present in the middle ear and proliferate in the secretions, resulting in a suppurative and symptomatic otitis media. The acute onset of otitis media with effusion, although relatively asymptomatic in children, most likely has a similar sequence of events. For children with recurrent episodes of acute otitis media or otitis media with effusion, anatomical or physiological abnormality of the eustachian tube appears to be an important, if not the most important, factor. The child with such an underlying abnormality of the eustachian tube may be subject to recurrent episodes of otitis media or persistent fluid in the middle ear. This chapter discusses present considerations of the physiology of the middle ear system, including the nasal cavities, eustachian tube, middle ear, and mastoid air cells, and the pathophysiology

and pathogenesis of acute otitis media and otitis media with effusion. The reader is also referred to a review of eustachian tube function and its role in otitis media, edited by Bluestone and Doyle (1985). Other features of physiology, pathophysiology, and pathogenesis are discussed in chapters on anatomy (Chapter Two), epidemiology (Four), microbiology (Five), and immunology (Six).

Abnormal function of the eustachian tube appears to be the most important factor in the pathogenesis of middle ear disease. This hypothesis was first suggested more than 100 years ago by Politzer (1862). However, later studies (such as Zollner, 1942; Suehs, 1952; Senturia et al., 1958; and Sade, 1966) suggested that otitis media was a disease primarily of the middle ear mucous membrane and due to infection or allergic reactions in this tissue, rather than to dysfunction of the eustachian tube. Related to this hypothesis is the concept that nasopharyngeal infection spreads up the mucosa of the eustachian tube. Figure 3–1 is an attempt to incorporate these hypotheses.

The vast majority of patients with otitis media and related conditions have (or have had in the past) abnormal function of the eustachian tube that may cause secondary mucosal disease of the middle ear, such as inflammation (Bluestone et al., 1972a). Infection is secondary to reflux, aspiration, or

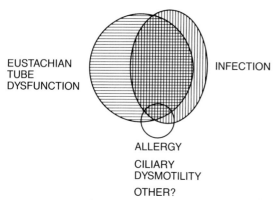

Figure 3–1. Etiology and pathogenesis of otitis media.

insufflation of nasopharyngeal bacteria up the eustachian tube and into the middle ear (Bluestone and Beery, 1976). Inflammation due to infection or possibly allergy may also cause intrinsic mechanical obstruction of the eustachian tube (Bluestone et al., 1977). Hematogenous spread of bacteria into the middle ear may also result in otitis media, but this is probably an uncommon event. A much smaller number of patients may have primary mucosal disease of the middle ear as a result of allergy (although this has not been proved) or, more rarely, an abnormality of

cilia, such as in Kartagener syndrome (Fisher et al., 1978).

PHYSIOLOGY AND PATHOPHYSIOLOGY OF THE EUSTACHIAN TUBE

The eustachian tube has at least three physiologic functions with respect to the middle ear (Fig. 3–2): (1) *protection* from nasopharyngeal sound pressure and secretions; (2) *drainage* into the nasopharynx of secretions produced within the middle ear; and (3) *ventilation* of the middle ear to equilibrate air pressure in the middle ear with atmospheric pressure and to replenish oxygen that has been absorbed. Clearance of secretions from the middle ear is provided by the mucociliary system of the eustachian tube and some of the middle ear mucous membrane. In ideal tubal function, intermittent active opening of the eustachian tube, due only to contraction of the tensor veli palatini muscle during swallowing, maintains nearly ambient pressures in the middle ear (Cantekin et al., 1979; Honjo et al., 1979; Rich, 1920). Assessment of these functions has been helpful in understanding the physiology and pathophysiology

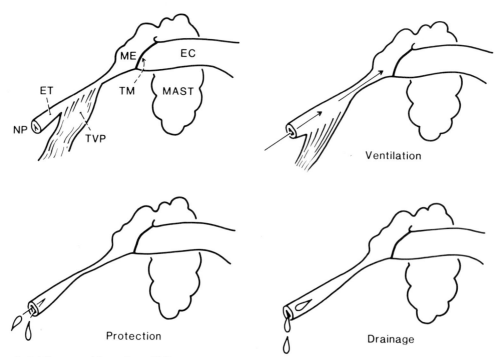

Figure 3–2. The eustachian tube–middle ear system. Note the three physiologic functions of the eustachian tube related to the middle ear, and that active dilation of the tube is by contraction of the tensor veli palatini muscle. *NP*, nasopharynx; *ET*, eustachian tube; *TVP*, tensor veli palatini muscle; *ME*, middle ear; *TM*, tympanic membrane; *EC*, external canal; *MAST*, mastoid air cells.

of the eustachian tube, as well as in the diagnosis and management of children with middle ear disease.

Protective and Drainage Functions

The protective and drainage functions of the eustachian tube and middle ear have been studied in children by using radiographic techniques (Bluestone, 1971; Bluestone et al., 1972a; Bluestone et al., 1972c; Honjo et al., 1981). Understanding of these radiographic studies can be best shown by a model of the system (Bluestone and Beery, 1976). The eustachian tube, middle ear, and mastoid air cell system can be likened to a flask with a long, narrow neck (Fig. 3–3). The mouth of the flask represents the nasopharyngeal end; the narrow neck, the isthmus of the eustachian tube; and the bulbous portion, the middle ear and mastoid air chamber. Fluid flow through the neck would be dependent upon the pressure at either end, the radius and length of the neck, and the viscosity of the liquid. When a small amount of liquid is instilled into the mouth of the flask, liquid flow stops somewhere in the narrow neck owing to capillarity within the neck and the relative positive air pressure that develops in the chamber of the flask. This basic geometric design is considered to be critical for the protective function of the eustachian tube–middle ear system. Reflux of liquid into the body of the flask occurs if the neck is excessively wide. This is analagous to an

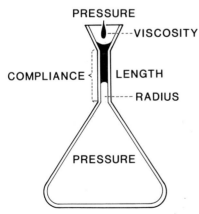

Figure 3–3. Flask model of eustachian tube–middle ear system. Eustachian tube, middle ear, and mastoid air cell system is compared to a flask in which the mouth of the flask represents the nasopharyngeal end of the eustachian tube, the neck is the cartilaginous portion of the tube, and the bulbous portion, the middle ear and mastoid air cells (see text).

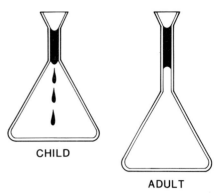

Figure 3–4. Flask model used to show how the shorter length of the eustachian tube can adversely affect the protective function in the child, as compared with the case in the adult.

abnormally patent human eustachian tube, in which there is not only free flow of air from the nasopharynx into the middle ear but also free flow of nasopharyngeal secretions, which can result in "reflux otitis media." Figure 3–4 shows that a flask with a short neck would not be as protective as a flask with a long neck. Since infants have a shorter eustachian tube than adults, reflux is more likely in the baby. The position of the flask in relation to the liquid is another important factor. In humans, the supine position enhances flow of liquid into the middle ear; thus, infants might be at particular risk for developing reflux otitis media because they are frequently supine.

Figure 3–5 shows that reflux of a liquid into the vessel can also occur if a hole is made in the bulbous portion of the flask, since this prevents the creation of the slight positive pressure in the bottom of the flask that deters reflux; that is, in this situation the middle ear and mastoid physiological cushion of air is lost. This hole is analogous to a perforation of the tympanic membrane or the presence of a tympanostomy tube that could allow reflux of nasopharyngeal secretions as a result of the loss of the middle ear–mastoid air cushion. Similarly, following a radical mastoidectomy, a patent eustachian tube could cause troublesome otorrhea (Bluestone et al., 1978).

If negative pressure is applied to the bottom of the flask, the liquid is aspirated into the vessel. In the clinical situation represented by the model, high negative middle ear air pressure could lead to the aspiration of nasopharyngeal secretions into the middle ear. If positive pressure is applied to the mouth of the flask, the liquid is insufflated into the vessel. Nose blowing, crying, closed

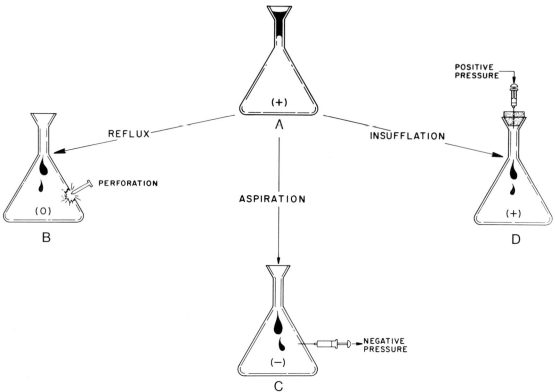

Figure 3–5. The flask model of the middle ear system for fluid flow. *A*, Model of normal function. *B*, Effect of perforation. *C*, Effect of negative pressure on the bottom of the flask. *D*, Effect of positive pressure on the mouth of the flask (see text).

nose swallowing, diving, or ascent in an airplane could create high positive nasopharyngeal pressure and result in a similar condition in the human system.

One of the major differences between a flask with a rigid neck and a biological tube such as the eustachian tube is that the isthmus (neck) of the human tube is *compliant*. Application of positive pressure at the mouth of a flask with a compliant neck distends the neck, enhancing fluid flow into the vessel. Thus, less positive pressure is required to insufflate liquid into the vessel. In humans, insufflation of nasopharyngeal secretions into the middle ear occurs more readily if the eustachian tube is abnormally distensible (has increased compliance). The effect of applied negative pressure in a flask with a compliant neck is shown in Figure 3–6; liquid flow through the neck does not occur until a negative pressure is slowly applied to the bottom of the flask. In this case, fluid flow occurs even if the neck is collapsed. If the negative pressure is applied suddenly, however, temporary locking of the compliant neck prevents flow of the liquid. Therefore, the speed with which the negative pressure is applied as well as the compliance

in such a system appears to be a critical factor in the results obtained. Clinically, aspiration of gas into the middle ear is possible, since negative middle ear pressure develops slowly as gas is absorbed by the middle ear mucous membrane. On the other hand, sudden application of negative middle ear pressure such as occurs with rapid alterations in atmospheric pressure (as in the descent in an airplane, in a descent after diving, or during an attempt to test the ventilatory function of the eustachian tube) could lock the tube, thus preventing the flow of air.

Certain aspects of fluid flow from the middle ear into the nasopharynx can be demonstrated by inverting the flask of the model (Fig. 3–7). In this case the liquid trapped in the bulbous portion of the flask does not flow out of the vessel because of the relative negative pressure that develops inside the chamber. However, if a hole is made in the vessel, the liquid drains out of the flask because the suction is broken. Clinically, these conditions occur in cases of middle ear effusion; pressure is relieved by spontaneous rupture of the tympanic membrane or by myringotomy. Inflation of air into the flask could also relieve

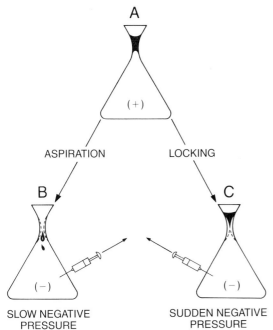

Figure 3–6. The flask model of the middle ear system for fluid flow through a flask with a compliant neck. *A*, Fluid stopped in the neck of the flask. *B*, Effect of negative pressure applied slowly to the bottom of the flask. *C*, Effect of negative pressure applied suddenly to the bottom of the flask.

the pressure, which may explain the frequent success of the Politzer or Valsalva method in clearing a middle ear effusion.

The example of fluid flow through a flask (Figs. 3–6 and 3–7) presents some of the mechanical aspects of the physiology of the human middle ear system. Other factors that probably affect flow of liquid and air through the middle ear include (1) the mucociliary transport system of the eustachian tube and middle ear (i.e., clearance); (2) active tubal opening and closing, acting to pump liquid out of the middle ear (Honjo et al., 1985); and (3) surface tension factors.

Ventilatory Function

The normal eustachian tube is functionally obstructed or collapsed at rest; there is probably a slight negative pressure in the middle ear. When the eustachian tube functions ideally, intermittent active dilation (opening) of the tube maintains near-ambient pressures in the middle ear. It is suspected that when active function is inefficient in opening the eustachian tube, functional collapse of the tube persists, which results in negative pressure in the middle ear. When tubal opening

does occur, a large bolus of air could enter the middle ear, which could eventually result in even higher negative pressure (Cantekin et al., 1980). This type of ventilation appears to be quite common in children, as moderate to high negative middle ear pressures have been identified by tympanometry in many children who have no apparent ear disease (Beery et al., 1975).

In an effort to describe normal eustachian tube function by using the microflow technique inside a pressure chamber, Elner and coworkers (1971) studied 102 adults with intact tympanic membranes and apparently no history of otologic disorder. The patients were divided into four groups according to their abilities to equilibrate static relative positive and negative pressures of 100 mm H_2O in the middle ear. The patients in Group 1 were able to equilibrate pressure differences across the tympanic membrane completely. Those in Group 2 equilibrated positive pressure, but a small residual negative pressure remained in the middle ear. The subjects in Group 3 were capable of equilibrating only relative positive pressure with a small residual remaining, but not negative pressure, and those in Group 4 were incapable of equilibrating any pressure. These data probably

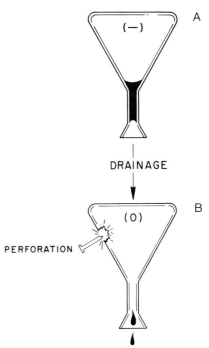

Figure 3–7. The flask model of the middle ear system for fluid flow from an inverted flask. *A*, Fluid trapped by relative negative pressure in the chamber. *B*, Effect of perforation of the chamber.

indicate decreased stiffness of the eustachian tube in the subjects in Groups 2 to 4 when compared with those in Group 1. This study also showed that 95 percent of normal adults could equilibrate an applied positive pressure and that 93 percent could equilibrate applied negative pressure to some extent by active swallowing. However, 28 percent of the subjects could not completely equilibrate either applied positive or negative pressure or both.

Children have less efficient eustachian tube ventilatory function than adults. Bylander (1980) compared the eustachian tube function of 53 children with that of 55 adults, all of whom had intact tympanic membranes and who were apparently otologically healthy. Employing a pressure chamber, Bylander reported that 35.8 percent of the children could not equilibrate applied negative intratympanic pressure (-100 mm H_2O) by swallowing, whereas only 5 percent of the adults were unable to perform this function. Children between three and six years of age had worse function than those of ages seven to 12. In this study and a subsequent one conducted by the same research group (Bylander, Tjernstrom, and Ivarsson, 1983), children who had tympanometric evidence of negative pressure within the middle ear had poor eustachian tube function.

From these two studies, it can be concluded that even in apparently otologically normal children, eustachian tube function is not as good as in adults, which would contribute to the higher incidence of middle ear disease in children.

Many children without apparent middle ear disease have high negative ear pressure. However, in children eustachian tube function does improve with advancing age, which is consistent with the decreasing incidence of otitis media from infancy to adolescence (Bylander and Tjernstrom, 1983).

Another explanation for the finding of high negative middle ear pressure in children is the possibility that some individuals who are habitual "sniffers" actually create underpressure within the middle ear by this act (Falk and Magnuson, 1984). However, this mechanism is uncommon in children.

In studying the parameters of middle ear pressure, Brooks (1969) determined by tympanometry that the resting middle ear pressure in a large group of apparently normal children was between 0 and -175 mm H_2O. However, pressures outside this range have been reported as normal for large populations of apparently asymptomatic children who were measured for middle ear pressure by screening (Jerger, 1970). High negative middle ear pressure does not necessarily indicate disease; it may indicate only physiological tubal obstruction. Ventilation occurs, but only after the nasopharynx–middle ear pressure gradient reaches an opening pressure. It has been suggested that these children probably should be considered at risk for middle ear problems until more is learned about the normal and abnormal physiology of the eustchian tube (Bluestone et al., 1973). In normal adults, Alberti and Kristensen (1970) obtained resting middle ear pressures of between 50 and -50 mm H_2O. Again, a pressure outside this range does not necessarily mean the patient has ear disease.

The *rate of gas absorption* from the middle ear has been reported by several investigators to be approximately 1 ml in a 24-hour period (Elner, 1972, 1977; Ingelstedt et al., 1967b; and Riu et al., 1966). However, since values taken over a short period were extrapolated to arrive at this figure, the true rate of gas absorption over 24 hours has yet to be determined in humans.

In a study by Cantekin and coworkers (1980), serial tympanograms were obtained in rhesus monkeys to determine the gas absorption process. During a four-hour observation period, the middle ear pressure was approximately normal in alert animals, whereas when the animals were anesthetized and swallowing was absent, the middle ear pressure dropped to -60 mm H_2O and remained at that level. The experiment indicated that, normally, middle ear gases are nearly in equilibrium with the mucosal blood-tissue gases or inner ear gas pressures. Under these circumstances, the gas absorption rate is small since the partial pressure gradients are not great. In the normally functioning eustachian tube, the frequent openings of the tube readily equilibrate the pressure differences between the middle ear and the nasopharynx with a small volume of air (1 to 5 μl) entering into the middle ear. However, an abnormally functioning eustachian tube may alter this mechanism.

The physiological role of the *mastoid air cell system* in relation to the middle ear is not fully understood, but the current concept is that it acts as a surge tank of gas (air) available to the relatively smaller middle ear cavity. During intervals of eustachian tube dysfunction, the compliance of the tympanic membrane and ossicular chain (which would affect hearing) would not be decreased due to reduced middle ear gas pressure since there is a reservoir of gas in the mastoid air cells. If this concept is correct, then a small mastoid air cell system could be detrimental to the middle ear if abnormal eustachian tube function is present.

Posture appears to have an effect on the function of the eustachian tube. The mean volume of air passing through the eustachian tube was found to be reduced by one third when the body was elevated 20° to the horizontal, and by two thirds when in the horizontal position (Ingelstedt et al., 1967a). This reduction in function with change in body position was found to be the result of venous engorgement of the eustachian tube (Jonson and Rundcrantz, 1969).

A *seasonal variation* in eustachian tube function occurs in children (Beery et al., 1979). Children who had had tympanostomy tubes inserted for recurrent or chronic otitis media with effusion and were evaluated using serial inflation-deflation studies had better eustachian tube function in the summer and fall than in the winter and spring.

EUSTACHIAN TUBE DYSFUNCTION RELATED TO PATHOGENESIS OF OTITIS MEDIA AND ATELECTASIS

The major types of abnormal function of the eustachian tube that can cause otitis media appear to be obstruction or abnormal patency (Fig. 3–8). Eustachian tube obstruction can be either *functional* or *mechanical*, or both. Functional obstruction results from persistent collapse of the eustachian tube due to increased tubal compliance, an abnormal active opening mechanism, or both. Functional eustachian tube obstruction is common in infants and younger children since the amount and stiffness of the cartilage support of the eustachian tube are less than in older children and adults. In addition, there appear to be marked age differences in the craniofacial base that render the tensor veli palatini muscle less efficient prior to puberty. In infants and young children, active tubal opening is probably impaired owing to lack of stiffness of the cartilage support during contraction of the tensor muscle. Mechanical obstruction of the eustachian tube may be intrinsic or extrinsic. *Intrinsic* obstruction could be the result of abnormal geometry or intraluminal or mural factors that compromise the lumen of the eustachian tube; the most common of these is inflammation due

to infection or possibly to allergy. *Extrinsic* obstruction could be the result of increased extramural pressure, such as occurs when the subject is supine or when there is peritubal compression secondary to a tumor or possibly an adenoid mass.

In extreme cases of abnormal patency of the eustachian tube, the tube is open even at rest (i.e., patulous). Lesser degrees of abnormal patency result in a semi-patulous eustachian tube that is closed at rest but has a lower resistance than the normal tube. Increased patency of the tube may be due to abnormal tube geometry or to a decrease in the extramural pressure, such as occurs as a result of weight loss or possibly as a result of mural or intraluminal factors.

Figure 3–9 depicts the chain of events in the pathogenesis of otitis media and atelectasis. Functional obstruction may result in persistent high negative middle ear pressure, and when associated with marked collapse or retraction of the tympanic membrane, it has been termed atelectasis. If ventilation occurs when there is high negative middle ear pressure, nasopharyngeal secretions can be aspirated into the middle ear and result in an acute bacterial otitis media.

If ventilation does not occur, persistent functional eustachian tube obstruction could result in sterile otitis media with effusion. Development of otitis media with effusion at this stage might be dependent upon the degree and duration of the negative pressure as well as middle ear hypoxia or hypercapnia. Since tubal opening is possible in a middle ear with an effusion, aspiration of nasopharyngeal secretions might occur, thus creating the clinical condition in which persistent otitis media with effusion and recurrent acute bacterial otitis media with effusion occur together. All infants with unrepaired palatal clefts and many children with repaired cleft palates have otitis media as a result of functional obstruction of the eustachian tube (Bluestone, 1971).

Intrinsic mechanical obstruction of the eustachian tube is most commonly the result of inflammation. Obstruction within the bony or middle ear portion of the tube is usually caused by acute or chronic inflammation of the mucosal lining, which may also be due to polyps or a cholesteatoma. Total obstruction may be present at the middle ear end of the tube. Stenosis of the eustachian tube has also been described but is a rare finding.

Most ears at risk for developing atelectasis or otitis media when inflammation is present

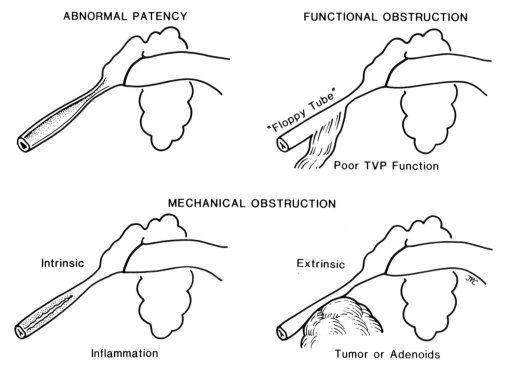

Figure 3–8. Eustachian tube dysfunction. The tube may be either abnormally patent or obstructed. When obstruction is present, it may be either functional or mechanical, or both.

probably have a significant degree of functional obstruction. An upper respiratory tract infection in children with this condition has been shown to significantly decrease eustachian tube function (Bluestone et al., 1977). Periods of upper respiratory tract infection may then result in atelectasis of the tympanic membrane–middle ear, acute otitis media, or otitis media with effusion due to swelling of the eustachian tube lumen. The mechanisms are similar to those described for functional eustachian tube obstruction. Allergy as a cause of intrinsic mechanical eustachian tube obstruction has not been demonstrated in children (Bluestone, 1978). However, in adult volunteers, eustachian tube obstruction has been produced by a challenge with antigen inhaled into the nasal cavity (Friedman et al., 1983).

Extrinsic mechanical obstruction of the eustachian tube may be the result of extrinsic compression by a nasopharyngeal tumor or adenoids. In an attempt to improve criteria for the preoperative selection of children for adenoidectomy to prevent otitis media with effusion, Bluestone and coworkers made radiographic studies of the nasopharynx and eustachian tube prior to and following adenoidectomy (1972c). The ventilatory function of the eustachian tube has also been studied by the inflation-deflation manometric technique both before and after adenoidectomy in a group of children with recurrent or chronic otitis media with effusion in whom tympanostomy tubes had been inserted (Bluestone et al., 1975). The results of these studies indicated that, following adenoidectomy, eustachian tube function improved in some, remained the same in others, and worsened in a few children. Improvement was related to a reduction of extrinsic mechanical obstruction of the eustachian tube.

Partial tube obstruction may result only in atelectasis of the tympanic membrane–middle ear or a bacterial otitis media with effusion, but more severe obstruction could result in a sterile otitis media with effusion. Otitis media with effusion has been produced in animal models when the eustachian tube was mechanically obstructed (Paparella et al., 1970).

Figure 3–9 also depicts the possible sequence of events that can cause an otitis media with effusion when the eustachian tube is abnormally patent. A patulous eustachian tube usually permits air to flow readily from the nasopharynx into the middle ear, which thus remains well ventilated; however,

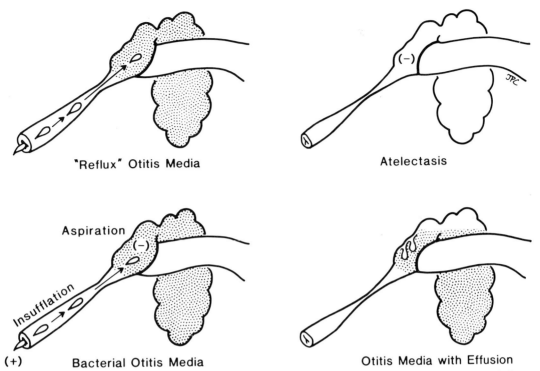

Figure 3–9. Pathogenesis of otitis media with effusion and atelectasis of the tympanic membrane. Shaded areas represent middle ear effusion.

unwanted nasopharyngeal secretions can also traverse the tube and result in reflux otitis media. A semipatulous eustachian tube may be obstructed functionally as the result of increased tubal compliance, and the middle ear may have negative pressure, or an effusion, or both. Since the tubal walls are abnormally distensible, nasopharyngeal secretions may readily be insufflated into the middle ear even with modest positive nasopharyngeal pressures, such as the results of nose-blowing, sneezing, crying, or closed-nose swallowing. If active tubal opening (tensor veli palatini contraction) occurs, resulting in an abnormally patent tube, reflux or insufflation of nasopharyngeal secretions is also likely.

If the eustachian tube has lower resistance than normal but remains functionally obstructed even during attempts at active tubal opening, it is conceivable that nasopharyngeal secretions would enter the middle ear more readily than would air. Certain American Indians have been shown to have tubal resistances that are lower than those in the average white population (Beery et al., 1980). They seem to have an increased incidence of reflux of nasopharyngeal secretion into the middle ear and frequently suffer from recur-

rent acute otitis media that is often associated with perforation and discharge. However, American Indians have a low incidence of cholesteatoma. This type of eustachian tube function and middle ear disease is different from the types of disease seen in individuals who have a cleft palate.

Nasal Obstruction Related to Eustachian Tube Function

Nasal obstruction may also be involved in the pathogenesis of otitis media with effusion. Swallowing when the nose is obstructed (as a result of inflammation or obstructed adenoids) results in an initial positive nasopharyngeal air pressure, followed by a negative pressure phase. When the eustachian tube is pliant, positive nasopharyngeal pressure might insufflate infected secretions into the middle ear, especially when the middle ear has a high negative pressure (Fig. 3–10); with negative nasopharyngeal pressure, such a tube could be prevented from opening and be further obstructed functionally. This mechanism has been termed the Toynbee phenomenon (Bluestone et al., 1974, 1975; Jorgensen and Holmquist, 1984).

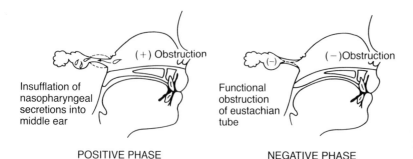

POSITIVE PHASE   NEGATIVE PHASE

Figure 3–10. The "Toynbee phenomenon."

Allergy and Eustachian Tube Function

Allergy is thought to be one of the etiologic factors in otitis media because otitis media occurs frequently in allergic individuals (Draper, 1967). The mechanism by which allergy might cause otitis media remains hypothetical and controversial. Figure 3–11 illustrates the role of allergy in the etiology and pathogenesis of otitis media by one or more of the following mechanisms: (1) middle ear mucosa functioning as a "shock organ," (2) inflammatory swelling of the mucosa of the eustachian tube, (3) inflammatory obstruction of the nose, or (4) aspiration of bacteria-laden allergic nasopharyngeal secretions into the middle ear cavity. In studies by Bernstein and coworkers (1984), a small percentage of children with proven allergy did have some evidence that the middle ear may be a "shock organ," but they considered this condition to be rare. A more likely explanation for the role of allergy in the pathogenesis and etiology of otitis media is related to allergic inflammation of the eustachian tube.

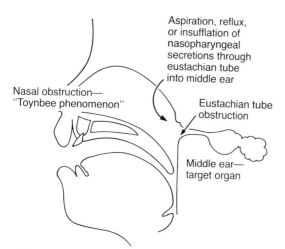

Figure 3–11. Possible roles of allergy in otitis media.

Recent studies in Pittsburgh involving adult volunteers demonstrated a relationship between intranasal antigen challenge, allergic rhinitis, and eustachian tube obstruction (Ackerman et al., 1984; Doyle et al., 1984a; Friedman et al., 1983). It seems reasonable that children with signs and symptoms of upper respiratory allergy may have otitis media as a result of the allergic condition.

Eustachian Tube Function Related to Cleft Palate

Otitis media with effusion is universally present in infants with an unrepaired cleft palate (i.e., functional obstruction of the eustachian tube) (Paradise et al., 1969; Stool and Randall, 1967). Palate repair appears to improve middle ear status, but middle ear disease nonetheless often continues or recurs even after palate repair (Paradise and Bluestone, 1974). Radiographic assessment has shown that infants and children with both unrepaired and repaired cleft palate have abnormal eustachian tube function, which suggests an abnormal opening mechanism in the infants with an unrepaired cleft palate, that is, functional obstruction of the eustachian tube (Bluestone, 1971; Bluestone et al., 1972d), and either a persistent failure of the eustachian tube to open actively or increased distensibility of the eustachian tube, or both, after repair of the soft palate (Bluestone et al., 1972b). Histopathological temporal bone studies have confirmed that the eustachian tube of cleft palate patients is not anatomically obstructed, which would give credence to functional, as opposed to mechanical, obstruction as the underlying defect (Kitajiri et al., 1984).

Inflation-deflation manometric eustachian tube function tests have shown that infants with unrepaired cleft palates have variable degrees of difficulty equilibrating increased middle ear pressure and are unable to equilibrate negative pressure by active function (swallowing) (Bluestone et al., 1975). Children with repaired cleft palates had either the same type of test results as did children with unrepaired palates or had lower opening pressures. Doyle, Cantekin, and Bluestone (1980), employing the forced-response eustachian tube function test, found that the eustachian tubes of infants and children with cleft palates constricted instead of dilated during swallowing. Animal subjects in which the palate has been surgically split have developed otitis media with effusion (Doyle et al., 1980, 1984b; Odoi et al., 1971).

All of these studies indicate that the eustachian tube is functionally obstructed in children with cleft palates, and this condition results in middle ear disease characterized by either persistent or recurrent high negative middle ear pressure, effusion, or both. Cholesteatoma is a frequent sequela in such children; this is not the case in American Indians, in whom the eustachian tube has been shown to be abnormally patent (i.e., to have low tubal resistance).

Patients with a submucous cleft of the palate appear to have the same risk of developing middle ear disease as those with an overt cleft. In addition, the presence of a bifid uvula has also been associated with a high incidence of otitis media (Taylor, 1972). Both of these conditions are probably associated with the same pathogenic mechanism for otitis media as is found in patients with overt cleft palates (i.e., functional obstruction of the eustachian tube).

Other Causes of Eustachian Tube Dysfunction

There are many other etiologic factors responsible for abnormal function of the eustachian tube. In addition to inflammation of the mucosa of the nose–nasopharynx–eustachian tube–middle ear system, there are congenital, traumatic, and neoplastic (Myers et al., 1984) conditions that also can result in tubal abnormalities.

Since a cleft of the palate results in functional obstruction of the eustachian tube, any child with a craniofacial malformation that has an associated cleft of the palate (one of the more common examples being Pierre Robin syndrome) will have recurrent and persistent otitis media. However, children with craniofacial anomalies that do not include an overt cleft of the palate also have an increased incidence of middle ear disease. Eustachian tube dysfunction has been described in children with Down syndrome and otitis media (White et al., 1984). Even though there have been no reports of formal eustachian tube function studies in individuals with other disorders such as Turner or Apert syndrome or Crouzon disease, dysfunction of the eustachian tube is the most likely cause of ear disease in these patients. Also, presumably, a defect related to the abnormal craniofacial complex, most often at the base of the skull, influences the relationship between the eustachian tube and the tensor veli palatini muscle.

Even in the absence of an obvious craniofacial malformation that is associated with otitis media, there is some evidence that children and adults with significant middle ear disease have a congenital anatomical or physiological abnormality that results in a dysfunction of the tube. Such a dysfunction could be abnormal patency or functional obstruction of the tube that is the result of an abnormal relationship between the eustachian tube and the tensor veli palatini muscle. Such an assumption is supported by apparent racial differences in the prevalence and incidence of otitis media; Eskimos and American Indians have a higher incidence of otitis media than do whites, whereas blacks have an incidence of otitis media that is less than that in whites. There is some evidence that otitis media is more prevalent in certain families.

It has been observed that patients with dentofacial abnormalities may have otitis media or develop middle ear disease as a result of these abnormalities. Correction of the defect to relieve the eustachian tube dysfunction would appear to be indicated.

In certain patients with a deviated nasal septum, impaired eustachian tube function has been reported. This dysfunction is especially apparent during attempts to equilibrate middle ear pressure by the Valsalva maneuver during periods of wide fluctuations in barometric pressure, such as occur when flying in an airplane or diving. In such cases, successful inflation of the middle ear by the Valsalva maneuver has been reported following repair of the deviated nasal septum (McNicholl, 1982; McNicoll and Scanlan, 1979).

Trauma to the palate, the pterygoid bone, the tensor veli palatini muscle, or the eustachian tube itself can also result in abnormal eustachian tube function. Injury to the tri-geminal nerve, or more specifically to the mandibular branch of this nerve, can result in either functional obstruction of the eusta-chian tube or a patulous tube, since the innervation of the tensor veli palatini is from this nerve (Cantekin et al., 1979; Perlman, 1951). The trauma may be associated with surgical procedures, such as palate or maxil-lary resection for tumor (Myers et al., 1984).

Neoplastic disease, either benign or malig-nant, that invades the palate and pterygoid bone can interfere with the function of the tensor veli palatini muscle and result in func-tional obstruction of the tube. Functional obstruction or abnormal patency of the tube can also occur from involvement of the in-nervation of the tensor veli palatini muscle. Mechanical obstruction of the eustachian tube can result from direct invasion by neo-plasm.

NONSPECIFIC FACTORS PRESENT IN THE MIDDLE EAR

Tissue Factors

A variety of nonspecific factors are present in the middle ear that may play roles in defense against infection. The epithelium of the eustachian tube and middle ear is cili-ated with mucus-producing cells that are equipped to trap and expel inhaled particles. The network of fibrin that is present in middle ear effusions, particularly in mucoid and purulent effusions, restricts movement of organisms and facilitates phagocytosis. De-struction of white blood cells and cells lining the mucosa produces lactic acid and a de-crease in pH sufficient to kill or inhibit growth of many bacteria.

Oxidative and Hydrolytic Enzymes

Biochemical studies of middle ear fluids reveal the presence of a variety of oxidative and hydrolytic enzymes. Oxidative enzymes include lactic, malic, and succinic dehydro-genases. Hydrolytic enzymes include lyso-zyme, acid and alkaline phosphatases, non-specific esterase, and leucine and alanine amino-peptidases. The enzymes in the mid-dle ear effusion may have a host cell origin derived from the blood or the inflamed mu-cosa. In some studies, concentrations of spe-cific enzymes differed, depending on the

quality (mucoid or serous) of the fluid. At present, most of the information about en-zymes in middle ear effusions is descriptive, but the increasing data may lead to hy-potheses about the role of tissue and cell products in initiation and maintenance of the middle ear effusion.

Lysozyme is a hydrolytic enzyme with bac-teriolytic activity that is present in blood, urine, tears, middle ear effusions, and other body fluids. Lysozyme is found in the lyso-somes of neutrophils, monocytes, and phago-cytic cells of the reticuloendothelial system. The bacteriolytic activity of lysozyme is the result of its ability to solubilize the rigid cell wall common to all bacteria. Lysozyme acts synergistically with complement and specific antibodies to achieve its antibacterial effect. High levels of lysozyme have been found in the middle ear effusions of patients with otitis media with effusion (Juhn and Huff, 1976; Liu et al., 1975; Veltri and Sprinkle, 1973). Lysozyme concentrations in middle ear ef-fusions are higher than those in serum and are higher in mucoid than in serous effusions (Lang et al., 1976). The high concentration of this antimicrobial substance may explain the bactericidal and virucidal effects of mid-dle ear effusion identified by Siirala and colleagues (1952, 1961).

Significant concentrations in middle ear effusions of lactic dehydrogenase, malate hy-drogenase, leucine aminopeptidase, and al-kaline phosphatase were identified by Juhn and Huff (1976). Lactic dehydrogenase is an intracellular enzyme liberated during the de-struction of tissue. Malate dehydrogenase and the other dehydrogenases of the Krebs cycle are believed to be bound to the inner mitochondrial membrane. In otitis media, proliferation of ciliated cells in the middle ear mucosa occurs. The increase in number of cells and increase in mitochondria may result in higher activity of the enzyme in the middle ear fluid than in serum (Juhn and Huff, 1976). Leucine aminopeptidase is a proteolytic enzyme that is present in various tissues and concentrated in leukocytes. His-tochemical studies of the location of the enzyme in the middle ear mucosa show increased activity throughout the mucoper-iosteum. The concentrations of all enzymes are higher in middle ear effusions than they are in simultaneously obtained serum, and they are higher in mucoid than in serous middle ear effusions. Glew and colleagues also found that there were higher concentra-tions of selected hydrolytic and oxidative enzymes in mucoid middle ear fluids than there were in serous ones (Glew et al., 1981). The specific activity of alpha-glucosidase, alpha-mannosidase, beta-glucuronidase, hexosaminidase, acid phosphatase, beta-galactosidase, alkaline phosphatase, and lactic dehydrogenase was three to 10 times greater in the mucoid effusions.

Collagenase activity was identified in middle ear effusions by Ganstrom and coworkers (1985). The enzyme had characteristics similar to those of granulocyte-derived collagenase. The authors hypothesized a role for the enzyme in tissue destruction and development of fluid in the middle ear.

Granulocyte proteases and protease inhibitors have been identified in middle ear effusions (Carlsson et al., 1983). The proteases may play a role in enhancing the inflammatory response. Protease inhibitors, alpha$_1$-antitrypsin, alpha$_1$-antichymotrypsin, and alpha$_2$-macroglobulin, alone or in complex with proteases, were identified in middle ear effusions of patients with acute otitis media and otitis media with effusion (Carlsson et al., 1983). The relative importance of the proteases and the inhibitors in the evolution and resolution of middle ear effusion is uncertain.

Recently Described Factors with Possible Roles in Pathogenesis

We are still in very early stages of our understanding of the pathogenesis of acute otitis media and otitis media with effusion. The limited insight into modes of pathogenesis restricts rational and appropriate therapy. Therapy is now based on pragmatic responses; acute infection is treated with antimicrobial agents; persistent fluid is drained. Further understanding of the pathogenesis of middle ear infection and its sequelae should yield more effective therapy.

In addition to the major issues discussed in this chapter and the chapters on anatomy (defects in the integrity of the middle ear system), epidemiology (genetic susceptibility), microbiology (products of microorganisms that elicit inflammation), and immunology (response to various antigens that lead to tissue injury), the following factors may play roles in the pathogenesis of middle ear infection and its sequelae:

Mucosal Damage. Damage to the epithelium of the upper respiratory tract, including nasal cavity, eustachian tube, and middle ear, may subject the individual to further damage from infectious or environmental agents. This theory suggests that early infection results in more disease because of damage caused by the agent, instead of genetic predisposition to disease that is identified by early infection.

Ciliary Dyskinesia. Intact mechanical processes of the mucosa of the respiratory tract prevent particulate antigens from reaching immunocompetent cells in the middle ear. Coordinated function of ciliated and secretory cells entraps and clears the airways of excess secretions, foreign particles, and cellular debris. A defect in ciliary activity may result in impairment of these functions. The ciliary defect may be on a genetic basis or due to acquired infectious or environmental factors. Children with the immotile cilia syndrome have recurrent pulmonary disease but also have chronic sinusitis and otitis media with effusion (Mygind and Pedersen, 1983). Infections by respiratory viruses are associated with transient abnormalities of cilia in nasal epithelium (Carson et al., 1985). Thus, antecedent viral infection may lead to compromise in mucociliary clearance, leading to pooling of secretions in the middle ear and multiplication of bacteria, and resulting in acute suppurative infection in the middle ear.

Bacterial Adherence. Biochemical factors of the mucosal membrane may inhibit or promote attachment of bacteria to respiratory mucosa. Preliminary studies of Jorgensen and colleagues identified increased receptivity for bacteria to nasopharyngeal epithelial cells in patients with acute otitis media, compared with healthy controls (Jorgensen et al., 1984).

Drug Factors. Drugs used for general or specific signs or symptoms may alter defense mechanisms and make the patient more or less prone to infection. Prostaglandins increase bronchial fluid secretions, whereas prostaglandin inhibitors decrease the output of serous and mucous cells. Salicylates, however, may also decrease lung mucociliary clearance and tracheal mucociliary transport rate (Gerrity et al., 1983). Similar mechanisms may occur in the eustachian tube and may result in development and persistence of effusion in the middle ear.

These factors are of speculative interest in developing pathogenic models for middle ear infection. Future investigations will identify whether or not they are important.

References

Ackerman, M. N., Friedman, R. A., Doyle, W. J., Bluestone, C. D., and Fireman, P.: Antigen-induced eustachian tube obstruction: An intranasal provocative challenge test. J. Allergy Clin. Immunol. 73:604–609, 1984.

Alberti, P. R., and Kristensen, R.: The clinical application of impedance audiometry. Laryngoscope 80:735–746, 1970.

Beery, Q. C., Bluestone, C. D., and Cantekin, E. I.: Otologic history, audiometry and tympanometry as a case finding procedure for school screening. Laryngoscope 85:1976–1985, 1975.

Beery, Q. C., Doyle, W. J., Cantekin, E. I., and Bluestone, C. D.: Longitudinal assessment of ventilatory function of the eustachian tube in children. Laryngoscope 89:1446–1456, 1979.

Beery, Q. C., Doyle, W. J., Cantekin, E. I., Bluestone, C. D., and Wiet, R.: Eustachian tube function in an American Indian population. Ann. Otol. Rhinol. Laryngol. 89(68):28–33, 1980.

Bernstein, J. M.: Immunologic reactivity in otitis media with effusion. Clin. Rev. Allergy 2:303–318, 1984.

Bluestone, C. D.: Eustachian tube obstruction in the infant with cleft palate. Ann. Otol. Rhinol. Laryngol. 80(2):1–30, 1971.

Bluestone, C. D.: Eustachian tube function and allergy in otitis media. Pediatrics 61:753–760, 1978.

Bluestone, C. D., Paradise, J. L., and Beery, Q. C.: Physiology of the eustachian tube in the pathogenesis and management of middle ear effusions. Laryngoscope 82:1654–1670, 1972a.

Bluestone, C. D., Paradise, J. L., Beery, Q. C., and Wittel, R.: Certain effects of cleft palate repair on eustachian tube function. Cleft Pal. J. 9:183–189, 1972b.

Bluestone, C. D., Wittel, R., Paradise, J. L., and Felder, H.: Eustachian tube function as related to adenoidectomy for otitis media. Trans. AAOO 76:1325–1339, 1972c.

Bluestone, C. D., Wittel, R., and Paradise, J. L.: Roentgenographic evaluation of eustachian tube function in infants with cleft and normal palates. Cleft Pal. J. 9:93–100, 1972d.

Bluestone, C. D., Beery, Q. C., and Paradise, J. L.: Audiometry and tympanometry in relation to middle ear effusions in children. Laryngoscope 83:594–604, 1973.

Bluestone, C. D., Beery, Q. C., and Andrus, W.: Mechanics of the eustachian tube as it influences susceptibility to and persistence of middle ear effusions in children. Ann. Otol. Rhinol. Laryngol. 83(11):27–34, 1974.

Bluestone, C. D., Cantekin, E. I., and Beery, Q. C.: Certain effects of adenoidectomy on eustachian tube ventilatory function. Laryngoscope 85:113–127, 1975.

Bluestone, C. D., and Beery, Q. C.: Concepts on the pathogenesis of middle ear effusions. Ann. Otol. Rhinol. Laryngol. 85(25):182–186, 1976.

Bluestone, C. D., Cantekin, E. I., and Beery, Q. C.: Effect of inflammation on the ventilatory function of the eustachian tube. Laryngoscope 87:493–507, 1977.

Bluestone, C. D., Cantekin, E. I., Beery, Q. C., and Stool, S. E.: Function of the eustachian tube related to surgical management of acquired aural cholesteatoma in children. Laryngoscope 88:1155–1163, 1978.

Bluestone, C. D., and Doyle, W. J. (Eds.): Eustachian tube function: Physiology and role in otitis media: Workshop report. Ann. Otol. Rhinol. Laryngol. 94 (Suppl 120):1–60, 1985.

Brooks, D.: The use of the electroacoustic impedance bridge in the assessment of middle ear function. Int. Audiol. 8:563–569, 1969.

Bylander, A.: Comparison of eustachian tube function in children and adults with normal ears. Ann. Otol. Rhinol. Laryngol. 89(68):20–24, 1980.

Bylander, A., and Tjernstrom, O.: Changes in eustachian tube function with age in children with normal ears. A longitudinal study. Acta Otolaryngol. (Stockh.) 96:467–477, 1983.

Bylander, A., Tjernstrom, O., and Ivarsson, A.: Pressure opening and closing functions of the eustachian tube by inflation and deflation in children and adults with normal ears. Acta Otolaryngol. (Stockh.) 96:255–268, 1983.

Cantekin, E. I., Doyle, W. J., Reichert, T. J., Phillips, D. C., and Bluestone, C. D.: Dilation of the eustachian tube by electrical stimulation of the mandibular nerve. Ann. Otol. Rhinol. Laryngol. 88:40–51, 1979.

Cantekin, E. I., Doyle, W. J., Phillips, D. C., and Bluestone, C. D.: Gas absorption in the middle ear. Ann. Otol. Rhinol. Laryngol. 68(89):71–75, 1980.

Carlsson, B., Lundberg, C., and Ohlsson, K.: Granulocyte protease inhibition in acute and chronic middle ear effusion. Acta Otolaryngol. (Stockh.) 95:341–349, 1983.

Carson, J. L., Collier, A. M., and Hu, S. S.: Acquired ciliary defects in nasal epithelium of children with acute viral upper respiratory infections. N. Engl. J. Med. 312:463–468, 1985.

Doyle, W. J., Cantekin, E. I., and Bluestone, C. D.: Eustachian tube function in cleft palate children. Ann. Otol. Rhinol. Laryngol. 89(68):34–40, 1980.

Doyle, W. J., Cantekin, E. I., Bluestone, C. D., Phillips, D. C., Kimes, K. K., and Siegel, M.: A nonhuman primate model of cleft palate and its implications for middle ear pathology. Ann. Otol. Rhinol. Laryngol. 89(68):41–46, 1980.

Doyle, W. J., Friedman, R., Fireman, P., and Bluestone, C. D.: Eustachian tube obstruction after provocative nasal antigen challenge. Arch. Otolaryngol. 110:508–511, 1984a.

Doyle, W. J., Ingraham, A. S., Saad, M., and Cantekin, E. I.: A primate model of cleft palate and middle ear disease: Results of a one-year postcleft follow-up. In Lim, D. J., Bluestone, C. D., Klein, J. O., and Nelson, J. D. (Eds.): Recent Advances in Otitis Media with Effusion. Proceedings of the Third International Symposium. Burlington, Ontario, B.C. Decker Inc., 1984b, pp. 215–218.

Draper, W. L.: Secretory otitis media in children: A study of 540 children. Laryngoscope 77:636–653, 1967.

Elner, A.: Indirect determination of gas absorption from the middle ear. Acta Otolaryngol. (Stockh.) 74:191–196, 1972.

Elner, A.: Quantitative studies of gas absorption from the normal middle ear. Acta Otolaryngol. (Stockh.) 83:25–28, 1977.

Elner, A., Ingelstedt, S., and Ivarsson, A.: The normal function of the eustachian tube. Acta Otolaryngol. (Stockh.) 72:320–328, 1971.

Falk, B., and Magnuson, B.: Eustachian tube closing failure in children with persistent middle ear effusion. Int. J. Pediatr. Otorhinolaryngol. 7:97–106, 1984.

Fisher, R., McManus, J., Entis, G., Cotton, R., Ghory, J., and Avsden-Moore, R.: Middle ear ciliary defect in Kartagener's syndrome. Pediatrics 62:443–445, 1978.

Friedman, R. A., Doyle, W. J., Casselbrant, M. L., Bluestone, C. D., and Fireman, P.: Immunologic-mediated eustachian tube obstruction: A double blind crossover study. J. Allergy Clin. Immunol. 71:442–447, 1983.

Ganstrom, G., Holmquist, J., Jarlstedt, J., and Renvall, U.: Collagenase activity in middle ear effusion. Acta Otolaryngol. (Stockh.) 100:405–413, 1985.

Gerrity, T. R., Cotromanes, E., Garrard, C. S., Yeates, D. B., and Lourenco, R. V.: The effect of aspirin on lung mucociliary clearance. N. Engl. J. Med. 308:139–141, 1983.

Glew, R. H., Diven, W. F., and Bluestone, C. D.: Lysosomal hydrolases in middle ear effusions. Ann. Otol. Rhinol. Laryngol. 90:148, 1981.

Honjo, I., Okazaki, N., and Kumazawa, T.: Experimental study of the eustachian tube function with regard to its related muscles. Acta Otolaryngol. (Stockh.) 87:84–89, 1979.

Honjo, I., Ushiro, K., Okazaki, N., and Kumazawa, T.: Evaluation of eustachian tube function by contrast roentgenography. Arch. Otolaryngol. 107:350–352, 1981.

Honjo, I., Hayashi, M., Ito, S., Takahashi, H.: Pumping and clearance function of the eustachian tube. Am. J. Otolaryngol. 6:241–244, 1985.

Ingelstedt, S., Ivarsson, A., and Jonson, B.: Mechanics of the human middle ear; pressure regulation in aviation and diving, a nontraumatic method. Acta Otolaryngol. (Stockh.) Suppl. 228:1–58, 1967a.

Ingelstedt, S., Ivarsson, A., and Jonson, B.: Quantitative determination of tubal ventilation during changes in ambient pressure as during ascent and descent in aviation. Acta Otolaryngol. (Stockh.) Suppl. 228:31–34, 1967b.

Jerger, J.: Clinical experience with impedance audiometry. Arch. Otolaryngol. 92:311–324, 1970.

Jonson, B., and Rundcrantz, H.: Posture and pressure within the internal jugular vein. Acta Otolaryngol. (Stockh.) 68:271–275, 1969.

Jorgensen, F., Andersson, B., Larsson, S. H., Nylen, O., and Svanborg Eden, C.: Children with frequent attacks of acute otitis media: A re-examination after eight years concerning middle ear changes, hearing, tubal function, and bacterial adhesion to pharyngeal epithelial cells. In Lim, D. J., Bluestone, C. D., Klein, J. O., and Nelson, J. D. (Eds.): Recent Advances in Otitis Media with Effusion. Proceedings of the Third International Symposium. Burlington, Ontario, B.C. Decker Inc., 1984, pp. 141–144.

Jorgensen, F., and Holmquist, J.: Toynbee phenomenon and middle ear disease. Am. J. Otolaryngol. 4:291–294, 1984.

Juhn, S. K., and Huff, J. S.: Biochemical characteristics of middle ear effusions. Ann. Otol. Rhinol. Laryngol. 85(25):110–116, 1976.

Kitajiri, M., Sando, I., Hashida, Y., and Doyle, W.: Histopathology of otitis media in infants with cleft and high arched palates. In Lim, D. J., Bluestone, C. D., Klein, J. O., and Nelson, J. D. (Eds.): Recent Advances in Otitis Media with Effusion. Proceedings of the Third International Symposium. Burlington, Ontario, B.C. Decker Inc., 1984, pp. 195–198.

Lang, R. W., Liu, Y. S., Lim, D. J., and Birck, H. G.: Antimicrobial factors and bacterial correlation in chronic otitis media with effusion. Ann. Otol. Rhinol. Laryngol. 85(25):145–151, 1976.

Liu, Y. S., Lim, D. J., Lang, R. W., and Birck, H. G.: Chronic middle ear effusions: Immunochemical and bacteriological investigations. Arch. Otolaryngol. 101:278–286, 1975.

McNicoll, W. D.: Remediable eustachian tube dysfunc-

tion in diving recruits: Assessment, investigation, and management. Undersea Biomed. Res. 9:37–43, 1982.

McNicoll, W. D., and Scanlon, S. G.: Submucous resection: The treatment of choice in the nose-ear distress syndrome. J. Laryngol. Otol. 93:357–367, 1979.

Myers, E. N., Beery, Q. C., Bluestone, C. D., Rood, S. R., and Sigler, B. A.: Effect of certain head and neck tumors and their management on the ventilatory function of the eustachian tube. Ann. Otol. Rhinol. Laryngol. 93(Suppl 114):3–16, 1984.

Mygind, N., and Pedersen, M.: Nose, sinus and ear symptoms in 27 patients with primary ciliary dyskinesia. Eur. J. Respir. Dis. 64(Suppl. 127):96–101, 1983.

Odoi, H., Proud, G. O., and Toledo, P. S.: Effects of pterygoid hamulotomy upon eustachian tube function. Laryngoscope 81:1242–1244, 1971.

Paparella, M., Hiraida, F., Juhn, S., and Kaneko, Y.: Cellular events involved in middle ear fluid production. Ann. Otol. Rhinol. Laryngol. 79:766–779, 1970.

Paradise, J. L., Bluestone, C. D., and Felder, H.: The universality of otitis media in fifty infants with cleft palate. Pediatrics 44:35–42, 1969.

Paradise, J. L., and Bluestone, C. D.: Early treatment of the universal otitis media of infants with cleft palate. Pediatrics 53:48–54, 1974.

Perlman, H. B.: Observations on the eustachian tube. Arch. Otolaryngol. 55:370–385, 1951.

Politzer, A.: Ueber die willkurlichen Bewegungen des Trommelfells. Weiner Med. Halle. Nr. 18:103, 1862.

Rich, A.: A physiological study of the eustachian tube and its related muscles. Bull. J. Hopkins Hosp. 31:206–214, 1920.

Riu, R., Flottes, L., Bouche, J., and Le Den, R.: La Physiologie de la Trompe d'Eustache. Paris, Librairie Anette, 1966.

Sade, J.: Pathology and pathogenesis of serous otitis media. Arch. Otolaryngol. 84:297–305, 1966.

Senturia, B. H., Gessert, C. F., Carr, C. D., and Bauman, E. S.: Studies concerned with tubotympanitis. Ann. Otol. Rhinol. Laryngol. 67:440–467, 1958.

Siirala, U., and Lahikainen, E. A.: Some observations on the bacteriostatic effect of the exudate in otitis media. Acta Otolaryngol. (Stockh.) Suppl. 100:20–25, 1952.

Siirala, U., Tarpila, S., and Halonen, P.: Inhibitory effect of sterile otitis media exudates on the cytopathogenicity of herpes simplex, poliomyelitis, and adenoviruses in HeLa cells. Acta Otolaryngol. (Stockh.) 53:230–236, 1961.

Stool, S., and Randall, P.: Unexpected ear disease in infants with cleft palate. Cleft Pal. J. 4:99–103, 1967.

Suehs, O. W.: Secretory otitis media. Laryngoscope 62:998–1027, 1952.

Taylor, G. D.: The bifid uvula. Laryngoscope 82:771–778, 1972.

Veltri, R. W., and Sprinkle, P. M.: Serous otitis media: Immunoglobulin and lysozyme levels in middle ear fluids and serum. Ann. Otol. Rhinol. Laryngol. 82:297–301, 1973.

White, B. L., Doyle, W. J., and Bluestone, C. D.: Eustachian tube function in infants and children with Down's syndrome. In Lim, D. J., Bluestone, C. D., Klein, J. O., and Nelson, J. D. (Eds.): Recent Advances in Otitis Media with Effusion. Proceedings of the Third International Symposium. Burlington, Ontario, B.C. Decker, Inc., 1984, pp. 62–66.

Zollner, R.: Anatomie, Physiologie und Klinik der Ohrtrompete. Berlin, Springer Verlag, 1942.

4

Epidemiology

Until recently, few studies were designed specifically to provide epidemiological information about middle ear disease in children. Reports of clinical experience, therapeutic trials, and microbiological studies of otitis media have provided some information that can be used to calculate incidence and prevalence rates, but the data are less complete than that obtained from studies designed for specifically epidemiological purposes. *Incidence* is the frequency of occurrence of new or separate episodes of illness in a defined population over a specific period of time. New cases of otitis media in children observed in a physician's practice in one year would be representative of an incidence study. *Prevalence* is the frequency of illness in a defined population at a given time. A survey of children for middle ear disease in a school or village performed by a team in one or a few days would be an example of a prevalence study. Recent longitudinal studies provide information about children over a long period of time and are an excellent source of information about the epidemiology of otitis media: These include the Arctic Health Research Center study of middle ear disease in Alaskan Eskimo children (Kaplan et al., 1973; Reed, et al., 1967); studies by two pediatricians, Virgil Howie and John Ploussard of Huntsville, Alabama, of the natural history of otitis media in children seen in their office practice (Howie, 1975; Howie et al., 1975); a prospective study of otitis media in 2565 children observed from birth by pediatricians in the greater Boston area (Teele et al., 1980); studies by members of the Department of Pediatrics, University of North Carolina School of Medicine, of res-

piratory disease in children attending the Frank Porter Graham Child Development Center, a day-care project (Henderson et al., 1982; Loda et al., 1972; Sanyal et al., 1980); a prospective study of 2404 children born in Malmo, Sweden, in 1977 (Lundgren et al., 1984); studies of Finnish children and adults (Pukander et al., 1982; Pukander, 1982); and a study of 210 Nashville children observed from birth to two years of age (Wright et al., 1985). The results of these longitudinal studies and selected data from other reports are the basis for this review of the epidemiology of otitis media in children.

HISTORICAL PERSPECTIVE

It is likely that humans have always suffered from acute infection of the middle ear and its suppurative complications. Studies of 2600-year-old Egyptian mummies reveal perforations of the tympanic membrane and destruction of the mastoid (Lynn and Benitez, 1974). Evidence of middle ear disease was also apparent in skeletal material from a prehistoric Iranian population (1900 to 800 B.C.) (Rathbun and Mallin, 1977). Prior to the introduction of antimicrobial agents, otitis media either resolved spontaneously (via central perforation of the tympanic membrane or evacuation of the middle ear contents through the eustachian tube) or came to the attention of a physician who drained the middle ear by means of myringotomy. Purulent otitis media was a frequent reason for admission to a hospital. In 1932, purulent otitis media accounted for 27 percent of all pediatric admissions to Bellevue Hospital

(Bakwin and Jacobinzer, 1939). Mastoiditis and intracranial complications were common. The introduction of sulfonamides in 1935 and subsequent antibacterial drugs limited the course of otitis media and reduced the incidence of suppurative complications. Otitis media in children from developing countries today resembles the disease seen in the United States and Western Europe before the era of chemotherapy.

INCIDENCE OF OTITIS MEDIA

Acute Otitis Media

Otitis media is one of the most common infectious diseases of childhood. A survey of the office practice of physicians who provide medical care to children showed that otitis media was the most frequent diagnosis for illness and the most frequent reason, after well-baby and child care, for office visits (Koch and Dennison, 1974). A survey of the frequency of infectious diseases during the first year of life in 246 Rochester children indicated that otitis media was second only to the common cold as a cause of infectious illness (Hoekelman, 1977). Otitis media was the most frequent diagnosis (22 percent) for visits of children to the Medical Emergency Clinic at Children's Hospital in Boston in a six-week survey from March through April, 1960 (Bergman and Haggerty, 1962). A review of the causes of visits to the Ambulatory Clinic of the Boston City Hospital in the fall of 1973 revealed that 19 percent of children between four and 24 months of age had otitis media (J.O. Klein and L. Bratton, unpublished data). In addition to visits for acute episodes of otitis media, visits for observation subsequent to a diagnosis of otitis media add substantially to the number of visits to physicians for the child.

The proportion of office visits of young children for otitis media was further elucidated by Teele and colleagues (1983) (Table 4–1): Disease of the middle ear accounted for a large proportion of visits during the first five years of age, rising from 22.7 percent in the first year to approximately 40 percent in years four and five; about one visit in three made for illness of any kind resulted in the diagnosis of middle ear disease; approximately three quarters of all visits to follow up any illness were made to follow up disease of the middle ear; and

Table 4–1. **PROPORTION OF VISITS ATTRIBUTABLE TO DISEASE OF THE MIDDLE EAR IN CHILDREN IN GREATER BOSTON (1975–1982)**[*]

Purpose of Visit[†]	Mean Number of Visits	Percentage of Visits for or with Middle Ear Disease
First Year of Life (2176 child-years of observation)		
Illness	2.19	34.0
Follow-up illness	1.18	69.9
Well-baby visit	4.73	5.7
Totals	8.10	22.7
Second Year of Life (1720 child-years of observation)		
Illness	2.10	34.7
Follow-up illness	1.10	75.7
Well-baby visit	1.77	7.1
Totals	4.96	33.9
Third Year of Life (1317 child-years of observation)		
Illness	1.75	29.5
Follow-up illness	0.77	74.1
Well-baby visit	1.07	5.7
Totals	3.58	34.6
Fourth Year of Life (660 child-years of observation)		
Illness	1.84	35.4
Follow-up illness	1.00	76.6
Well-baby visit	0.71	9.6
Totals	3.55	41.8
Fifth Year of Life (529 child-years of observation)		
Illness	1.39	34.2
Follow-up illness	0.66	72.1
Well-baby visit	0.59	9.0
Totals	2.64	38.1

[*]From Teele, D. W., et al.: Burden and the practice of pediatrics: Middle ear disease during the first five years of life. JAMA 249:1026–1029, 1983.
[†]According to patients.

either acute otitis media or asymptomatic middle ear effusion was diagnosed at 5 to 10 percent of all well-child visits.

Howie, Ploussard, and Sloyer (1975) found that two thirds of children seen in their office practice had at least one episode of otitis media by their second birthday, and one in seven children had more than six episodes. The Boston study showed similar trends: 71 percent of children had one or more episodes, and 33 percent had three or more episodes of otitis media by three years of age (Table 4–2).

These studies suggest that by three years of age children may be categorized into three groups of approximately equal size relative to acute infections of the middle ear. One group is free of ear infections, a second group may have occasional episodes of otitis, and a third group is "otitis prone," subject to repeated episodes of acute middle ear infections.

Table 4–2. **INCIDENCE OF ACUTE OTITIS MEDIA IN BOSTON CHILDREN***

Age (months)	Cumulative Percentage of Children Observed with Indicated Number of Episodes of Otitis Media†		
	0	1 or 2	3
≤3	91	9	0
6	75	25	0
12	53	38	9
24	35	40	24
36	29	38	33

*From Teele, D. W., et al., in preparation.
†2565 children enrolled at birth.

Persistent and Asymptomatic Middle Ear Effusions

The incidence or prevalence of otitis media with effusion that is apparently asymptomatic and unrecognized by parents (and therefore not brought to medical attention) has been the subject of recent studies in the United States and in Scandinavia. Persistence of middle ear effusion for weeks to months after onset of acute otitis media was frequent in Boston children (Teele et al., 1980): 70 percent of children still had effusion at two weeks, 40 percent had effusion at one month, 20 percent had effusion at two months, and 10 percent had effusion at three months (Fig. 4–1). The means of periods of time spent with middle ear effusion after the first, second, and third episode of acute otitis media were almost identical, ranging from 39 to 44 days. Multiple logistic regression analysis of 26 variables, including age at diagnosis of otitis, site of health care, duration of breast-feeding, duration of bottle-feeding in bed,

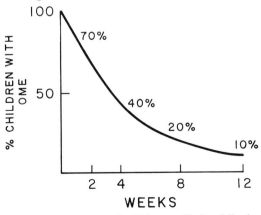

Figure 4–1. Persistence of middle ear effusion following onset of acute otitis media. (Modified from Teele, D. W., Klein, J. O., and Rosner, B. A.: Epidemiology of otitis media in children. Ann. Otol. Rhinol. Laryngol. 89(68):5–6, 1980.)

sex, race, birth weight, family history of allergy, or season at time of diagnosis did not affect time spent with effusion. After the first and second episode of acute infection, only presence of a sibling in the home was significantly associated with prolonged time of middle ear effusion. Similar results of persistent middle ear effusion after an episode of acute otitis media have been noted in recent studies from other centers (Table 4–3).

Surveys of healthy children for presence of middle ear fluid have identified a surprisingly high incidence of apparently asymptomatic middle ear effusion (Fiellau-Nikolajsen et al., 1977; Lous and Fiellau-Nikolajsen, 1981; Poulson and Tos, 1978; Sly et al., 1980; Tos, 1980; Tos et al., 1978, 1979) (Table 4–4). All surveys used tympanometry to assess the status of the middle ear. The prevalence of effusion varied with age and the time of year. Incidence of effusion peaked during the second year of life and was more prevalent in winter than in summer months. Repeated examinations (Lous and Fiellau-Nikolajsen, 1981; Sly et al., 1980; Tos, 1980) revealed that the middle ear fluid cleared spontaneously in most children within a few months. In Pittsburgh children two to six years of age observed monthly over a two-year period, approximately two thirds of the episodes of otitis media with effusion cleared within a month (Casselbrant et al., 1985). In many children, the duration of effusion may be as short as one or several days; a novel investigation of daily impedance screening of children three to six years of age in a day-care center revealed that many children had tympanometric evidence of effusion (B curves) for one day only (Birch and Elbrond, 1985). Some children, however, had fluid for six months or longer, and it often was seen first in one ear and then in the other on subsequent examinations. Thus, asymptomatic middle ear effusion is relatively frequent in healthy children but usually resolves without medical or surgical intervention.

AGE

Newborn Infant

In the newborn infant otitis media may be an isolated infection, or it may be associated with sepsis, pneumonia, or meningitis. The incidence of otitis media in newborn infants is uncertain, but the few available studies

Table 4–3. **PERCENTAGE OF PERSISTENT MIDDLE EAR EFFUSION AFTER INITIATING ANTIBIOTIC TREATMENT FOR ACUTE OTITIS MEDIA**

Investigators	Antibiotics	Percentage with Middle Ear Effusions After				
		10 to 14 Days	4	Weeks 6	8	12
Puhakka et al., 1979	Ampicillin*	58	29			
Teele et al., 1980		70	40		29	10
Thomsen et al., 1980		50	33			25
Schwartz et al., 1981		50	23		12	8
Mandel et al., 1982	Amoxicillin	56		33		
	Cefaclor	41		31		
Marchant et al., 1984a	Cefaclor	84	73			
	TMP–SMZ†	85	67			
Odio et al., 1985	Cefaclor	72	48		29	7
	Amoxicillin + clavulanic acid	70	44		13	5

*Ampicillin in all but small numbers of children who received various alternative regimens.
†Trimethoprim-sulfamethoxazole.

suggest that the incidence is high in both normal infants and infants with underlying factors, such as prematurity, that place them in intensive care units. Otitis media with effusion was identified in 24 of 70 Cleveland infants (34 percent) recruited from normal newborn nurseries observed at or before two months of age. Approximately half of the children at two months of age with otitis media with effusion were asymptomatic

(Marchant et al., 1984b). Warren and Stool (1971) consecutively examined 127 infants whose birth weights were under 2300 gm, and they found three with infections of the middle ear (at two, seven, and 26 days). Jaffe, Hurtado, and Hurtado (1970) examined 101 Navajo infants within 48 hours of birth and identified 18 with impaired mobility of the tympanic membrane. Balkany and coworkers identified effusion in the middle ear of 30

Table 4–4. **PREVALENCE AND MORBIDITY OF OTITIS MEDIA WITH EFFUSION AND HIGH NEGATIVE PRESSURE IN CHILDREN OF AGES 0 TO 7 YEARS IN DENMARK**

Investigators	Age	Months of Evaluation	Presence of Negative Pressure (%)	Presence of Middle Ear Effusions (%)
Poulsen and Tos, 1978	2 to 4 days	Jan 1977	10.6	—
	3 months	Apr 1977	17.9	—
	6 months	Jul 1977	36.9	1.3
Tos et al., 1979	9 months	Oct 1978	48.3	4.2
	12 months	Jan 1978	46.6	13.1
Tos and Poulsen, 1979	2 years	Nov 1977	39.4	12.0
		Feb 1978	38.5	14.6
		May 1978	36.7	77.3
		Aug 1978	29.7	7.2
Fiellau-Nikolajsen, 1979	3 years	Jan 1978	27.4	9.8
		Aug 1978	22.1	8.2
Thomsen and Tos, 1981		Feb 1979	39.0	11.0
Tos et al., 1982	4 years	Feb 1979	48.6	14.2
		May 1979	47.4	11.3
		Aug 1979	51.2	10.2
		Nov 1979	53.8	14.4
		Feb 1980	56.2	18.1
Lous and Fiellau-Nikolajsen, 1981	7 years	Aug–Sep 1978	15.0	5.7
		Nov–Apr 1979	20.0	9.0
		May–June 1979	18.0	6.0
		Aug 1979	9.0	2.4

percent of 125 consecutively examined infants who were admitted to a neonatal intensive care unit. The clinical diagnosis was corroborated by aspiration of middle ear fluid. Nasotracheal intubation for more than seven days was correlated with presence of effusion (Balkany et al., 1978). Pestalozza observed 970 newborn infants, two to 25 days of age, who were on the neonatal pathology ward; 205 infants (21.1 percent) were diagnosed to have otitis media by otoscopy, corroborated in two consecutive visits within 48 hours (Pestalozza, 1984).

Infants and Toddlers

Otitis media is very common in infants beyond the neonatal period (after 28 days of age). In the study of children in Boston, 9 percent had at least one episode of otitis media by three months of age, 25 percent had one or more episodes by six months of age, and 65 percent experienced otitis media by 24 months of age (Table 4–2). The highest age-specific incidence for all episodes of acute otitis media (first and subsequent episodes) occurred between six and 13 months of age. Similar results were identified in Nashville children observed from birth; by three months of age 7 percent had an episode of acute otitis media, and the peak incidence of middle ear infection was seven to nine months of age (Wright et al., 1985).

School-Age Children and Adults

The incidence of otitis media declines with age after the first year of life except for a limited reversal of the downward trend between five and six years of age, the time of entrance into school. Otitis media is less common in children seven years of age and older. Although the incidence of acute otitis media is limited in adults, a survey by the National Disease and Therapeutic Index published in 1970 found that there are almost four million visits by adults each year to private physicians for this infection (NDTI Review, 1970). Approximately 20 percent of young Swedish adult males (20 to 30 years old) and 30 percent of older males (50 to 60 years old) had pathological changes of the tympanic membrane; most with serious pathological findings had histories of otitis and otorrhea of long duration (Rudin et al., 1985).

Age at First Episode and Recurrent Acute Otitis Media

Age at first episode of acute otitis media is significantly associated with recurrent episodes. In the Boston study (Teele et al.) the peak incidence for first episodes of acute otitis media occurred at six months of age. Age at first episode of acute otitis media was significantly and inversely associated with risk for one or more or two or more episodes of acute otitis media in the 12 months after initial diagnosis. Cleveland infants with onset of otitis media with effusion before age two months had a mean of 3.5 total months of bilateral effusion, compared with 1.2 months for those with later onset. Bilateral middle ear effusion in these infants at age two months was highly predictive of subsequent bilateral persistent otitis media with effusion (effusion for a continuous period of three months or longer) (Marchant et al., 1984b). Navajo infants with otitis media during the first months of life had more recurrences than those infants free of disease early in life (Jaffe et al., 1970). Alaskan Eskimo children who had onset of disease during the first two years of life had many more middle ear infections in later life than did children who escaped middle ear infections early in life (Kaplan et al., 1973). Howie and colleagues (1975) called children with two or more episodes in the first year of life "otitis-prone"; the children had twice as many subsequent episodes of otitis media than children who had no or one episode in the first year. The reasons that children with episodes of acute otitis media early in life are at risk for recurrent disease are uncertain. These children may have an underlying anatomical or physiological predisposition to middle ear infection, most likely due to the structure or function of the eustachian tube. Alternatively, infection early in life may cause changes in the mucosa of the middle ear system that make children more susceptible to subsequent infection.

Age and Middle Ear Effusion

The age-specific incidence of otitis media with effusion parallels that of acute infection; the peak was at ages six to 13 months in Boston children (Teele et al.) and 10 to 12 months in Nashville children (Wright et al., 1985). Persistent effusions of the middle ear were more likely in young children. Pelton, Shurin, and Klein (1977) found that approximately 50 percent of children two years of age or younger had effusions that lasted for four weeks or more after an episode of acute otitis media, whereas only 20 percent of children older than two years had effusions of this duration. Asymptomatic middle ear effusion identified in surveys of healthy children is more frequent in children one to four years of age than in children aged seven years and older (see Table 4–4).

SEX

In most studies the incidence of acute episodes of otitis media was not significantly different in boys and girls. However, in the Boston study, males had significantly more single and recurrent (three or more) episodes (Teele et al., 1980). Finnish males had significantly more episodes than did females in eight communities studied in a one-year period beginning June, 1978 (Pukander et al., 1982). Males have more myringotomies and tympanoplasties than do females, a fact suggesting that chronic or severe infections of the middle ear may be more common among males (Solomon and Harris, 1976).

RACE

Studies of American Indians and Alaskan and Canadian Eskimos indicate that there is an extraordinary incidence of infection of the middle ear and that the disease is severe in these groups. Otorrhea is frequent, but chronic otitis and persistent effusion are uncommon. The following examples illustrate the extent and severity of ear disease in these populations. Zonis performed a prevalence study of an Apache community of 500 people of all ages; evidence of present or past ear infection was found in 23 percent (draining ear = 5.6 percent; perforation = 2.8 percent; healed perforation or tympanosclerosis or both = 13.1 percent; serous otitis = 1 percent; and acute otitis media = 0.4 percent) (Zonis, 1968). Arctic Health Research investigators found a high rate of otorrhea in Alaskan Eskimo children. By one year of age, 38 percent had at least one episode and 20 percent of all children had two or more episodes; by four years of age, 62 percent of children had one or more episodes of otor-

rhea and 40 percent of the children had two or more episodes (Reed et al., 1967). Ling, McCoy, and Levinson (1969) found that 31 percent of Canadian Eskimo children 10 years of age or younger living on Baffin Island had draining ears at the time of examination. None of the children were febrile or had evidence of acute otitis media (Ling et al., 1969).

The severity of middle ear infection has also been noted in African children and in Australian aboriginal children. Perforated eardrums are common. The prevalence of perforated eardrums in an aboriginal settlement in Queensland was 25 percent of children four to 12 months of age and approximately 10 percent in children six to 12 years of age (Dugdale et al., 1982). A prevalence survey in a Nigerian village identified wet or dry perforation in 4.2 percent of 170 children under 15 years of age (Miller et al., 1983). In a prevalence study of children and adults in Micronesia, approximately one half of the infants under one year had otitis media with effusion, and 4 percent of ears examined of persons ages two months to 25 years had a perforation (Dever et al., 1985). A form of the disease, termed necrotizing otitis media, is seen in these children that is rarely seen in children living in developed areas. An episode of acute middle ear infection progresses to perforation of the tympanic membrane with profuse discharge. Necrosis of the tympanic membrane follows, leaving a large central perforation that may persist for many years. This ear is called a "safe ear" because the perforation allows for drainage of the middle ear infection, and intracranial complications rarely occur, even without use of antimicrobial agents. However, there may be destruction of the ossicular chain and deafness may result (Clements, 1968; Dugdale et al., 1978; Pisacane and Ruas, 1982). Parents in these areas accept otorrhea as a way of life.

Timmermans and Gerson (1980) described a more indolent form of otitis media in Inuit Eskimo children that they termed chronic granulomatous otitis media. After one or more episodes of acute otitis media (usually treated with antimicrobial agents), there is a sudden onset of otorrhea without pain or fever. The discharge may persist for years, interspersed with periods of variable length in which the ear is dry. A large central perforation of the tympanic membrane is present, and granulomatous tissue fills the middle ear cavity. Resolution occurs with a scarred tympanic membrane and a mild to moderate hearing deficit.

Thus, the studies of children in different geographical and climatic areas suggest that the severity of disease, represented by chronic otorrhea, destruction of the tympanic membrane and ossicles, and other forms of a necrotizing process in the middle ear, is much more frequent (at present, almost unique) in underdeveloped areas.

American black children appear to have less disease due to middle ear infection than do white American children. The incidence of pathological ear disorders and hearing impairment was higher in white children than in black children aged six months through 11 years who lived in Washington, D.C. (Kessner et al., 1974). Ear disease was noted in 35 percent of 112 white children and 18 percent of 2031 black children. Hearing was tested in children four to 11 years of age; 20 percent of 82 white children and 6 percent of 1545 black children had significant impairment of hearing. The predominance of ear disease in white children was not readily explained. The results may be related to the relatively small size of the sample of white children or to socioeconomic factors unique to the white children living in a predominantly black community. In a second study in the Washington, D.C., area, investigators observed a tenfold difference in the incidence of acute otitis media in white and black children. The disease rate in children less than 15 years of age with at least one encounter for acute otitis media was 155 per 1000 children attending a clinic in an affluent, predominantly white suburb; it was 15 per 1000 children attending a clinic in a blue-collar area of northeast Washington, D.C., in which nearly all of the patients were black. Acute otitis media during the first year of life occurred in significantly more white (38 of 44 [86 percent]) than black (16 of 26 [62 percent]) Cleveland children observed in a uniform protocol (Marchant et al., 1984b). In the study of persistence of middle ear effusions after acute episodes of otitis media, Pelton and coworkers (1977) also noted a higher incidence of persistent effusions in white or Hispanic children than that seen in black children (21 percent of 42 black children and 51 percent of 51 white children).

The higher incidence of ear disease in white children (or lower incidence in black children) is not readily explained. Of interest

are the studies of Doyle of the position of the bony eustachian tube in skulls of American blacks, Americans of Caucasian ancestry, and American Indians (Doyle, 1977). Significant differences among the racial groups were present in the length, width, and angle of the tube in the groups, implicating an anatomical basis for racial predisposition to, or protection from, otitis media.

Further information about possible mechanisms was provided by Beery and associates, who studied eustachian tube function in Apache Indians living in Arizona (Beery et al., 1980). The results of inflation-deflation tests indicated that American Indians had lower forced opening pressures than had been measured previously in a group of Caucasians (with perforations secondary to chronic otitis media). The eustachian tube of the American Indian was functionally different from that of the Caucasians previously studied and was characterized by comparatively abnormal, low passive tubal resistance, which may be considered to facilitate ventilatory activity but to impair the protective function of the tube. The authors speculated that the difference may account for the high prevalence of otitis media with perforation (and the low incidence of cholesteatoma) in this population.

Few interracial studies have been done, and we cannot therefore fully evaluate the significance of the extent and severity of ear disease in different racial groups. Poverty is a common factor among many of the nonwhite populations that have been studied. Other variables include extremes of climate (temperature, humidity, altitude), crowding in the homes, inadequate hygiene, poor sanitation, and lack of medical care. Although the difference in disease incidence for different racial groups may be real, other explanations must be considered, including differences in the perception of signs of ear infection by parents, the basis for visits to the physician, the basis of payment for medical services, and the diagnostic acumen or style of the clinic physicians (Bush and Rabin, 1980).

SOCIAL AND ECONOMIC CONDITIONS

Cambon, Galbraith, and Kong (1965) noted a strong relationship between middle ear disease and poor social conditions among

American Indians of British Columbia. The specific reasons for the high incidence and severity of disease were not identified. Factors suggested include crowded living conditions, poor sanitation, and inadequate medical care. "The running ear is the heritage of the poor" (Cambon et al., 1965) may be true today as in the past, but we still do not understand the reasons for the high incidence and marked severity of disease among the underprivileged.

Children living in households with many members are more likely to have otitis media than are children living in smaller households. Canadian Eskimo children living in camps have less disease than do children living in villages and towns (Schaefer, 1971). Finnish children living in rural areas have fewer episodes of acute otitis media than do children living in towns (Pukander, 1982).

DAY-CARE CENTERS

The number of American children who receive some form of day care is large and growing. Current estimates are that more than 11 million children receive full or part-time day care. More than 50 percent of mothers who have children younger than six years of age work outside the home. Day-care centers vary in size from small groups in the responsibility of one or two adults to large, organized group centers. Similarly, some facilities have adequate room and ventilation, whereas others are crowded and poorly ventilated. In the day-care setting, coughing and sneezing at close range are common. Rhinovirus and respiratory syncytial virus can remain infective for hours to days in moist or dried secretions on nonporous materials such as toys, and the organisms can survive for more than 30 minutes on cloth or paper tissues saturated with secretions. Epidemics of disease due to respiratory viruses are common. Thus, there is ample opportunity for spread of respiratory infections among children in day care and for higher incidence of infection in children attending day care than children who receive care at home.

In urban areas of Finland, community day-care centers are common and children have a higher incidence of otitis than do children living in the Finnish countryside, who are more likely to be cared for in their homes (Pukander et al., 1984). Similarly, Danish

children cared for outside the home have shown a history of otitis media that is 25 percent higher than that for children cared for in the home; in addition, effusion, identified by tympanometry, occurs more frequently in children cared for outside the home than at home (Vinther et al., 1982). Approximately three or more episodes of otitis media occurred in 10 percent of 150 Swedish children aged six to 24 months in family day care (42) or in day-care centers (108) and in none of 57 children who received care at home (Strangert, 1977).

Although the data from Scandinavia suggest that the incidence of otitis media is higher in children who attend day care, problems of bias are present that may account for all or part of the difference in incidence. The estimate of acute otitis media in children cared for at home may be low. Parents of children in day care may seek medical attention for illness at a lesser degree of severity because of concern for loss of parent time at work if needed to stay home to care for a sick child. Alternately, the higher incidence of febrile illnesses in children in day care may result in more examinations by physicians and more observations of ears. Until studies of appropriate design using comparable observations of children in day care and in home care are performed, we must consider conclusions based on the Scandinavian data as tentative.

SEASON

The seasonal incidence of infections of the middle ear parallels the seasonal variations of upper respiratory tract infections. Acute episodes peak during the winter but are also frequent in the fall and spring; they are least frequent in the summer. In observations during three years in the Boston study, 27 percent of children had an episode of otitis in the summer, compared with 48 percent in the spring and fall and 51 percent in the winter (Teele et al., 1984). The incidence of episodes of otitis media also increases during outbreaks of viral infections of the respiratory tract in children; these are most likely to occur in the winter and spring seasons (Henderson et al., 1982).

The prevalence of middle ear effusion in asymptomatic children of various ages has been determined by use of tympanometry combined, in some cases, with physical examination. Four- to five-year-old children in New Orleans had different prevalence of middle ear effusion in winter and fall: 29 percent of children tested in February and 6 percent of those tested in September had effusion (Sly et al., 1980). Examination of Pittsburgh preschool-aged children attending a day-care center identified a prevalence of zero for otitis media with effusion in August, 7 percent in September, and 25 percent in January and February (Casselbrant et al., 1984). A one-year study of 389 seven-year-old Danish schoolchildren used tympanometry on eight to 10 occasions during the year to test for the presence of middle ear effusions. Twenty-six percent of the children had evidence of middle ear effusion on one or more tests during the year. The prevalence varied from 5.7 percent in August, 1978, to 9 percent in November through April and returned to 2.4 percent in August, 1979. Middle ear effusion occurring in the winter months persisted longer than effusion occurring in the summer months (Lous and Fiellau-Nikolajsen, 1981).

GENETIC FACTORS

Genetic predisposition to middle ear infection was suggested by data from the Boston study (Teele et al., 1980) and in a study of Apache children living on a reservation as well as those who were adopted and living outside the Indian community (Spivey and Hirschhorn, 1977). Children enrolled in the Boston study who had single or recurrent episodes of otitis media were more likely to have siblings with histories of significant middle ear infections than were children who had had no episodes of otitis media. Adopted Apache children had more episodes of acute otitis media than did their non-Apache siblings, and they had an illness rate similar to that of Apache children who remained on the reservation.

Low responses to pneumococcal polysaccharides were associated in some adults with lack of certain genetic markers of immunoglobulins (Ambrosino et al., 1985, 1986). Immunoglobulin allotypes were investigated in children with recurrent episodes of acute otitis media and in their parents by Prellner and associates (1985); the results did not identify differences among children with recurrent otitis media and controls for markers of genetic loci involved in antibody responses

to pneumococcal polysaccharide antigens. The epidemiological data suggest that genetic susceptibility to middle ear disease does exist and that further investigation of genetic markers is likely to yield useful information.

BREAST-FEEDING

Breast-feeding has been suggested as an important factor in prevention of respiratory and gastrointestinal infections in infancy. Does breast-feeding prevent otitis media? Various investigators have attempted to answer the question in different geographical areas and different cultural populations. Schaefer (1971) surveyed Canadian Eskimo children in five areas, including an urban center (Frobisher Bay), village settlements, and hunting camps. There was an increase in the incidence of middle ear disease in children who lived in urban centers, compared with those living in villages or camps, but in each area there was an inverse relationship of incidence of middle ear disease and duration of breast-feeding. Children who were breast-fed for 12 or more months had significantly less ear disease related to otitis media than did infants who were bottle-fed at birth, or within the first month.

Timmermans and Gerson (1980) conducted a prevalence study of ear disease in a small Inuit Eskimo community in Labrador. The number of children with evidence of otitis media (defined as acute otitis media, or wet or dry perforation) was inversely related to the age at onset of bottle-feeding. History of infant feeding was obtained by interview of the mother at the time of the prevalence study. Children who were bottle-fed at or soon after birth had significantly more disease (67 of 160 children, 42 percent) than did children who had been bottle-fed only after six months of breast-feeding (0 of 21 children).

Chandra reported a significant decrease in episodes of otorrhea (observed or recorded by a nurse midwife) among 35 infants who lived in a rural community in India and were breast-fed for at least two months, when they were compared with 35 bottle-fed infants matched for socioeconomic status and family size (Chandra, 1979).

Cunningham (1977) reviewed the medical records of infants who were born at the Mary Imogene Bassett Hospital in Cooperstown, New York, and who were seen regularly in the pediatric clinic in the first year of life. A significant difference in acute lower respiratory tract infections occurred in infants who were breast-fed for at least four and one-half months, when compared with infants who were bottle-fed. The incidence of otitis media was lower in the breast-fed infants, but the difference was not statistically significant.

These studies suggest that breast-feeding does have a protective effect against infections of the middle ear in some populations. But results are not conclusive because one or more significant defects in design is present in each of the studies, including retrospective analysis of records, otoscopic examination at one point in time to determine prior disease history, lack of uniform criteria for diagnosis, lack of standardization, absence of multivariable analysis or failure to control adequately for other variables, and insufficient sample size to provide appropriate analysis of confounding variables.

Saarinen followed 256 healthy term infants from birth through the first three years of life. Breast-feeding was categorized as long (only source of milk until six or more months), intermediate (two to six months), and little or none (two months). The incidence of otitis media was inversely associated with the duration of breast-feeding. The differences persisted up to age three. No differences were associated with other respiratory infections (Saarinen, 1982).

In the Boston Study (Teele et al., 1984) children were followed from birth, with frequent examinations and frequent assessments of the mode of feeding. A large number of children were studied (692), and multivariable analysis was performed; 31.2 percent of children were breast-fed at some time. Breast-feeding was associated significantly with decreased risk of recurrent acute otitis media (three or more episodes) by age one year but not by three years of age. Since the first year of life appears to be the most critical period in which middle ear disease contributes to morbidity, method of feeding may be important, as it alters the risk for recurrent disease during the first year of life.

These studies do not provide reasons for the effect of feeding method on disease resulting from middle ear infection. Is breast-feeding beneficial or is bottle-feeding harmful? A number of hypotheses have been suggested:

1. Immunological factors of value are provided in breast milk, and these prevent various bacterial and viral infections. Breast milk contains important anti-infective agents, including immunoglobulins (secretory IgA and IgG), various leukocytes (B-cells, T-cells, macrophages, and neutrophils), and components of complement. Although there is an abundant literature about specific factors in breast milk that may protect against enteric infection, there is a paucity of information about materials in breast milk that might protect against respiratory infections. Colostrum and, to a lesser extent, breast milk have neutralizing activity to respiratory syncytial virus, but the clinical importance of this immune factor is uncertain (Downham et al., 1976).

2. Allergy to one or more components in cow or formula milk may result in alteration of the mucosa of the eustachian tube and middle ear.

3. Nonimmune components in breast milk may also play a role, including antiviral factors (interferon) and antibacterial factors (lactoferrin and lysozyme). Breast milk prevents the attachment of pneumococci and *Haemophilus influenzae* to epithelial cells. The anti-attachment capability for pneumococci was identified in a high- and a low-molecular-weight fraction of breast milk without detectable antibody. These studies suggest that breast milk prevents adhesion of these organisms to respiratory mucosa, the initial factor in infection in the respiratory tract (Hanson et al., 1985).

4. The facial musculature of breast-fed infants develops differently from that of bottle-fed infants. The muscles may affect eustachian tube function and assist in promoting the drainage of middle ear fluids.

5. Aspiration of fluids into the middle ear occurs during bottle-feeding because the bottle-fed infant is required to produce high negative, intraoral pressure, whereas breast-feeding involves nipple massage and reflex "let-down" of milk.

6. The breast-fed infant is maintained in a vertical or semivertical reclining position, whereas the bottle-fed infant is placed in a reclining or horizontal position. The horizontal position may result in reflux of milk through the wide and horizontal eustachian tube. The practice of propping a bottle in bed has been criticized because fluids are forced under pressure into the oral cavity, with possible reflux into the middle ear.

The results of a study of children with cleft palate appear to diminish the importance of the positional advantage of breast-feeding (Paradise and Elster, 1984). None of the 222 infants fed formula only was free of ear effusion at any examination during the first 18 months of life, whereas in 11 of 30 infants fed breast milk, one or both ears were free of effusion at one or more examinations. The results suggest that breast milk protected infants in spite of the severe anatomical disability. Since all feedings, of breast milk or formula, were given via an artificial feeder, the protection afforded the infants was more likely to be a quality of the milk rather than the mode of feeding.

EFFECT OF ALTERED HOST DEFENSES OR UNDERLYING DISEASE

Although the vast majority of children have no obvious defect responsible for chronic otitis media with effusion, a small number may have altered host defenses, including anatomical changes (cleft palate, cleft uvula, submucous cleft), alteration of normal physiological defenses (patulous eustachian tube or barotrauma), congenital or acquired immunological deficiencies (immunoglobulin deficiencies, chronic granulomatous disease), or presence of malignancies or use of drugs that suppress immune processes. Active middle ear disease is almost a constant event in children with cleft palate (see Chapter 8). Some patients may have disease states, such as nasopharyngeal tumors or connective tissue disorders, that lead to otitis media. An increased incidence of otitis media occurs in children with Down syndrome (Schwartz and Schwartz, 1978). These conditions are too infrequent to affect epidemiological studies but should be considered in management of individual patients.

Local and systemic bacterial infections, including otitis media, are early manifestations of acquired immunodeficiency syndrome (AIDS) in infants. Recurrent episodes of acute otitis media are seen in 10 to 50 percent of these infants (Ammann and Shannon, 1985). Data about pediatric AIDS are increasing with such rapidity that the interested physician requires current information. The most valuable resource for such information is Morbidity and Mortality Weekly Reports prepared by the Centers for Disease Control, Atlanta, Georgia, available through the Mas-

sachusetts Medical Society C.S.P.O., Box 9120, Waltham, Massachusetts 02254-9120.

Various procedures in the nose, throat, or airway may increase susceptibility to infection in the middle ear. Nasotracheal intubation was identified as a factor in development of middle ear effusion in neonates (Balkany et al., 1978). A similar observation was made in children two days to five years of age in an intensive care unit; nasotracheal, but not nasogastric, intubation was associated with development of middle ear effusion. Effusion was identified within four days of intubation and appeared earlier in the ear on the side of intubation than in the contralateral ear (Persico et al., 1985).

References

Ambrosino, D. M., Schiffman, G., Gotschlisch, E. C., Schur, P. H., Rosenberg, G. A., DeLange, G. G., van Loghem, E., and Siber, G. R.: Correlation between G2 MCr) immunoglobin allotype and human antibody response and susceptibility to polysaccharide encapsulated bacteria. J. Clin. Invest. 75:1935–1942, 1985.

Ambrosino, D. M., Barrus, V. A., DeLange, G. G., and Siber, G. R.: Correlation of the Km (1) immunoglobin allotypes with human anti-polysaccharide antibody concentrations. J. Clin. Invest. 78:361–365, 1986.

Ammann, A. J., and Shannon, K.: Recognition of acquired immunodeficiency syndrome (AIDS) in children. Ped. Rev. 7:101–107, 1985.

Bakwin, H., and Jacobinzer, H.: Prevention of purulent otitis media in infants. J. Pediatr. 14:730–736, 1939.

Balkany, T. J., Berman, S. A., Simmons, M. A., and Jafek, B. W.: Middle ear effusions in neonates. Laryngoscope 88:398–405, 1978.

Beery, Q. C., Doyle, W. J., Cantekin, E. I., Bluestone, C. D., and Wiet, R. J.: Eustachian tube function in an American Indian population. Ann. Otol. Rhinol. Laryngol. 89(68):28–33, 1980.

Bergman, A. B., and Haggerty, R. J.: The emergency clinic: A study of its role in a teaching hospital. Am. J. Dis. Child. 104:36–44, 1962.

Birch, L., and Elbrond, O.: Daily impedance audiometric screening of children in a day-care institution: Changes through one month. Scand. Audiol. 14:5–8, 1985.

Bush, P. J., and Rabin, D. L.: Racial differences in encounter rate for otitis media. Pediatr. Res. 14:1115–1117, 1980.

Cambon, K., Galbraith, J. D., and Kong, G.: Middle-ear disease in Indians of the Mount Currie reservation, British Columbia. Can. Med. Assoc. J. 93:1301–1305, 1965.

Casselbrant, M. L., Okeowo, P. A., Flaherty, M. R., Feldman, R. M., Doyle, W. J., Bluestone, C. D., Rogers, K. D., and Hanley, T.: Prevalence and incidence of otitis media in a group of preschool children in the United States. *In* Lim, D. J., Bluestone, C. D., Klein, J. O., and Nelson, J. D. (Eds.): *Recent Advances in Otitis Media with Effusion.* Burlington, Ontario, B. C. Decker Inc., 1984, pp. 16–19.

Casselbrant, M. L., Brostoff, L. M., Cantekin, E. I.,

Flaherty, M. R., Doyle, W. J., Bluestone, C. D., and Fria, T. J.: Otitis media with effusion in preschool children. Laryngoscope 95:428–436, 1985.

Chandra, R. K.: Prospective studies of the effect of breast feeding on incidence of infection and allergy. Acta Paediatr. Scand. 68:691–694, 1979.

Clements, D. A.: Otitis media and hearing loss in a small aboriginal community. Med. J. Aust. 1:665–667, 1968.

Cunningham, A. S.: Morbidity in breast-fed and artificially fed infants. J. Pediatr. 90:726–729, 1977.

Dever, G. J., Stewart, J. L., and Davis, A.: Prevalence of otitis media in selected populations on Pohnpei; A preliminary study. Int. J. Pediatr. Otorhinolaryngol. 10:143–152, 1985.

Downham, M. A., Scott, R., Sims, D. G., Webb, J. K. G., and Gardner, P. S.: Breast-feeding protects against respiratory syncytial virus infections. Br. Med. J. 2:274–276, 1976.

Doyle, W. J.: A functiono-anatomic description of eustachian tube vector relations in four ethnic populations—an osteologic study. Ph.D. Dissertation, University of Pittsburgh, 1977.

Dugdale, A. E., Canty, A., Lewis, A. J., and Lovell, S.: The natural history of chronic middle ear disease in Australian aboriginals: A cross-sectional study. Med. J. Aust. Spec. Suppl. 1:6–8, 1978.

Dugdale, A. E., Lewis, A. N., and Canty, A. A.: The natural history of chronic otitis media. N. Engl. J. Med. 307:1459–1460, 1982.

Fiellau-Nikolajsen, M.: Tympanometry in three year old children. II. Seasonal influence on tympanometric results in nonselected groups of three-year-old children. Scand. Audiol. 8:181–185, 1979.

Fiellau-Nikolajsen, M., Lous, J., Vang Pedersen, S., and Schousboe, H. H.: Tympanometry in three year old children. I. A regional prevalence study on the distribution of tympanometric results in a nonselected population of three-year-old children. Scand. Audiol. 6:99–124, 1977.

Hanson, L. A., Andersson, B., Carlsson, B., Dahlgren, U., Mellander, L., Porras, O., Soderstrom, T., and Svanborg, E. D.: Defense of mucous membranes by antibodies, receptor analogues and nonspecific host factors. Infection 13(2):S166–170, 1985.

Henderson, F. W., Collier, A. M., Sanyal, M. A., Watkins, J. M., Fairclough, O. L., Clyde, W. A., Jr., and Denny, F. W.: A longitudinal study of respiratory viruses and bacteria in the etiology of acute otitis media with effusion. N. Engl. J. Med. 306:1377–1383, 1982.

Hoekelman, R. A.: Infectious illness during the first year of life. Pediatrics 59:119–121, 1977.

Howie, V. M.: Natural history of otitis media. Ann. Otol. Rhinol. Laryngol. 84(19):67–72, 1975.

Howie, V. M., Ploussard, J. H., and Sloyer, J.: The "otitis-prone" condition. Am. J. Dis. Child. 129:676–678, 1975.

Jaffe, B. F., Hurtado, F., and Hurtado, E.: Tympanic membrane mobility in the newborn (with seven months' follow-up). Laryngoscope 80:36–48, 1970.

Kaplan, G. J., Fleshman, J. K., Bender, T. R., Baum, C., and Clark, P. S.: Long-term effects of otitis media. A ten-year cohort study of Alaskan Eskimo children. Pediatrics 52:577–585, 1973.

Kessner, D. M., Snow, C. K., and Singer, J.: *Assessment of Medical Care for Children*, Vol. 3. Washington, D.C., Institute of Medicine, National Academy of Sciences, 1974.

Koch, H., and Dennison, N. J.: *Office Visits to Pediatricians.* Hyattsville, Md., National Ambulatory Medical Care Service, National Center for Health Statistics, 1974.

Ling, D., McCoy, R. H., and Levinson, E. D.: The

incidence of middle ear disease and its educational implications among Baffin Island Eskimo children. Can. J. Public Health 60:385–390, 1969.

Loda, F. A., Glezen, W. P., and Clyde, W. A.: Respiratory disease in group day care. Pediatrics 49(3):428–437, 1972.

Lous, J., and Fiellau-Nikolajsen, M.: Epidemiology of middle ear effusion and tubal dysfunction: A one-year prospective study comprising monthly tympanometry in 387 nonselected seven-year-old children. Int. J. Pediatr. Otorhinolaryngol. 3:303–317, 1981.

Lundgren, K., Ingvarsson, L., and Olofsson, B.: Epidemiologic aspects in children with recurrent otitis media. *In* Lim, D. J., Bluestone, C. D., Klein, J. O., and Nelson, J. D. (Eds.): *Recent Advances in Otitis Media with Effusion.* Burlington, Ontario, B. C. Decker Inc., 1984, pp. 22–25.

Lynn, G. E., and Benitez, J. T.: Temporal bone preservation in a 2600-year-old Egyptian mummy. Science 183:200–202, 1974.

Mandel, E. M., Bluestone, C. D., Rockette, H. E., Blatter, M. D., Reisinger, K. S., Wucher, F. R., and Harper, J.: Duration of effusion after antibiotic treatment for acute otitis media: Comparison of cefaclor and amoxicillin. Pediatr. Infect. Dis. 1:310–316, 1982.

Marchant, C. D., Shurin, P. A., Turcyzk, V. A., Feinstein, J. C., Johnson, C. E., Wasikowski, D. E., Knapp, L. J., and Tutihasi, M. A.: A randomized controlled trial of cefaclor compared with trimethoprim-sulfamethoxazole for treatment of acute otitis media. J. Pediatr. 105:633–638, 1984a.

Marchant, C. D., Shurin, P. A., Turcyzk, V. A., Wasikowski, D. E., Tutihasa, M. A., and Kinney, S. E.: Course and outcome of otitis media in early infancy: A prospective study. J. Pediatr. 104:826–831, 1984b.

Miller, S. A., Omene, J. A., Bluestone, C. D., and Torkelson, D. W.: A point prevalence of otitis media in a Nigerian village. Int. J. Pediatr. Otorhinolaryngol. 5:19–29, 1983.

NDTI Review: Leading diagnoses and reasons for patient visits. 1:18–23, 1970.

Odio, C. M., Kusmiesz, H., Shelton, S., and Nelson, J. D.: Comparative treatment trial of Augmentin versus cefaclor for acute otitis media with effusion. Pediatrics 75:819–826, 1985.

Paradise, J. L., and Elster, B. A.: Breast milk protects against otitis media with effusion. Pediatr. Res. 18:283A, 1984.

Pelton, S. I., Shurin, P. A., and Klein, J. O.: Persistence of middle ear effusion after otitis media. Pediatr. Res. 11:504, 1977.

Persico, M., Barker, G. A., and Mitchell, D. P.: Purulent otitis media—a "silent" source of sepsis in the pediatric intensive care unit. Otolaryngol. Head Neck Surg. 93:330–334, 1985.

Pestalozza, G.: Otitis media in newborn infants. Int. J. Pediatr. Otorhinolaryngol. 8:109–124, 1984.

Pisacane, A., and Ruas, I.: Bacteriology of otitis media in Mozambique. Lancet 1:1305, 1982.

Poulson, G., and Tos, M.: Screening tympanometry in newborn infants and during the first six months of life. Scand. Audiol. 7:159–166, 1978.

Prellner, K., Hallberg, T., Kalm, O., and Mansson, B.: Recurrent otitis media: Genetic immunoglobulin markers in children and their parents. Int. J. Pediatr. Otorhinolaryngol. 9:219–225, 1985.

Puhakka, H., Virolainen, E., Aantaa, E., Tuohimaa, P., Eskola, J., and Ruuskanen, O.: Myringotomy in the treatment of acute otitis media in children. Acta Otolaryngol. (Stockh.) 88:122–126, 1979.

Pukander, J.: Occurrence of acute otitis media. Academic Dissertation. Acta Universitatis Tamperensis Ser. A vol., 135, 1982.

Pukander, J., Luotonen, J., Sipila, M., and Karma, P.: Incidence of acute otitis media. Acta Otolaryngol. (Stockh.) 93:447–453, 1982.

Pukander, J., Sipila, M., and Karma, P.: Occurrence of and risk factors in acute otitis media. *In* Lim, D. J., Bluestone, C. D., Klein, J. O., and Nelson, J. D. (Eds.): *Recent Advances in Otitis Media with Effusion.* Burlington, Ontario, B. C. Decker Inc., 1984, pp. 9–13.

Rathbun, T. A., and Mallin, R.: Middle ear disease in a prehistoric Iranian population. Bull. N.Y. Acad. Med. 53:901–905, 1977.

Reed, D., Struve, S., and Maynard, J. E.: Otitis media and hearing deficiency among Eskimo children: A cohort study. Am. J. Publ. Health 57:1657–1662, 1967.

Rudin, R., Welin, L., Svardsudd, K., and Tibblin, G.: Middle ear disease in samples from the general population. II. History of otitis and otorrhea in relation to tympanic membrane pathology, the study of men born in 1913 and 1923. Acta Otolaryngol. (Stockh.) 99:53–59, 1985.

Saarinen, U. M.: Prolonged breast feeding as prophylaxis for recurrent otitis media. Acta Pediatr. Scand. 71:567–571, 1982.

Sanyal, M. A., Henderson, F. W., Stempel, E. C., Collier, A. M., and Denny, F. W.: Effect of upper respiratory tract infection on eustachian tube ventilatory function in the preschool child. J. Pediatr. 97:11–15, 1980.

Schaefer, O.: Otitis media and bottle-feeding. An epidemiological study of infant feeding habits and incidence of recurrent and chronic middle ear disease in Canadian Eskimos. Can. J. Public Health 62:478–489, 1971.

Schwartz, D. M., and Schwartz, R. H.: Acoustic impedance and otoscopic findings in young children with Down's syndrome. Arch. Otolaryngol. 104:652–656, 1978.

Schwartz, R. H., Rodriguez, W. J., and Schwartz, D. M.: Office myringotomy for acute otitis media: Its value in preventing middle ear effusion. Laryngoscope 91:616–619, 1981.

Sly, R. M., Zambie, M. F., Fernandes, D. A., and Fraser, M.: Tympanometry in kindergarten children. Ann. Allergy 44:1–7, 1980.

Solomon, N. E., and Harris, L. J.: *Otitis Media In Children. Assessing the Quality of Medical Care Using Short-Term Outcome Measures. Quality of Medical Care Assessment Using Outcome Measures: Eight Disease-Specific Applications.* Santa Monica, Ca., Rand Corp., 1976.

Spivey, G. H., and Hirschhorn, N.: A migrant study of adopted Apache children. Johns Hopkins Med. J. 140:43–46, 1977.

Strangert, K.: Otitis media in young children in different types of day-care. Scand. J. Infect. Dis. 9:119–123, 1977.

Teele, D. W., Klein, J. O., and Rosner, B. A.: Epidemiology of otitis media in children. Ann. Otol. Rhinol. Laryngol. 89(68):5–6, 1980.

Teele, D. W., Klein, J. O., Rosner, B., Bratton, L., Fisch, G. R., Mathieu, O. R., Porter, P. J., Starobin, S. G., Tarlin, L. O., and Younes, M. D.: Burden and the practice of pediatrics: Middle ear disease during the first five years of life. JAMA 249:1026–1029, 1983.

Teele, D. W., Klein, J. O., and Rosner, B.: Otitis media with effusion during the first three years of life and development of speech and language. Pediatrics 74:282–287, 1984.

Teele, D. W., Klein, J. O., and Rosner, B.: The Greater Boston Otitis Media Study Group: In preparation.

Thomsen, J., Meistrup-Larson, K. I., Sorensen, H., Larsen, P. K., and Mygind, N.: Penicillin and acute otitis: Short and long term results. Ann. Otol. Rhinol. Laryngol. 89(68):271–274, 1980.

Thomsen, J., and Tos, M.: Spontaneous improvement of secretory otitis. A long-term study. Acta Otolaryngol. (Stockh.) 92:493–499, 1981.

Timmermans, F. J., and Gerson, S.: Chronic granulomatous otitis media in bottle-fed Inuit children. Can. Med. Assoc. J. 122:545–547, 1980.

Tos, M.: Spontaneous improvement of secretory otitis and impedance screening. Arch. Otolaryngol. 106:345–349, 1980.

Tos, M., Poulsen, G., and Borch, J.: Tympanometry in two-year-old children. ORL 40:77–85, 1978.

Tos, M., and Poulsen, G.: Tympanometry in two-year-old children. Seasonal influence on frequency of secretory otitis and tubal function. ORL 41:1–10, 1979.

Tos, M., Poulsen, G., and Hancke, A. B.: Screening tympanometry during the first year of life. Acta Otolaryngol. (Stockh.) 88:388–394, 1979.

Tos, M., Holm-Jensen, S., Hjort Sorensen, C., and Mogensen, C.: Spontaneous course and frequency of secretory otitis in four-year-old children. Arch. Otolaryngol. 108:4–10, 1982.

Vinther, B., Elbrond, O., and Pedersen, C. B.: Otitis media in childhood, socio-medical aspects with special reference to day-care and housing conditions. Acta Otolaryngol. (Stockh.) 386:121–123, 1982.

Warren, W. S., and Stool, S. E.: Otitis media in low-birth-weight infants. J. Pediatr. 79:740–743, 1971.

Wright, P. F., McConnell, K. B., Thompson, J. M., Vaughn, W. K., and Sell, S. H.: A longitudinal study of the detection of otitis media in the first two years of life. Int. J. Pediatr. Otorhinolaryngol. 10:245–252, 1985.

Zonis, R. D.: Chronic otitis media in the southwestern American Indian. Arch. Otolaryngol. 88:360–365, 1968.

5

Microbiology

The microbiological causes of otitis media have been documented by appropriate cultures of middle ear effusions obtained by needle aspiration. Many bacteriological studies of acute otitis media have been performed, and the results are remarkably consistent in demonstrating the importance of *Streptococcus pneumoniae* and *Haemophilus influenzae*. Recent investigations identify an increased incidence of infection due to *Branhamella catarrhalis*. Studies of asymptomatic children with middle ear effusion indicate that bacterial pathogens are also present in these fluids, suggesting that bacteria may be a factor in the development and persistence of the effusion. Epidemiological evidence associates viral infection with otitis media, but viruses have been isolated or identified by detection of antigen in relatively few episodes of acute otitis media. *Chlamydia trachomatis* is responsible for some episodes of otitis media in infants six months of age and younger. The purpose of this chapter is to review the results of these microbiological studies and to consider various aspects of the infectious process in the middle ear. The microbiological complications of otitis media are discussed in Chapters Nine and Ten.

BACTERIOLOGY

The results of bacteriological studies of otitis media in children from Sweden, Finland, and the United States during the period 1952 to 1981 are very similar from country to country and over time (Table 5–1). Microbiological results of middle ear aspirates of Pittsburgh children with acute "severe" otitis media during the period 1981 to 1984 is presented in Figure 5–1. "Severe" was defined as body temperature greater than 38.5° C, acute otalgia, or headache and irritability. Recent investigations in Japan (Sugita et al., 1983) and Colombia, South America (Trujillo et al., 1981) report similar bacteriological results. *S. pneumoniae* and *H. influenzae* are the most frequent agents in all age groups. *B. catarrhalis*, group A streptococcus, *Staphylococcus aureus*, and gram-negative enteric bacilli are less frequent causes of otitis. No growth (or isolation of an organism considered to be a contaminant, such as *Staphylococcus epidermidis* or diphtheroids) occurs in approximately one third of effusions that are cultured for bacteria.

Table 5–1. **BACTERIAL PATHOGENS ISOLATED FROM MIDDLE EAR FLUID IN 4675 CHILDREN WITH ACUTE OTITIS MEDIA***

Bacterial Pathogen	Percentage of Children with Pathogen	
	Mean	Range
Streptococcus pneumoniae	33	26–53
Haemophilus influenzae	21	14–31
Streptococcus, group A	8	0.3–24
Staphylococcus aureus	2	0–3
Branhamella catarrhalis	3	0–4
Gram-negative enteric bacilli	1	0–4
Miscellaneous bacteria	1	0–2
None or nonpathogens	31	2–47

*Twelve reports from centers in United States, Finland, and Sweden, 1952–1981: Bjuggren and Tunevall, 1952; Lahikainen, 1953; Mortimer and Watterson, 1956; Groonroos et al., 1964; Coffey, 1966; Feingold et al., 1966; Halstead et al., 1968; Nilson et al., 1969; Howie et al., 1970; Kamme et al., 1970; Howard et al., 1976; Schwartz, 1981.

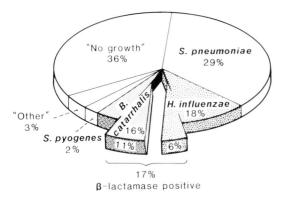

Figure 5–1. Microbiologic results of 247 middle ear aspirates of infants and children with acute "severe" otitis media from the Pittsburgh Otitis Media Research Center, 1981–1984.

Streptococcus pneumoniae

Because *S. pneumoniae* is the most important cause of otitis media, investigators have carefully studied the types responsible for infections of the middle ear. The results of studies of 1837 episodes of acute otitis media due to *S. pneumoniae* indicate that relatively few types are responsible for most disease. The most common types in order of decreasing frequency are 19, 23, 6, 14, 3, and 18 (Austrian et al., 1977; Gray et al., 1979; Kamme et al., 1970) (Table 5–2). All are included in the currently available 23-type pneumococcal vaccine. Capsular polysaccharide antigens have been identified in most middle ear fluids from which pneumococci can be cultured and also in some fluids that

Table 5–2. **DISTRIBUTION OF SEROTYPES OF 1837 STRAINS OF *STREPTOCOCCUS PNEUMONIAE* ISOLATED FROM MIDDLE EAR EFFUSIONS OF CHILDREN WITH ACUTE OTITIS MEDIA***

Serotype	Percentage of Strains
1	2.1
3	8.5
4	3.4
6	12.0
7	2.3
8	1.5
9	2.9
14	10.3
18	5.8
19	23.0
23	12.5
Others	15.7

*Data from Austrian et al., 1977; Gray et al., 1979; Kamme et al., 1970.

are sterile. Detection of bacterial antigens is discussed below.

Studies of bacterial adherence of pneumococci to mucosal surfaces suggest mechanisms of pathogenicity for respiratory infections. Pneumococci isolated from patients with recurrent episodes of acute otitis media adhered in larger numbers to epithelial cells from the nasopharynx than did strains from cases of bacteremia or meningitis (Andersson et al., 1981). More bacteria attached to epithelial cells from patients with recurrent episodes of acute otitis media than to cells obtained from controls (Jorgensen et al., 1984).

A change in the ecology of *S. pneumoniae* is reflected in altered patterns of susceptibility to antimicrobial agents. Multiresistant strains of *S. pneumoniae* that are highly resistant to penicillin G (minimum inhibitory concentration [MIC], more than 4 µg/ml) were first noted in South Africa in 1977 (Applebaum et al., 1977) and have remained restricted to that area. Few of these strains have been identified in the United States and Western Europe (Cates et al., 1978; Ward, 1981). However, many strains of *S. pneumoniae* that have been isolated from cases of otitis media in recent years have had decreased susceptibility to penicillin G (MIC 0.1 to 1.0 µg/ml) (Ward, 1981).

Haemophilus influenzae

Otitis media due to *H. influenzae* is associated with nontypable strains in the vast majority of patients. In approximately 10 percent of cases due to *H. influenzae* the isolate is type b; some of these children appear to have severe infection, and about one quarter have concomitant bacteremia or meningitis (Harding et al., 1973). Cases of otitis due to types a, e, and f have been reported but are very infrequent.

Until recently, no markers were available to distinguish among the nonencapsulated types of *H. influenzae*. We now know that the group is heterogeneous and may be classified by biochemical and antigenic markers. Biochemical profiles have been used to classify strains of nontypable *H. influenzae* isolated from middle ear fluids; the majority of strains belong to two biotypes based on assays of indole, urease, and ornithine decarboxylase (DeMaria et al., 1984b). Current studies of outer membrane proteins also aim at a means of classifying the nonencapsulated strains;

eight major proteins have been identified (Loeb and Smith, 1980). A serotyping system based on antigenic patterns of outer membranes has been suggested (Murphy and Apicella, 1985). Thus, outer membrane protein patterns may be used to evaluate the relatedness of nontypable *H. influenzae* isolated from middle ear fluids.

H. influenzae was considered to be restricted in importance to otitis media occurring in preschool children; however, the organism is a significant cause of otitis media in older children, adolescents, and adults. *H. influenzae* was isolated from middle ear fluids of 36 percent of children, aged five to nine years, with acute otitis media (Schwartz et al., 1977). *H. influenzae* was the cause of otitis media in 33 percent of 18 children aged eight through 17 years (Schwartz and Rodriguez, 1981). *H. influenzae* was also isolated from 15 of 45 patients over 16 years of age (Herberts et al., 1971). In a survey of cases of acute otitis seen in primary care hospitals in metropolitan Tokyo for the year beginning July, 1979, 28 percent of 31 bacteria isolated from middle ear effusions of patients 10 to 15 years of age and 15 percent of 76 bacteria found in patients 16 to 70 years of age were *H. influenzae* (Sugita et al., 1983). Thus, the proportion of acute otitis media due to *H. influenzae* is approximately the same in all age groups.

Fifteen to 30 percent of nontypable strains of *H. influenzae* isolated from middle ear effusions of children with acute otitis media produce a beta-lactamase that hydrolyzes ampicillin, amoxicillin, and penicillins G and V. The incidence of beta-lactamase–producing strains has been relatively stable since 1977.

Branhamella catarrhalis

Before 1983, *B. catarrhalis* was isolated infrequently from purulent middle ear fluids (Coffey et al., 1967), and many considered the organism a commensal with limited potential for causing disease. In 1983, reports from Pittsburgh (Kovatch et al., 1983) and Cleveland (Shurin et al., 1983) noted a marked increase in incidence; the organism was isolated from middle ear fluids of 22 percent and 27 percent, respectively, of a consecutive series of children enrolled in studies of acute otitis media. In Dallas, during a similar time period, the incidence of *B. catarrhalis* in middle ear fluids was lower: 6 percent of 150 children (Odio et al., 1985).

We now must consider *B. catarrhalis* a respiratory pathogen capable of causing acute otitis media. The data from Pittsburgh and Cleveland make it the third most likely bacterium responsible for acute otitis media, behind *S. pneumoniae* and *H. influenzae*. Future studies will determine whether or not the Cleveland and Pittsburgh experiences were isolated or presage a uniform increase in importance of *B. catarrhalis* in otitis media.

Prior to 1970 almost all strains of *B. catarrhalis* were sensitive to penicillin and ampicillin. Today, a majority of strains of *B. catarrhalis* isolated from middle ear fluids produce beta-lactamase. The increased incidence of infection due to this organism may require a change in initial therapy from the ampicillins, which are susceptible to beta-lactamases. We will need to add the proportion of cases of otitis media caused by beta-lactamase–producing *B. catarrhalis* and *H. influenzae* to determine the need for a change in initial therapy.

Leiononen and colleagues (1981) provided serological evidence for a pathogenic role of *B. catarrhalis* in children with acute otitis media. The presence of IgG and IgA antibodies to *B. catarrhalis* in serum or middle ear fluid, or both, was correlated with isolation of the organism from the middle ear. An increase in titer of antibodies to the organisms was found between acute and convalescent serums in 10 of 19 children with acute otitis media whose middle ear fluid yielded *B. catarrhalis* alone, and no increase was seen in 14 children with acute otitis media whose middle ear fluids yielded other pathogens.

Groups A and B Streptococci

During the preantibiotic era, otitis due to group A streptococcus was frequently associated with scarlet fever and was often of a very destructive form (Clarke, 1962). *Streptococcus hemolyticus* (presumably group A streptococcus) was the most prevalent organism in cultures taken at myringotomy for acute otitis media and the most frequent cause of mastoid infection in patients undergoing mastoidectomy at the Manhattan Eye, Ear, and Throat Hospital during 1934 (Page, 1935). Recently, group A streptococcus has been a significant pathogen in some studies of otitis media from Scandinavia, but this has not been the case in most studies from the United States. Otitis media due to group A streptococcus now seems to be less frequent and less virulent.

Group B streptococcus is, with *Escherichia coli*, the leading cause of sepsis and meningitis in the newborn infant, as reported by surveys in the United States and Western Europe (Klein and Marcy, 1983). Group B streptococci have been isolated from various body fluids, including middle ear fluid in neonates with otitis media. Bacteremia is frequently associated with otitis media in these infants.

Staphylococcus aureus

S. aureus is an uncommon cause of acute otitis media; the organism was isolated in fewer than 3 percent of samples of middle ear fluids from children with acute infection (Table 5–1). Studies from Japan indicate a higher incidence of middle ear infection, approximately 10 percent, due to *S. aureus* (Baba, 1985).

Staphylococcus epidermidis and Diphtheroids

The roles of coagulase-negative staphylococci (Feigin et al., 1973) and diphtheroids in acute otitis media are uncertain. These organisms are considered commensals and are part of the skin flora of the external ear canal. Isolation of pure cultures of coagulase-negative staphylococci from cases of purulent middle ear effusions after adequate cleansing of the external canal suggest a pathogenic role in a limited number of cases. Nine different species of coagulase-negative staphylococci have been isolated from middle ear fluids; *S. epidermidis* is the most common (Bernstein et al., 1984).

Specific antibody to diphtheroids was identified in middle ear effusions and serums of children undergoing myringotomy for chronic otitis media with effusion (Lewis et al., 1979). Bernstein and colleagues (1980) found antibody-coated *S. epidermidis* and diphtheroids in the middle ears of children with otitis media with effusion. The fluids contained specific antibody, and in several cases of otitis due to *S. epidermidis*, antibody was present in middle ear fluid but absent from serum. These data indicate that diphtheroids and *S. epidermidis* may elicit an immune response in the middle ear. The role of these organisms in middle ear disease,

however, remains uncertain. It is possible that they are opportunistic bacteria that invade the middle ear only under certain circumstances, such as persistent effusion.

Gram-negative Bacilli

Gram-negative bacilli are responsible for about 20 percent of cases of otitis media in young infants, but these organisms are rarely present in the middle ear effusions of older children with acute otitis media (Table 5–3). Gram-negative bacteria, particularly *Pseudomonas aeruginosa*, are frequently associated with chronic suppurative otitis media.

A report from Israel described 33 patients of varying ages with acute otitis media caused by gram-negative bacilli (Ostfeld and Rubinstein, 1980). *P. aeruginosa* was isolated from middle ear fluids of 23 patients, and an indole-positive *Proteus* species was isolated from the fluids in six patients. Seven of the patients were three months of age or younger, 16 were four to 24 months of age, and 10 were two to 80 years of age. Four adult patients had diabetes mellitus, but there were no other patients with significant underlying diseases. The patients had a high rate of other disease manifestations due to the organism isolated from the middle ear effusion; of these patients, five had acute mastoiditis, three had accompanying bacter-

Table 5–3. **BACTERIAL PATHOGENS ISOLATED FROM 169 INFANTS WITH OTITIS MEDIA DURING THE FIRST SIX WEEKS OF LIFE**[*]

Microorganism	Percentage of Infants with Pathogen
Respiratory bacteria	
Streptococcus pneumoniae	18.3
Haemophilus influenzae	12.4
S. pneumoniae and *H. influenzae*	3.0
Staphylococcus aureus	7.7
Streptococcus, groups A and B	3.0
Branhamella catarrhalis	5.3
Enteric bacteria	
Escherichia coli	5.9
Klebsiella and *Enterobacter* species	5.3
Pseudomonas aeruginosa	1.8
Miscellaneous	5.3
None or nonpathogens	32.0

[*]Data from Berman et al., 1978; Bland, 1972; Shurin et al., 1978; Tetzlaff et al., 1977.

emia, and four adult patients showed extensive osteomyelitis of the base of the skull. Culture material was obtained from purulent drainage from the middle ear in cases with perforated tympanic membranes, and the bacteriological results may represent contaminants from the external ear. In addition, some patients had prolonged courses that might be better described as chronic suppurative otitis media. Nevertheless, this series indicates a potential danger of acute middle ear infection due to gram-negative bacilli.

Anaerobic Bacteria

Recent improvements in techniques for isolation and identification of anaerobic bacteria have provided a better understanding of the anaerobic flora of humans and the roles of these organisms in disease. The studies of Brook, Anthony, and Finegold (1978) suggest that anaerobic bacteria may cause otitis media. Anaerobic bacteria were isolated from the middle ear effusions of 28 percent of 62 children with acute otitis media. *Peptococcus*, an organism that colonizes the upper respiratory tract and may cause lower respiratory tract disease, and *Propionibacterium acnes*, a part of normal skin flora, were the anaerobic organisms most frequently isolated. However, these investigators did not cleanse the external canal prior to aspiration, and it is possible that the organisms isolated represented contaminants from the external canal rather than pathogens in the middle ear fluid. A subsequent study by one of the authors (Brook and Schwartz, 1981) indicated a more limited role for anaerobic bacteria in acute otitis media. Twenty-eight infants with acute infection were studied: aerobic bacteria were isolated from the middle ear fluids of 20 children; cultures from two children yielded mixtures of aerobic and anaerobic bacteria. Luotonen and coworkers (1982) failed to isolate anaerobic bacteria from 71 middle ear aspirates from 59 subjects. These data suggest that anaerobic organisms are relatively uncommon in middle ear effusions of children who have acute otitis media.

Mixed and Disparate Cultures

Disparate results of cultures of middle ear fluids occur when cultures of the two ears in

bilateral disease yield different information: effusion from one ear is sterile but a bacterial pathogen is isolated from the other ear, or a different bacterial pathogen is isolated from each of the two ears. Mixed cultures may also occur: two types or two species of bacteria are found in the same middle ear fluid. Groonroos and colleagues (1964) reported 31.6 percent disparate results of cultures from children with bilateral otitis media. All children had either *S. pneumoniae, H. influenzae,* or group A streptococci in fluid from one middle ear and sterile fluid in the other. Van Dishoeck, Derks, and Voorhorst (1959) found that 19 percent of cultures from children with bilateral otitis media yielded different results. The majority of children had a pathogen recovered from one ear and sterile fluid in the other. Also included were six cases in which cultures of one middle ear fluid yielded a single pathogen but in the opposite middle ear fluid, two pathogens were found. Austrian, Howie, and Ploussard (1977) recovered different serotypes of *S. pneumoniae* from middle ear fluids in 18 children, which represented 1.5 percent of the cases of bilateral pneumococcal otitis media. Pelton and coworkers (1980) cultured middle ear fluid from both ears of 122 children with bilateral acute otitis media. Disparate results were found in 31 (25 percent) of the children: in 25 children a pathogen was present in one ear and the fluid from the other ear was sterile or yielded a nonpathogen; in six children different pathogens (*H. influenzae* and *S. pneumoniae* in each case) were isolated from the two fluids. Howard and colleagues (1976) noted *S. pneumoniae* and *H. influenzae* together in 20 effusions (5 percent of those studied).

These data indicate that investigative microbiological studies of bilateral otitis media must include aspiration of both ears to determine the efficacy of methods of treatment (i.e., trials of antimicrobial agents) or prevention (i.e., evaluation of vaccines or drugs). In addition, the complete bacteriological assessment of the middle ear for a child undergoing tympanocentesis for diagnostic purposes can only be accomplished by aspirating both middle ear effusions when the disease is bilateral.

Sterile Cultures

In all studies of acute otitis media, a significant proportion (approximately one third) of middle ear fluids are sterile after appropriate and usual cultures for bacteria have been made. The cause of these cases of otitis media may be one or more of the following:

1. A nonbacterial organism such as a virus, chlamydia, or mycoplasma.

2. A fastidious bacterial organism, such as an anaerobic bacterium, that is not isolated by usual laboratory techniques.

3. An immune response to a noninfectious agent such as pollen or other antigen.

4. Prior administration of an antimicrobial agent that would suppress growth of bacteria.

5. Presence of antimicrobial enzymes, such as lysozymes, alone or in combination with immunoglobulins in middle ear fluid, that would suppress growth of bacteria.

6. An acute illness in a child who has persistent middle ear effusion from an episode of otitis media some time in the past. Since children may have middle ear effusion for weeks to months after the onset of acute otitis media (Teele et al., 1980b), an illness due to a subsequent infectious episode, during the time spent with middle ear effusion persisting from a prior episode of otitis, might be assumed by the physician to be a recurrence of acute otitis media.

Use of the Gram stain is of value in identification of fastidious bacterial organisms and may provide evidence of bacterial infection, although antibiotics or antimicrobial substances inhibit growth of bacteria. Techniques for identification of bacterial and viral antigens are also likely to decrease the number of episodes of otitis that are now categorized as "no growth."

Identification of Bacterial Antigens

Results of studies using techniques for identification of bacterial antigens provide new insights into the infectious process. Countercurrent immunoelectrophoresis (CIE), latex agglutination, and enzyme-linked immunosorbent assay (ELISA) have been used to detect bacterial antigens such as capsular polysaccharides of *S. pneumoniae*, *H. influenzae* type b, *Neisseria meningitidis*, and group B streptococci in blood, urine, cerebrospinal fluid, and other body fluids. These methods are advantageous because of ease of performance, rapidity, specificity, sensitivity (as little as 0.2 ng of polysaccharide capsular antigens can be detected), and ability to identify bacteria that do not grow in culture media.

S. pneumoniae is identified by CIE in most middle ear fluids in which the organism is cultured and in many specimens that have no bacterial growth (Luotonen et al., 1981; Ostfeld and Altmann, 1980). Luotonen and colleagues identified pneumococcal capsular polysaccharide in 83 percent of middle ear fluids from which *S. pneumoniae* was cultured and in about one third of middle ear effusions from which no bacteria was grown. Type-specific pneumococcal antigens may persist for periods in excess of six months (Karma et al., 1985). Different serotypes have differing sensitivity of antigen detection. Thus, sensitivity for detection in culture-positive samples of types 1, 15, and 19 was high, whereas sensitivity for type 23 was low; the sensitivity for type 6A was higher than that for 6B (Herva et al., 1984). These methods used to detect bacterial antigen add information about the large number of patients who have negative results of bacterial cultures.

VIRUSES

Epidemiological data suggest that viral infection is frequently associated with acute otitis media. In a longitudinal study of respiratory illnesses and complications in children six weeks to six years of age attending a day-care and school program, Henderson and colleagues (1982) demonstrated a correlation between isolation of viruses from the upper respiratory tract and clinical diagnosis of otitis media. Concurrent or antecedent (within 14 days) viral infection was identified in 26.3 percent of episodes of otitis media in children under three years of age. Viral outbreaks coincided with epidemics of otitis media. Otitis media was increased in the 14 days after upper respiratory tract isolation of respiratory syncytial viruses, adenoviruses (usually types 1, 2, and 5), influenza virus types A and B, parainfluenza and mumps viruses, and enteroviruses. Rhinoviruses were not significantly associated with the occurrence of otitis media.

Viruses are infrequently isolated from the middle ear effusions of children with acute infection of the middle ear; a virus was isolated from only 4.4 percent of 663 patients (Klein and Teele, 1976) (Table 5–4). Respiratory syncytial virus and influenza virus were isolated most frequently. The isolation of these two agents was usually made during periods of epidemic infection in the com-

Table 5–4. **ISOLATION OF VIRUSES IN 663 PATIENTS WITH OTITIS MEDIA***†

Virus	Number of Patients
Respiratory syncytial virus (RSV)	22
Influenza viruses	4
Coxsackievirus B4	1
Adenovirus 3	1
Parainfluenza 2	1
Totals	29 (4.4%)
No Growth	634

*622 patients had acute and 41 had chronic otitis media.

†From Klein, J. O., and Teele, D. W.: Isolation of viruses and mycoplasmas from middle ear effusions: A review. Ann. Otol. Rhinol. Laryngol. 85(Suppl. 25):140–144, 1976.

munity. Isolation rates of viruses have not improved with current techniques. Howie and coworkers (1982) isolated viruses from four of 88 middle ear fluids obtained from patients with acute otitis media: two specimens yielded adenovirus; influenza B virus and respiratory syncytial virus were each present in one specimen.

Studies of viral antigens yield more information about their role in otitis media (Klein et al., 1982). Klein and colleagues found evidence of viral antigen by means of ELISA in middle ear fluids obtained from approximately one quarter of children with acute otitis media. Of 13 children with viral antigen in the middle ear, respiratory syncytial virus (RSV) was most frequently identified (10 children); influenza virus (two children) and rotavirus (one child) were also identified but were uncommon. The ELISA measures viral antigens rather than replicating virions and may detect viral materials that grow poorly or not at all in tissue culture or animal systems. Failure to identify viruses in middle ear fluids may be due to inadequate sensitivity of available techniques. During an epidemic of RSV, Sarkkinen and colleagues identified RSV antigen in the middle ear effusions of 15 percent of children with otitis media; adenovirus antigen was found in an additional 3 percent of patients (Sarkkinen et al., 1985). Interferon was identified in four of eight middle ear fluids that had positive results for RSV antigen (Salonen et al., 1984). Bacterial isolations were similar in middle ear fluids, regardless of whether the results were positive or negative for viruses. Thus, antibacterial agents may successfully eradicate the bacterial agent from the middle ear ef-

fusion, but signs of disease may persist because of the concurrent viral infection.

As in studies of isolation of viruses from middle ear fluids, RSV antigen was identified in the majority of fluids, and other viral antigens were identified infrequently. Richman and colleagues believe that current ELISA techniques have reached the limit of their sensitivity for identification of viral antigens and that rapid viral diagnosis will require new approaches. They discuss two useful techniques: detection of viral antigen by visual localization of virus-specific immunoenzyme staining, and detection of viral nucleic acids in clinical specimens by hybridization with nucleic-acid probes (Richman et al., 1984).

Otitis media may accompany exanthematous viral infections, such as measles and infectious mononucleosis caused by Epstein-Barr virus (Sumaya and Ench, 1985). Invasion of the middle ear by smallpox virus has been demonstrated. Guarnieri bodies were present in the tympanic membrane of a three-month-old Indian child who died of smallpox (Bordley and Kapur, 1972).

Viral studies of children with acute otitis media suggest an important role for RSV, a lesser role for adenoviruses and influenza viruses, but an uncertain role for other respiratory viruses. The small number of viruses other than RSV that have been isolated from middle ear fluids may indicate that (1) viruses were present early in the course of the disease and were no longer present when the patients sought medical attention; (2) these viruses were present in low concentrations and not readily isolated from the ear fluids; (3) inhibitory materials such as antibody, interferon, or lysozymes prevented successful isolation; (4) viruses produced inflammatory changes in the upper respiratory tract but were not present in the effusion fluid; or (5) these viruses have not been associated with many episodes of otitis media.

MYCOPLASMA

The isolation and identification of mycoplasma from secretions obtained from the upper respiratory tract are now readily accomplished in solid and liquid media. An initial report of a volunteer study suggested a role for these organisms in otitis media. Myringitis, associated with hemorrhage and bleb formation in the more severe cases, was observed in nonimmune volunteers inoculated with *Mycoplasma pneumoniae* (Rifkind et al., 1962). Bullous myringitis in children may result from various bacterial pathogens responsible for otitis media; its presence does not indicate mycoplasma infection (Roberts, 1980). However, the middle ear fluid of a large number of patients (771) has been studied (Klein and Teele, 1976), and *M. pneumoniae* was isolated in only one case (Sobeslavsky et al., 1965).

During an investigation of a community outbreak of pneumonia due to mycoplasma, 59 percent of children with otitis media were shown (by isolation of the organism from the pharynx or by antibody responses) to have had an infection with *M. pneumoniae* (Jensen et al., 1967). Thus, it is likely that mycoplasma infection causes disease in all parts of the respiratory tract, including the middle ear. Patients with respiratory disease due to *M. pneumoniae* may have accompanying otitis media, but the organism appears to play a limited role in the overall picture of acute otitis media in children.

CHLAMYDIA

C. trachomatis is the etiologic agent of a mild but prolonged pneumonitis in infants. Many infants with pneumonia due to *C. trachomatis* have otitis media (Schachter et al., 1979; Tipple et al., 1979). Tipple, Beem, and Saxon (1979) isolated the organism from ear aspirates of three of 11 infants with chlamydial pneumonia. Chang and colleagues (1982) recovered *C. trachomatis* from the middle ear effusions of two of 12 children with acute otitis media and one of 14 children with persistent middle ear effusion. One of the children with acute infection was 10 months of age, but the report did not provide ages for the other two children. *C. trachomatis* was not isolated from middle ear fluids obtained at the time of placement of tympanostomy tubes in 68 children, nine months to eight years of age (Hammerschlag et al., 1980). Thus, *C. trachomatis* is associated with acute respiratory infections, including otitis media, in young infants (under age six months).

UNCOMMON MICROORGANISMS

Corynebacterium diphtheriae

Diphtheritic otitis may accompany diphtheritic croup and nasopharyngitis. Although many cases cannot be differentiated from other forms of purulent otitis, diphtheritic membranes may form and be recognized in the middle ear. Complications are frequent, including destruction of the tympanic membrane and ossicles and invasive infection of contiguous structures leading to necrosis of the mastoid process, temporal bone, and labyrinth (Downes, 1959; Drury, 1925). Thirteen cases of otitis media due to *C. diphtheriae* were among 3916 cases reported to the Centers for Disease Control of the U.S. Public Health Service for the years 1959 to 1970. Five cases of diphtheritic otitis occurred among 1433 cases of diphtheria seen at the Los Angeles County Hospital during the 10-year period beginning June, 1941 (Naiditch and Bower, 1954).

Mycobacterium tuberculosis

At the turn of the century, tuberculous otitis was an occasional cause of severe middle ear disease, particularly in the very young. Turner and Fraser (1915) reported a series of cases at the Royal Infirmary in Edinburgh for the period 1907 to 1914; 51, or 2.8 percent, were due to tuberculosis, and 84 percent of these cases occurred in the first year of life. Today, the disease is seen in underdeveloped areas of the world, but occasional cases occur in the United States: bovine tuberculosis was responsible for 29 cases of chronic otorrhea in children seen in Kampala between 1969 and 1972 (Raikundalia, 1975), 11 cases of tuberculous otitis were reported in Capetown children between 1967 and 1971 (Sellars and Seid, 1973), and three patients with tuberculous otitis were seen at the Children's Memorial Hospital in Oklahoma City in the same period as the Capetown cases (MacAdam and Rubio, 1977). Tuberculous infection should be considered when chronic otorrhea occurs in recent immigrants from areas with high rates of infection. Skolnik and colleagues recently reviewed the literature of tuberculosis of the middle ear (Skolnik et al., 1986).

When otitis occurs as the only apparent focus of tuberculous infection, the disease is usually due to ingestion of infected cow's milk. The infection may also occur in patients with active pulmonary disease; the middle ear is infected from the upper respiratory tract.

Tuberculous otitis is characterized by a painless, watery otorrhea through single or multiple perforations of the tympanic membrane; enlarged periauricular lymph nodes; and a high incidence of facial paralysis and early hearing loss. Mastoiditis is a frequent complication (Mumtaz et al., 1983). The diagnosis of tuberculous otitis media is based on demonstration of acid-fast bacilli within granuloma in biopsy materials, with or without the culture of *M. tuberculosis* from the biopsy, aural drainage, or aspirate of middle ear fluid. Chemotherapy shortens the course and severity of the disease, but persistent hearing loss is frequent.

Clostridium tetani

Otogenous tetanus usually occurs as a sequela of chronic otitis media. *C. tetani* multiplies in the purulent drainage in the external ear canal and may gain access to the middle ear (Deinard et al., 1980). The organism may be present also in the oropharynx, and it is possible that infection in the middle ear occurs via the eustachian tube. *C. tetani* was isolated from swabs of middle ear fluid of eight children admitted to Children's Hospital in Bangkok with otitis media, otorrhea, and trismus and other signs of tetanus (Fischer et al., 1977).

Ascaris lumbricoides

The only parasitic infection that has been associated with otitis media is *Ascaris lumbricoides*. Roundworms may be vomited through the mouth or nostrils, enter the eustachian tube, and produce an inflammatory reaction in the middle ear. The worm perforates the tympanic membrane and emerges through the external canal. A case report described infection in a one-and-a-half-year-old child who was brought to a Bombay clinic with a worm emerging from the ear. A 7.5-cm-long roundworm, *A. lumbricoides*, was removed from the canal and middle ear (Shah and Desai, 1969).

MICROBIAL PRODUCTS

Endotoxin

Endotoxin has been detected in middle ear effusions that contain nontypable *H. influenzae*. Endotoxins are lipopolysaccharide complexes on the surface of gram-negative bacteria that have many biological effects, including production of fever and inflammation. Physiological activities persist after death of the organism. DeMaria and colleagues (1984c) detected endotoxin in 80 percent of 89 middle ear fluids obtained at placement of ventilating tubes. Endotoxin was not only present in all except one fluid from which *H. influenzae* was cultured but also was present (though in lesser concentrations) in fluids that had negative results at culture and fluids that cultured *S. pneumoniae* (which does not contain endotoxin). The source of endotoxin for the middle ear fluids that did not contain endotoxin-producing microorganisms is unknown. Endotoxin may play a role in the pathogenesis of inflammation in the middle ear; purified endotoxin from killed *H. influenzae* induced production of middle ear fluid (DeMaria et al., 1984a).

Interferon

Local production of interferon in the middle ear was suggested by findings of higher concentrations in specimens of middle ear fluid when compared with levels in serum (Howie et al., 1982). The presence of interferon suggests a current or antecedent viral infection; Salonen and colleagues recovered interferon in middle ear fluids positive for RSV antigen and failed to detect interferon in antigen-negative specimens (Salonen et al., 1984). In contrast, Howie and colleagues demonstrated the presence of interferon in middle ear fluids containing pathogenic bacteria in the absence of detectable viruses, suggesting bacterial induction of interferon (Howie et al., 1982). The role of interferon in middle ear infection remains to be elucidated.

Neuraminidase

Neuraminidase identified at neutral pH was found in middle ear fluids from patients with acute otitis media and otitis media with effusion. LaMarco and colleagues noted that almost all fluids that grew *S. pneumoniae* had neuraminidase activity, whereas only about one third of fluids that grew other bacteria or no bacteria had evidence of the enzyme (LaMarco et al., 1984). The plasma of patients lacked neuraminidase activity, indicating that the enzyme in the middle ear fluid originated in the middle ear and was not a transudate from blood. Since mammalian neuraminidases have optimal activity near pH 4, the authors conclude that the source of the neutral pH neuraminidase was microorganisms. The enzyme may be an important factor in the pathogenesis of disease caused by *S. pneumoniae*.

BACTERIOLOGICAL STUDIES OF CHRONIC OTITIS MEDIA WITH EFFUSION

Chronic effusions have in the past been assumed to be sterile, since several reports describe unsuccessful attempts to culture bacteria from them (Harcourt and Brown, 1953; Robinson and Nicholas, 1951; Siirala and Vuori, 1956). Senturia and coworkers (1958), however, were able to identify bacteria by means of smears and cultures from 42 percent of children with otitis media with effusion; since then other workers have reported similar results. The studies were performed by investigators in Columbus, Ohio (Liu et al., 1975), Boston (Healy and Teele, 1977), and Minneapolis (Giebink et al., 1979). The protocols were similar: most children were observed to have persistent effusion for at least two months; at the time of myringotomy or placement of tympanostomy tubes, fluid was obtained from the middle ear for culture of bacteria. In each study, 30 to 50 percent of the children had bacteria in the middle ear fluid. *S. pneumoniae*, *H. influenzae*, *B. catarrhalis*, or group A streptococcus were isolated from 10 to 22 percent of the fluids of these asymptomatic children.

These studies are cited because all included appropriate cleansing of the external canal prior to aspiration of the middle ear fluid. Other studies are not included because of failure to cleanse the canal and thus may include bacteriological results of middle ear fluids contaminated by external canal flora. A special problem is presented by obtaining appropriate sampling for bacteria of the chronically draining ear. Cultures of fluid from draining ears require, first, removal of debris and fluid in the canal, which includes material from the middle ear mixed with external canal flora, and second, careful aspiration of fluid from the middle ear as it emerges through the tympanic membrane or by means of tympanocentesis. Without use of techniques of direct aspiration of fluid from the middle ear, microbiological results must be considered of uncertain validity.

The bacteriological results of chronic middle ear effusions of 179 Pittsburgh children aged one to 16 years are given in Table 5–5 (Riding et al., 1978). Bacteria were cultured from 86 of 179 (48 percent) chronic middle ear effusions (see Table 5–5), and the organisms were present in serous, mucoid, and purulent effusions. The most common species were *H. influenzae*, *B. catarrhalis*, *S. pneumoniae*, and *S. aureus*. *S. epidermidis* was cultured from many middle ears when this organism was not cultured from the external canal of the same ear (a culture preceded sterilization and tympanocentesis). Bacteria were also cultured from 37 percent of chronic middle ear effusions found in Pittsburgh infants aged one to 12 months (Stanievich et al., 1981); *S. pneumoniae* and *H. influenzae* were present in 23 percent of the ears. *S. pneumoniae* and *H. influenzae* were cultured from 50 percent of 20 persistent middle ear

Table 5–5. **BACTERIOLOGICAL RESULTS OF 179 CHRONIC MIDDLE EAR EFFUSIONS IN CHILDREN ONE TO 16 YEARS OF AGE***

Type of Organism	Percentage of Ears with Middle Ear Effusion			
	Serous (48 ears)	Mucoid (112 ears)	Purulent (19 ears)	Total Ears (179 ears)
S. pneumoniae	4	4	—	4
H. influenzae	8†	11	16	11
Streptococcus	—	—	5	0.6
B. catarrhalis	2	4	16	4
S. aureus	4	3	—	3
S. epidermidis	15	12	5	12
Others‡	31	22	26	25
Percentage of ears with organism	52§	43	68	48

*Modified from Riding, K. H., et al.: Microbiology of recurrent and chronic otitis media with effusion. J. Pediatr. 93:739–743, 1978.

†Includes one effusion with *H. influenzae* type b; no ampicillin-resistant organisms were identified.

‡Alpha- or nonhemolytic streptococci, microaerophilic streptococci, *Moraxella*, *Propionibacterium*, *Escherichia coli*, diphtheroids, *Candida albicans*.

§This number is smaller than the sum of each percentage above because some ears contained more than one type of organism.

fluids of Pittsburgh infants with unrepaired cleft palates (Stanievich et al., 1981). More recent information from Pittsburgh contrasts the microbiological results of acute otitis media with those of chronic otitis media with effusion (Fig. 5–2).

Anaerobic bacteria were isolated from the middle ear fluids of most patients with chronic otitis media by Brook (1979), but the findings are of uncertain validity because of the failure to adequately cleanse the external canal prior to tympanocentesis. When the canal was adequately cleansed by other investigators (Giebink et al., 1979; Sipila et al., 1981; Teele et al., 1980a), anaerobic organisms were rarely isolated.

A higher incidence of respiratory pathogens was noted in children three years of age or younger in the Boston study.

Herpes simplex virus was isolated from fluid of one child with persistent middle ear effusion (Giebink et al., 1979), but use of an ELISA technique did not detect viral antigens in 96 such fluids (Sarkkinen et al., 1982).

Middle ear fluid of asymptomatic children may harbor bacterial pathogens similar to those identified in acute otitis media, including *S. pneumoniae* and *H. influenzae*. The significance of this finding is at present uncertain. There were only minimal differences in the rates of isolation of bacteria from serous, mucoid, or purulent fluids. The bacteria may be present without provoking an inflammatory response, or they may produce a low-grade or subclinical infection, or the effusion may represent an immune response to the

prolonged presence of the bacteria. Specific antibody to the bacteria isolated is present in the middle ear fluid of children with persistent effusion (Bernstein et al., 1980; Lewis et al., 1979). This finding suggests that the bacteria are not passive in chronic middle ear effusion but elicit an immunological response and may be involved in the production and persistence of fluid.

OTITIS MEDIA IN THE NEWBORN INFANT

Bacteriological data are available from aspiration of middle ear fluids of 169 neonates with otitis media (Berman et al., 1978; Bland, 1972; Shurin et al., 1978; Tetzlaff et al., 1977) (Table 5–3). *S. pneumoniae* and *H. influenzae* are the bacteria isolated most frequently in the very young, as is the case in older infants and children. However, organisms associated with local and systemic infection in the newborn infant, group B streptococcus, *S. aureus*, and gram-negative enteric bacilli, are important pathogens in the newborn infant within two weeks after birth or in older infants who have remained in the nursery because of risk features (low birth weight or prematurity) or disease (respiratory distress syndrome). When term infants who have had no problems with delivery or nursery experience develop otitis media two or more weeks after hospital discharge, the bacterial pathogens are most likely to be *S. pneumoniae* and *H. influenzae*.

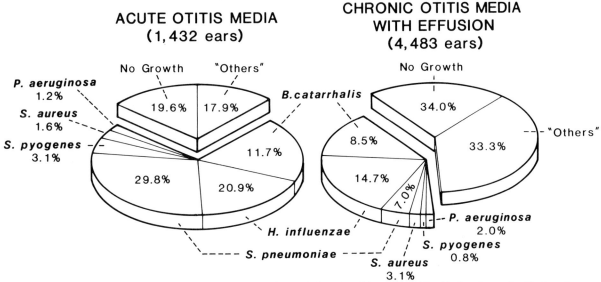

Figure 5–2. Microbiologic causes of acute otitis media and chronic otitis media with effusion from the Pittsburgh Otitis Media Research Center, 1980–1985.

BACTERIOLOGICAL STUDIES OF THE EXTERNAL EAR CANAL

The microbial flora of the external canal is similar to the flora of skin elsewhere on the body. In various microbiological studies (Brook and Schwartz, 1981; Pelton et al., 1980; Riding et al., 1978) there is a predominance of *S. epidermidis*, *S. aureus*, and diphtheroids and, to a lesser extent, anaerobic bacteria such as *P. acnes* and anaerobic cocci. Pathogens, responsible for infection of the middle ear, *S. pneumoniae*, *H. influenzae*, or *B. catarrhalis*, are uncommonly found in cultures of the external auditory canal when the tympanic membrane is intact. Isolation of *S. epidermidis*, *S. aureus*, diphtheroids, or certain anaerobic bacteria from cultures of middle ear fluids may represent contamination of the fluid by organisms present in the external canal. Adequate cleansing of the external canal is necessary before tympanocentesis is performed for the purpose of microbiological diagnosis.

Diseases of the external canal are not considered in this monograph. The interested reader is referred to a monograph by Senturia, Marcus, and Lucente (1980).

References

Andersson, B., Eriksson, B., Falsen, E., Fogh, A., Hanson, L. A., Nylen, O., Peterson, H., Svanborg, E. C.: Adhesion of *Streptococcus pneumoniae* to human pharyngeal epithelial cells in vitro: Differences in adhesive capacity among strains isolated from subjects with otitis media, septicemia, or meningitis or from healthy carriers. Infect. Immun. 32:311–317, 1981.

Applebaum, P. C., Bhamjee, A., Scragg, J. N., Hallett, A. F., Brown, A. J., and Cooper, R. C.: *Streptococcus pneumoniae* resistant to penicillin and chloramphenicol. Lancet 2:995–997, 1977.

Austrian, R., Howie, V. M., and Ploussard, J. H.: The bacteriology of pneumococcal otitis media. Johns Hopkins Med. J. 141:104–111, 1977.

Baba, S.: Recent aspects of clinical bacteriology in otitis media. Presented at Presymposium on Management of Otitis Media, January 12, 1985, Kyoto, Japan.

Berman, S. A., Balkany, T. J., and Simmons, M. A.: Otitis media in the neonatal intensive care unit. Pediatrics 62:198–201, 1978.

Bernstein, J. M., Myers, D., Kosinski, D., Nisengard, R., and Wicher, K.: Antibody coated bacteria in otitis media with effusion. Ann. Otol. Rhinol. Laryngol. 89(68):104–109, 1980.

Bernstein, J. M., Dryja, D., and Neter, E.: The clinical significance of coagulase negative staphylococci in otitis media with effusion. *In* Lim, D. J., Bluestone, C. D., Klein, J. O., and Nelson, J. D., (Eds.): *Recent Advances in Otitis Media with Effusion.* Burlington, Ontario, B. C. Decker Inc., 1984, pp. 114–116.

Bjuggren, G., and Tunevall, G.: Otitis in childhood: A clinical and serobacteriological study with special reference to the significance of *Haemophilus influenzae* in

relapses. Acta Otolaryngol. (Stockh.) 42:311–328, 1952.

Bland, R. D.: Otitis media in the first six weeks of life: Diagnosis, bacteriology, and management. Pediatrics 49:187–197, 1972.

Bordley, J. E., and Kapur, Y. P.: The histopathological changes in the temporal bone resulting from acute smallpox and chickenpox infection. Laryngoscope 82:1477–1490, 1972.

Brook, I.: Bacteriology and treatment of chronic otitis media. Laryngoscope 89:1129–1134, 1979.

Brook, I., Anthony, B. F., and Finegold, S. M.: Aerobic and anaerobic bacteriology of acute otitis media in children. J. Pediatr. 92:13–15, 1978.

Brook, I., and Schwartz, R.: Anaerobic bacteria in acute otitis media. Acta Otolaryngol. (Stockh.) 91:111–114, 1981.

Cates, K. L., Gerrard, J. M., Giebink, G. S., Lund, M. E., Bleeker, E. Z., O'Leary, M. C., Krivit, W., and Quie, P. G.: A penicillin-resistant pneumococcus. J. Pediatr. 93:624–626, 1978.

Chang, M. J., Rodriguez, W. J., and Mohla, C.: *Chlamydia trachomatis* in otitis media in children. Pediatr. Inf. Dis. 1:95–97, 1982.

Clarke, T. A.: Deafness in children: Otitis media and other causes; a selective survey of prevention and treatment and of educational problems. Proc. R. Soc. Med. 55:61–70, 1962.

Coffey, J. D., Jr.: Otitis media in the practice of pediatrics: Bacteriological and clinical observations. Pediatrics 38:25–32, 1966.

Coffey, J. D., Jr., Martin, A. D., and Booth, H. N.: *Neisseria catarrhalis* in exudative otitis media. Arch. Otolaryngol. 86:403–406, 1967.

Deinard, A. S., Dassenko, D., Kloster, B., Welle, P., and Zavoral, J.: Otogenous tetanus. JAMA 243:2156, 1980.

DeMaria, T. F., Briggs, B. R., Okazaki, N., and Lim, D. J.: Experimental otitis media with effusion following middle ear inoculation of nonviable *H. influenzae*. Ann. Otol. Rhinol. Laryngol. 93:52–56, 1984a.

DeMaria, T. F., Lim, D. J., Barnishan, J., Ayers, L. W., and Birck, H. G.: Biotypes of serologically nontypable *Hemophilus influenzae* isolated from the middle ears and nasopharynges of patients with otitis media with effusion. J. Clin. Microbiol. 20:1102–1104, 1984b.

DeMaria, T. F., Prior, R. B., Briggs, B. R., Lim, D. J., and Birck, H. G.: Endotoxin in middle ear effusions from patients with chronic otitis media with effusion. *In* Lim, D. J., Bluestone, C. D., Klein, J. O., and Nelson, J. D. (Eds.): *Recent Advances in Otitis Media with Effusion.* Burlington, Ontario, B. C. Decker Inc., 1984c, pp. 123–124.

Downes, J. J.: Primary diphtheritic otitis media. Arch. Otolaryngol. 70:27–31, 1959.

Drury, D. W.: Diphtheria of the ear. Arch. Otolaryngol. 1:221–230, 1925.

Feigin, R. D., Shackelford, P. G., Campbell, J., Lyles, T. O., Schechter, M., and Lins, R. S.: Assessment of the role of *Staphylococcus epidermidis* as a cause of otitis media. Pediatrics 52:569–575, 1973.

Feingold, M., Klein, J. O., Haslan, G. E., Tilles, J. G., Finland, M., and Gellis, S. S.: Acute otitis media in children: Bacteriological findings in middle ear fluid obtained by needle aspiration. Am. J. Dis. Child. 111:361–365, 1966.

Fischer, G. W., Sunakorn, P., and Duangman, C.: Otogenous tetanus: A sequela of chronic ear infections. Am. J. Dis. Child. 131:445–446, 1977.

Giebink, G. S., Mills, E. L., Huff, J. S., Edelman, C. K., Weber, M. L., Juhn, S. K., and Quie, P. G.: The microbiology of serous and mucoid otitis media. Pediatrics 63:915–919, 1979.

Gray, B. M., Converse, G. M., and Dillon, H. C., Jr.: Serotypes of *Streptococcus pneumoniae* causing disease. J. Infect. Dis. 140:979–983, 1979.

Gronroos, J. A., Kortekangas, A. E., Ojala, L., and Vuori, M.: The aetiology of acute middle ear infection. Acta Otolaryngol. (Stockh.) 58:149–158, 1964.

Halstead, C., Lepow, M. L., Balassanian, N., Emmerich, J., and Wolinsky, E.: Otitis media: Clinical observations, microbiology, and evaluation of therapy. Am. J. Dis. Child. 115:542–551, 1968.

Hammerschlag, M. R., Hammerschlag, P. E., and Alexander, E. R.: The role of *Chlamydia trachomatis* in middle ear effusion in children. Pediatrics 66:615, 1980.

Harcourt, F. L., and Brown, A. K.: Hydrotympanum (secretory otitis media). Arch. Otolaryngol. 57:12, 1953.

Harding, A. L., Anderson, P., Howie, V. M., Ploussard, J. H., and Smith, D. H.: *Haemophilus influenzae* isolated from children with otitis media. *In* Sell, S. H., and Karzon, D. T. (Eds.): *Haemophilus Influenzae.* Vanderbilt University Press, Nashville, 1973, pp. 21–28.

Healy, G. B., and Teele, D. W.: The microbiology of chronic middle ear effusions in young children. Laryngoscope 87:1472–1478, 1977.

Henderson, F. W., Collier, A. M., Sanyal, M. A., Watkins, J. M., Fairclough, D. L., Clyde, W. A., and Denny, F. W.: A longitudinal study of respiratory viruses and bacteria in the etiology of acute otitis media with effusion. N. Engl. J. Med. 306:1377–1383, 1982.

Herberts, G., Jeppson, P. H., Nylen, O., and Branefors-Helander, P.: Acute otitis media: Etiological and therapeutical aspects of acute otitis media. Prac. Otol. Rhinol. Laryngol. 33:191–202, 1971.

Herva, E., Haiva, V.-M., Koskela, M., Leinonen, M., Gronroos, P., Sipila, M., Karma, P., and Makela, P. H.: Pneumococci and their capsular polysaccharide antigens in middle ear effusion in acute otitis media. *In* Lim, D. J., Bluestone, C. D., Klein, J. O., and Nelson, J. D. (Eds.): *Recent Advances in Otitis Media with Effusion.* Burlington, Ontario, B. C. Decker Inc., 1984, pp. 120–122.

Howard, J. E., Nelson, J. D., Clashen, J., and Jackson, L. H.: Otitis media of infancy and early childhood: A double-blind study of four treatment regimens. Am. J. Dis. Child. 130:965–970, 1976.

Howie, V. M., Ploussard, J. H., and Lester, R. L.: Otitis media: A clinical and bacteriological correlation. Pediatrics 45:29–35, 1970.

Howie, V. M., Pollard, R. B., Kleyn, K., Lawrence, B., Peskuric, T., Paucker, K., and Baron, S.: Presence of interferon during bacterial otitis media. J. Infect. Dis. 145:811–814, 1982.

Jensen, K. J., Senterfit, L. B., Scully, W. E., Conway, T. J., West, R. F., and Drummy, W. W.: *Mycoplasma pneumoniae* infections in children. An epidemiologic appraisal in families treated with oxytetracycline. Am. J. Epidemiol. 86:419–432, 1967.

Jorgensen, F., Andersson, B., Larsson, S. H., Nylen, O., and Svanborg-Eden C.: Children with frequent attacks of acute otitis media: A re-examination after eight years concerning middle ear changes, hearing, tubal function, and bacterial adhesion to pharyngeal epithelial cells. *In* Lim, D. J., Bluestone, C. D., Klein, J. O., and Nelson, J. D. (Eds.): *Recent Advances in Otitis Media with Effusion.* Burlington, Ontario, B. C. Decker Inc., 1984, pp. 141–144.

Kamme, C., Ageberg, M., and Lundgren, K.: Distribution of *Diplococcus pneumoniae* types in acute otitis media in children and influence of the types on the clinical course in penicillin V therapy. Scand. J. Infect. Dis. 2:183–190, 1970.

Karma, P., Sipila, P., Virtanen, T., Luotonen, J., Sipila, M., and Haiva, V.-M.: Pneumococcal bacteriology after pneumococcal otitis media with special reference to pneumococcal antigens. Int. J. Pediatr. Otorhinolaryngol. 10:181–190, 1985.

Klein, J. O., and Teele, D. W.: Isolation of viruses and mycoplasmas from middle ear effusions: A review. Ann. Otol. Rhinol. Laryngol. 85(25):140–144, 1976.

Klein, B. S., Dollette, F. R., and Yolken, R. H.: The role of respiratory syncytial virus and other viral pathogens in acute otitis media. J. Pediatr. 101:16–20, 1982.

Klein, J. O., and Marcy, S. M.: Bacterial sepsis and meningitis. *In* Remington, J. S., and Klein, J. O. (Eds.): *Infectious Diseases of the Fetus and Newborn Infant.* Philadelphia, W. B. Saunders Co., 1983, pp. 679–735.

Kovatch, A. L., Wald, E. R., and Michaels, R. H.: β-Lactamase–producing *Branhamella catarrhalis* causing otitis media in children. J. Pediatr. 102:261–264, 1983.

Lahikainen, E. A.: Clinico-bacteriologic studies on acute otitis media: Aspiration of tympanum as diagnostic and therapeutic method. Acta Otolaryngol. (Stockh.) 107:1–82, 1953.

LaMarco, K. L., Diven, W. F., Glew, R. H., Doyle, W. J., and Cantekin, E. I.: Neuraminidase activity in middle ear effusion. Ann. Otol. Rhinol. Laryngol. 93:76–84, 1984.

Leinonen M., Luotonen, J., Herva, E., Valkonen, K., and Makela, P. H.: Preliminary serologic evidence for a pathogenic role of *Branhamella catarrhalis.* J. Infect. Dis., 144:570–574, 1981.

Lewis, D. M., Schram, J. L., Birck, H. G., and Lim, D. J.: Antibody activity in otitis media with effusion. Ann. Otol. Rhinol. Laryngol. 88:392–396, 1979.

Liu, Y. S., Lim, D. J., Lang, R. W., and Birck, H. G.: Chronic middle ear effusions: Immunochemical and bacteriological investigations. Arch. Otolaryngol. 101:278–286, 1975.

Loeb, M. R., and Smith, D. H.: Outer membrane protein composition in disease isolates of *Haemophilus influenzae*: Pathogenic and epidemiological implications. Infect. Immun. 30:710–717, 1980.

Luotonen, J., Herva, E., Karma, P., Timonen, M., Leinonen, M., and Makela, P. H.: The bacteriology of acute otitis media in children with special reference to *Streptococcus pneumoniae* as studied by bacteriological and antigen detection methods. Scand. J. Infect. Dis. 13:177–183, 1981.

Luotonen, J., Jokipii, A. M. M., Vayrynen, J., Jokipii, L., and Karma, P.: Aerobic and anaerobic bacteria in the middle ear and ear canal in acute otitis media. Acta Otolaryngol. (Stockh.) 386:100–102, 1982.

MacAdam, A. M., and Rubio, T.: Tuberculosis otomastoiditis in children. Am. J. Dis. Child. 131:152–156, 1977.

Mortimer, E. A., Jr., and Watterson, R. L., Jr.: A bacteriologic investigation of otitis media in infancy. Pediatrics 17:359–366, 1956.

Mumtaz, M. A., Schwartz, R. H., Grundfast, K. M., and Baumgartner, R. C.: Tuberculosis of the middle ear and mastoid. Pediatr. Infect. Dis. 2:234–236, 1983.

Murphy, T. F., and Apicella, M. A.: Antigenic heterogenicity of outer membrane proteins of nontypable *Haemophilus influenzae* as a basis for serotyping system. Infect. Immun. 50:15–21, 1985.

Naiditch, M. J., and Bower, A. G.: Diphtheria: A study of 1,433 cases observed during a ten-year period at Los Angeles County Hospital. Am. J. Med. 17:229–245, 1954.

Nilson, B. W., Poland, R. L., Thompson, R. S., Morehead, D., Baghdassarian, A., and Carver, D. H.: Acute otitis media: Treatment results in relation to bacterial etiology. Pediatrics 43:351–358, 1969.

Odio, C. M., Kusmiesz, H., Shelton, D., and Nelson, J. D.: Comparative treatment trial of Augmentin versus cefaclor for acute otitis media with effusion. Pediatrics 75:819–826, 1985.

Ostfeld, E., and Altmann, G. L.: Evaluation of countercurrent immunoelectrophoresis as a diagnostic tool in bacterial otitis media. Ann. Otol. Rhinol. Laryngol. 89(68):110–114, 1980.

Ostfeld, E., and Rubinstein, E.: Acute gram-negative bacillary infections of middle ear and mastoid. Ann. Otol. Rhinol. Laryngol. 89:33–36, 1980.

Page, J. R.: Report of acute infections of middle ear and mastoid process at Manhattan Eye, Ear, and Throat Hospital during 1934: Their prevalance and virulence. Laryngoscope 45:839–843, 1935.

Pelton, S. I., Teele, D. W., Shurin, P. A., and Klein, J. O.: Disparate cultures of middle ear fluids. Am. J. Dis. Child. 134:951–953, 1980.

Raikundalia, K. B.: Analysis of suppurative otitis media in children: Aetiology of nonsuppurative otitis media. Med. J. Aust. 1:749–750, 1975.

Richman, D. D., Cleveland, P. H., Redfield, D. C., Oxman, M. N., and Wahl, G. M.: Rapid viral diagnosis. Rev. Infect. Dis. 149:298–310, 1984.

Riding, K. H., Bluestone, C. D., Michaels, R. H., Cantekin, E. I., Doyle, W. J., and Poziviak, C.: Microbiology of recurrent and chronic otitis media with effusion. J. Pediatr. 93:739–743, 1978.

Rifkind, D. R., Chanock, R. M., Kravetz, H., Johnson, K., and Knight, V.: Ear involvement (myringitis) and primary atypical pneumonia following inoculation of volunteers with Eaton agent. Am. Rev. Respir. Dis. 85:479–489, 1962.

Roberts, D. B.: The etiology of bullous myringitis and the role of mycoplasmas in ear disease: A review. Pediatrics 65:761–766, 1980.

Robinson, J. M., and Nicholas, H. O.: Catarrhal otitis media with effusion—a disease of a retropharyngeal and lymphatic system. South. Med. J. 44:777, 1951.

Salonen, R., Sarkkinen, H., and Ruuskanen, O.: Presence of interferon in middle ear fluid during acute otitis media. J. Infect. Dis. 19:480, 1984.

Sarkkinen, H., Meurman, O., Puhakka, H., Suonpaa, J., and Virolainen, E.: Failure to detect viral antigens in the middle ear secretions of patients with secretory otitis media. Acta Otolaryngol. (Stockh.) 386:106–107, 1982.

Sarkkinen, H., Ruuskanen, O., Meurman, O., Puhakka, H., Virolainen, E., and Eskola, J.: Identification of respiratory virus antigens in middle ear fluids of children with acute otitis media. J. Infect. Dis. 151:444–448, 1985.

Schachter, J., Grossman, M., Holt, J., Sweet, R., Goodner, E., and Mills, J.: Prospective study of chlamydial infection in neonates. Lancet 2:377–379, 1979.

Schwartz, R. H.: Bacteriology of otitis media: A review. Otolaryngol. Head Neck Surg. 89:444–450, 1981.

Schwartz, R. H., Rodriguez, W. J., Khan, W. N., and Ross, S.: Acute purulent otitis media in children older than five years: Incidence of Haemophilus as a causative organism. JAMA 238:1032–1033, 1977.

Schwartz, R. H., and Rodriguez, W. J.: Acute otitis media in children eight years old and older: A reappraisal of the role of Haemophilus influenzae. Am. J. Otolaryngol. 2:19–21, 1981.

Sellars, S. L., and Seid, A. B.: Aural tuberculosis in childhood. S. Afr. Med. J. 47:216–218, 1973.

Senturia, B. H., Gessert, C. F., Carr, C. D., and Bauman, E. S.: Studies concerned with tubotympanitis. Ann. Otol. Rhinol. Laryngol. 67:440–467, 1958.

Senturia, B. H., Marcus, M. D., and Lucente, F. E.: Diseases of the External Ear: An Otologic-Dermatologic Manual. 2nd ed. New York, Grune & Stratton, 1980.

Shah, K. N., and Desai, M. P.: Ascaris lumbricoides from the right ear. Indian Pediatr. 6:92–93, 1969.

Shurin, P. A., Howie, V. M., Pelton, S. I., Ploussard, J. H., and Klein, J. O.: Bacterial etiology of otitis media during the first six weeks of life. J. Pediatr. 92:893–896, 1978.

Shurin, P. A., Marchant, C. D., Kim, C. H., VanHare, G. F., Johnson, C. E., Tutihasi, M. A., and Knapp, L. J.: Emergence of beta-lactamase–producing strains of Branhamella catarrhalis as important agents of acute otitis media. Pediatr. Infect. Dis. 2:34–38, 1983.

Siirala, U., and Vuori, M.: The problem of sterile otitis media. Prac. Otorhinolaryngol. 19:159, 1956.

Sipila, P., Jokipii, A. M. M., Jokipii, L., and Karma, P.: Bacteria in the middle ear and ear canal of patients with secretory otitis media and with noninflamed ears. Acta Otolaryngol. (Stockh.) 92:123–130, 1981.

Skolnik, P. R., Nadol, J. B., Jr., and Baker, A. S.: Tuberculosis of the middle ear: Review of the literature with an instructive case report. Rev. Infect. Dis. 8:403–410, 1986.

Sobeslavsky, O., Syrucek, L., Bruckoya, M., and Abrahamovic, M.: The etiological role of Mycoplasma pneumoniae in otitis media in children. Pediatrics 35:652–657, 1965.

Stanievich, J. F., Bluestone, C. D., Lima, J. A., Michaels, R. H., Rohn, D., and Effron, M. Z.: Microbiology of chronic and recurrent otitis media with effusion in young infants. Int. J. Pediatr. Otorhinolaryngol. 3:137–143, 1981.

Sugita, R., Kawamura, S., Ichikawa, G., Fujimaki, Y., and Deguchi, K.: Bacteriology of actue otitis media in Japan and chemotherapy, with special reference to Haemophilus influenzae. Int. J. Pediatr. Otorhinolaryngol. 6:135–144, 1983.

Sumaya, C. V., and Ench, Y.: Epstein-Barr virus infectious mononucleosis in children. I. Clinical and general laboratory findings. Pediatrics 75:1003–1010, 1985.

Teele, D. W., Healy, G. B., and Tally, F. P.: Persistent effusions of the middle ear: Cultures for anaerobic bacteria. Ann. Otol. Rhinol. Laryngol. 89(68):102–103, 1980a.

Teele, D. W., Klein, J. O., and Rosner, B. A.: Epidemiology of otitis media in children. Ann. Otol. Rhinol. Laryngol. 89(68):5–6, 1980b.

Tetzlaff, T. R., Ashworth, C., and Nelson, J. D.: Otitis media in children less than 12 weeks of age. Pediatrics 59:827–832, 1977.

Tipple, M. A., Beem, M. O., and Saxon, E. M.: Clinical characteristics of the afebrile pneumonia associated with Chlamydia trachomatis infection in infants less than six months of age. Pediatrics 63:192–197, 1979.

Trujillo, H., Callejas, R., Mejia de R, G. I.: Otitis media aguda. Medicina U.P.B. 1:31–38, 1981.

Turner, A. L., and Fraser, J. S.: Tuberculosis of the middle ear cleft in children: A clinical and pathological study. J. Laryngol. Rhinol. Otol. 30:209–247, 1915.

Van Dishoeck, H. A. E., Derks, A. C. W., and Voorhorst, R.: Bacteriology and treatment of acute otitis media in children. Acta Otolaryngol. (Stockh.) 50:250–262, 1959.

Ward, J.: Antibiotic-resistant Streptococcus pneumoniae: Clinical and epidemiological aspects. Rev. Infect. Dis. 3:254–266, 1981.

6

Immunology

The middle ear mucosa has a secretory immune system similar to those of other areas of the respiratory tract (see Fig. 2–9). Immunologically active antigen interacts with immunocompetent cells in the lamina propria to produce a local immune response. The middle ear effusion that results from acute or chronic infection contains the major classes of immunoglobulins, complement, cells, immune complexes of antigen and antibody, and various chemical mediators of inflammation (Table 6–1). The role of these substances in the course of otitis media with effusion is uncertain. The immune response to various antigens may prevent subsequent infection, assist in clearance of the middle ear effusion, or contribute to the accumulation and persistence of fluid in the middle ear cavity.

The immunological effect of otitis media with effusion is a relatively new area of investigation. Almost all reports of important studies have been published since 1967. At present, our understanding of immunological factors of otitis media is incomplete, but investigations are in progress in many centers in the United States, Scandinavia, and Japan, and the results should yield important new information.

PROBLEMS IN METHODOLOGY

Immunological studies of otitis media in the human are based on assays of serum, middle ear effusion (obtained by needle aspiration through the tympanic membrane), and middle ear mucosa (obtained by biopsy). Problems in methodology and limitations of data from human materials must be considered in evaluating results of these studies:

1. Effusion or mucosa is most readily obtained at operation. Therefore, most reports include patients with chronic disease who required an operative procedure. Only a few reports of materials obtained from patients with acute otitis media are available.

2. Without information gathered prospectively, the investigator cannot identify the stage of disease when material is obtained. In most reports the stage of otitis media is identified grossly as acute or chronic by the characteristic of the middle ear effusion (serous, mucoid, purulent, or hemorrhagic). Few studies have results from more than one specimen or one observation. Thus, there is a paucity of information on the sequence of immune events.

3. Techniques for assay of the same function vary in sensitivity and specificity. New techniques may provide results at variance with previously used methods.

Table 6–1. **SUBSTANCES IDENTIFIED IN MIDDLE EAR EFFUSION OF PATIENTS WITH ACUTE OR CHRONIC OTITIS MEDIA WITH EFFUSION**

Immunoglobulins	Oxidate Enzymes
G, A, M, E, D	Lactic dehydrogenase
Complement	Malic dehydrogenase
Rheumatoid Factor	Succinic dehydrogenase
Prostaglandins E and F	Hydrolytic enzymes
Chemotactic substances	Lysozyme
Macrophage inhibitory	Acid phosphatase
factor	Alkaline phosphatase
Lactoferrin	Esterase
Histamine	Leucine aminopeptidase
Granulocyte proteases	Alanine aminopeptidase
Protease inhibitors	
Collagenase	

4. The quality and quantity of middle ear fluid obtained by tympanocentesis is limited. The volume of most aspirates is 0.3 ml or less. Only a few studies can be performed with each sample. In addition, the liquid may be fibrinous, mucoid, or filled with cellular debris, making homogenization difficult.

5. Materials are not usually available from "normal" patients, and controls are difficult to define.

6. The investigator may not be able to identify the origin of the substance in the effusion. Trauma may occur during the course of aspiration and contaminate the effusion with products of blood and tissue. The liquid represents the sum of substances derived from serum, inflamed middle ear mucosa, degenerating white blood cells, or other cellular elements.

Experiments in animal models have provided important new information and stimulated new concepts. However, significant differences exist between species, and data derived from studies in animals must be viewed with caution. For the purposes of this chapter, only data derived from studies of humans will be presented.

IMMUNOLOGY OF THE PHARYNX

Immunocompetent lymphoid tissue is present in the mucosa of the upper respiratory tract, the site of initial exposure for ingested and inhaled antigens. The lymphoid tissue of the pharynx includes the palatine tonsils and adenoids, lymphoid tissue at the base of the tongue (lingual tonsil), lymphoid tissue on the posterior wall of the pharynx (pharyngeal tonsil), and a circular ring of lymphoid tissue (Waldeyer's ring). Plasma cells capable of producing all the major classes of immunoglobulins have been identified in the tonsils. The immunological aspects of the tonsils have been reviewed by Wong and Ogra (1980).

The specific immunological relationship of the tonsils and adenoids with the middle ear is unknown. The immunocompetent cells present in the tonsils and adenoids are an important defense in excluding microbial and environmental antigens from the systemic lymphoid system, thus performing a "gatekeeper" function. Since microbial organisms responsible for infection of the middle ear proliferate first in the throat or nasopharynx, the tonsils may play a signifi-

cant immunological role in the host's defense against otitis media.

HUMORAL FACTORS

Immunoglobulin A (IgA) and Secretory Immunoglobulin A (SIgA)

Immunoglobulin A (IgA) is secreted by plasma cells in lymphoid tissues lining the gastrointestinal, genitourinary, and respiratory tracts. Secretory component (SIgA) is a nonimmune glycoprotein, formed by local epithelial cells, that exists either in a bound state with IgA or in a free state in effusion fluids. Two IgA molecules combine with secretory component in the epithelium, and the complex (SIgA) is transported through the cell and into the lumen. The production of SIgA begins when antigen is presented to immunocompetent cells in the mucosa.

IgA is the predominant immunoglobulin in middle ear effusions. The ratio of IgA:IgG is higher in middle ear effusion than in serum in most patients, and some patients have IgA in middle ear fluid but not in serum. Fluorescent antibody staining of middle ear mucosa demonstrates SIgA in the epithelium. Small amounts of free SIgA are present, but most secretory component in middle ear effusions is bound to IgA (Mogi et al., 1973).

A specific IgA or SIgA response takes place in the middle ear mucosa following exposure to antigen. IgA and SIgA specific for adenovirus, respiratory syncytial virus (RSV), and parainfluenza viruses have been identified in middle ear fluids of children with otitis media with effusion (Meurman et al., 1980; Yamaguchi et al., 1984). The presence of specific IgA antibody for measles, mumps, rubella, and poliovirus in middle ear fluid and its absence in some specimens of simultaneously obtained serum indicate that local antibody production takes place (Sloyer et al., 1977).

Specific IgA can interfere with adhesion of bacteria to mucous membrane and can neutralize viruses. In the intestine IgA prevents absorption of toxic proteins and antigens. Which, if any, of these functions applies to IgA and SIgA in the middle ear is unknown.

Immunoglobulin G (IgG)

Immunoglobulin G (IgG) is present in the effusions of patients with both acute and chronic otitis media in concentrations suggesting that local development of IgG occurs in the middle ear. IgG is divided into subclasses IgG1, IgG2, IgG3, and IgG4 based on differences in structure of the gamma heavy polypeptide chain. Data presented by Freijd and coworkers (1985) suggest an association between plasma IgG2 concentrations and susceptibility to otitis media in children. Otitis-prone children (eight to 17 episodes by 30 months of age) had significantly lower plasma concentrations of IgG2 than did children who were not otitis-prone (fewer than two episodes by 30 months of age) at ages 12 and 32 months. Concentrations of IgG1, IgG3, and IgG4 were similar in the two groups.

Immunoglobulin M (IgM)

Immunoglobulin M (IgM) is produced in response to primary exposure to a microbial antigen; it is an effective mediator of complement fixation and regulates B-cell function. IgM is present in the middle ear effusions of patients with both acute and chronic otitis media with effusion, but concentrations are lower than in serum, and studies of middle ear mucosa obtained by biopsy in patients with chronic otitis media with effusion suggest that local synthesis of IgM does not occur.

Immunoglobulin D (IgD)

Immunoglobulin D (IgD) has been identified in middle ear effusions of patients with otitis media with effusion in excess of concentrations found in serum (Veltri and Sprinkle, 1973). IgD is found in serum in trace concentrations but has no identifiable function.

Immunoglobulin E (IgE)

Immunoglobulin E (IgE) is part of the external secretory system of antibody produced in the lymphoid tissue of the respiratory and gastrointestinal tracts. Increased concentration of IgE has been found in serum and secretions of patients with various atopic diseases. IgE antibody, when combined with appropriate antigen, causes release of histamine, slow-reacting substance,

and chemotactic substance from mast cells and basophilic granulocytes.

IgE-producing plasma cells have been identified in biopsy of mucosa of the middle ear, and IgE has been found in the middle ear effusions of patients with both acute and chronic otitis media. The source of IgE in the middle ear fluid of patients with otitis media with effusion may be middle ear mucosa in some patients (Bernstein, 1984; Phillips et al., 1974) and a transudate of serum in others (Lewis et al., 1978; Mogi et al., 1974).

Complement

The term *complement* represents a system that includes 11 discrete but interacting proteins and possesses a wide variety of activities, such as viral neutralization, phagocytosis, immune adherence, chemotaxis, anaphylatoxin activities on smooth muscle and blood vessels, and a cytotoxic effect that may serve a protective function leading to destruction of foreign cells (Ward and McLean, 1978). Activation of complement occurs by the classical or alternate pathways. The classical pathway is usually activated by antigen-antibody complexes and proceeds in sequence from C1 to C9. The alternate pathways do not require immune complex for activation but utilize materials such as endotoxin or bacterial polysaccharide. The early factors of the classical pathway (C1, C2, C4) are not required, but properdin and C3 are involved in activation.

Evidence for activation of complement in the middle ear effusions of patients with acute and chronic otitis media has been reviewed by Bernstein and colleagues (1978a) and Prellner and coworkers (1980). Studies of middle ear effusion indicate that levels of C2, C3, C4, and C5 are all significantly depressed when compared with corresponding levels in serum and that the amounts of C3 breakdown products are significantly elevated in the middle ear fluid of children with otitis media with effusion (Meri et al., 1984), indicating utilization of complement in the middle ear during the course of the disease. Meri and colleagues (1984) suggest that activation of complement in middle ear fluid may play a significant role in the pathogenesis of otitis media with effusion either by decreasing local defenses against bacterial infection or by generating breakdown products that maintain and prolong the inflammatory process.

Rheumatoid Factor

Rheumatoid factor is an IgM that has the capacity to react with IgG *in vitro* and has been identified in the serum of patients with rheumatoid arthritis and other chronic inflammatory diseases. Rheumatoid factors may participate in the inflammatory process stimulated by immune complexes. DeMaria and colleagues (1984) demonstrated rheumatoid factor in 85 percent of 156 middle ear fluids obtained from patients with otitis media with effusion; the factor was found in only 8 percent of serums from the same patients. The investigators suggest that rheumatoid factor is produced in the middle ear and may participate in the pathogenesis of middle ear effusion. These results were not corroborated by Bernstein; none of 21 middle ear fluids tested showed positive results for rheumatoid factor (Bernstein, 1984).

PRODUCTS OF IMMUNE AND INFLAMMATORY REACTIONS

A variety of other substances that take part in immune or inflammatory reactions have been identified in the middle ear effusions of patients with chronic otitis media with effusion.

1. A chemotactic factor for neutrophils has been found (Bernstein, 1976). Chemotactic substances alter the pattern of movement of neutrophils so that cells, which otherwise would migrate randomly, are directed to the vicinity of the chemotactic substance.

2. Macrophage inhibition factor inhibits the migration of macrophages *in vitro; in vivo* it serves to contain macrophages at the site of injury or inflammation (Bernstein, 1976). Macrophage inhibition factor augments the capacity of the macrophage to kill certain bacteria.

3. Lactoferrin inhibits growth of iron-dependent bacteria by competing for elemental iron. Bernstein and coworkers (1972) identified lactoferrin in mucoid but not serous effusions.

4. Prostaglandins have a wide range of biological activities, including increasing capillary permeability, contraction of smooth muscles, and release of lysozymal enzymes. Bernstein, Okazaki, and Reisman (1976) found prostaglandins E and F in middle ear fluids; in some patients the concentration in the fluid was higher than it was in serum.

The effect of prostaglandins on capillary permeability may play a role in development and persistence of middle ear effusion.

5. Histamine was identified in 104 of 131 middle ear fluids of patients with otitis media with effusion at time of placement of tympanostomy tubes. Berger and colleagues (1984) postulated that mast cells located in the middle ear mucosa were triggered to degranulate and release histamine by a product derived from activation of the complement system.

6. Products derived from microorganisms that participate in immune or inflammatory responses (endotoxins, interferon, neuraminidase) are discussed in Chapter Five, Microbiology.

CYTOLOGY OF THE MIDDLE EAR AND MIDDLE EAR EFFUSIONS

Neutrophils, macrophages, and lymphocytes are the predominant cell types in middle ear effusions (Sipila and Karma, 1982; Yamanaka et al., 1982). The proportion of B- and T-lymphocytes varies widely in published reports. Bernstein and colleagues (1978b) found that mucoid middle ear effusions contained many B-cells but few T-cells, whereas serous effusions contained mainly T-cells but no B-cells. Monocytes and phagocytes are present, but they occur in small numbers in most specimens. Occasionally, giant phagocytes with ingested cells, cell debris, and bacteria are seen. Eosinophils, mast cells, basophils, and plasma cells are rare. Epithelial cells include numerous flat endothelial cells and few ciliated and goblet cells.

After onset of acute otitis media, the middle ear effusion contains large numbers of neutrophils and few lymphocytes, monocytes, and phagocytes. Initially, polymorphonuclear leukocytes may defend the middle ear from bacterial infection, as well as contribute to the middle ear effusion by release of enzymes that stimulate an inflammatory response. After several weeks, the proportion of cells is reversed, and lymphocytes, monocytes, and phagocytes predominate (Qvarnberg et al., 1984).

Similar cell types are found in middle ear mucosa obtained by biopsy of patients with otitis media with effusion. Inflammatory cells in the submucosa are predominantly of the mononuclear type. Plasma cells and small lymphocytes predominate. The presence of

IgA and IgG was demonstrated by use of an immunofluorescent stain of mononuclear cells from middle ear effusions; IgM and IgE were infrequently detected (Palva et al., 1976).

IMMUNOLOGY OF ACUTE OTITIS MEDIA

Role of Serum Antibody

An immune response reflected in a rise in specific serum antibody occurs in some children after acute infection of the middle ear (Howie et al., 1973). The number of responders to pneumococcal infection is dependent on the age of the patient and the pneumococcal serotype: 18 percent of Finnish children less than one year old, 48 percent of one-year-olds, and 39 percent of children two to seven years old had a significant increase in type-specific antibody following pneumococcal otitis media. Types 3 and 18 induced very good antibody responses irrespective of age; types 4, 7, 8, and 9 were intermediate; and types 6, 19, and 23 were poor antigens, even in older children (Koskela et al., 1982). Similar results were found in Alabama children who had acute otitis media due to *Streptococcus pneumoniae;* only 12 percent of children under one year of age had a significant rise in type-specific antibody in the convalescent serum, whereas 48 percent of the children two years of age or older responded (Sloyer et al., 1974). The antibody responses to the type-specific pneumococcal infection were in general agreement with the responses to polysaccharide vaccine for children of similar ages.

A specific serum antibody response also occurs following acute otitis media due to nontypable *Haemophilus influenzae*. A majority of Alabama children two years of age or younger with *H. influenzae* infection had specific antibody in the convalescent serum (Sloyer et al., 1975). Shurin and coworkers (1980) found similar immune responses in children two months to 12 years of age with acute otitis media due to nontypable strains of *H. influenzae*. Eleven percent of the children had homotypic antibody in the acute serum, but 78 percent had antibody in the convalescent specimen. Thus, an immune response to nontypable *H. influenzae* occurred in infants as well as older children.

Children with recurrent episodes of otitis media have new middle ear infections due to the same spectrum of organisms that was responsible for the first episode. *S. pneumoniae* and nontypable *H. influenzae* are the most common bacteria in recurrent infections, but the new episodes are rarely due to the same serotype that infected the child in a prior episode. Austrian and colleagues (1977) found that approximately 1 percent of isolates of *S. pneumoniae* in recurrent episodes of pneumococcal otitis media were due to the same serotype responsible for a prior episode (Austrian et al., 1977). Recurrent episodes of otitis media due to nontypable *H. influenzae* are also associated with new types. Using outer membrane protein gel analysis and biotyping, Barenkamp and colleagues (1984) determined that episodes of early recurrence of otitis due to nontypable *H. influenzae* (less than 30 days after initial *H. influenzae* infection) had first and second isolates that were identical. In contrast, children with late recurrences of nontypable *H. influenzae* (more than 30 days after initial infection) had disease due to a different strain. These data suggest that infections due to *S. pneumoniae* or nontypable *H. influenzae* produce an immune response that protects the child against subsequent infection due to the same type. The specific protective mechanism, a serum or local antibody or other immune factor, is uncertain.

Role of Antibody in Clearance of the Middle Ear Effusion

Clearance of fluid from the middle ear in patients with acute otitis media due to *S. pneumoniae* and *H. influenzae* was significantly associated with the presence and concentration of specific antibody to the infecting strain in the middle ear fluid at the time of diagnosis (Sloyer et al., 1976). Clearing of the effusion by second visit (two to seven days following diagnosis) was associated with specific antibody in the middle ear effusion obtained at first visit and was directly associated with the concentration of specific antibody. Infection due to *H. influenzae* was cleared rapidly in more children (45.3 percent) than those with infection due to *S. pneumoniae* (13.6 percent), whether or not antibody was present. The source for the antibody in the effusion at the time of presentation of acute otitis media is uncertain; antibody may have developed after a prior infection, may have developed rapidly after a current infection, or may indicate a delay of presentation until the time when the specimen of middle ear fluid was obtained. If present from a prior infection, type-specific antibody did not protect the patient from a recurrent episode of acute otitis media but did reduce the duration of effusion. No other data are available to confirm or deny these findings.

Polymorphonuclear Leukocyte Response

Hill and coworkers (1977) identified defective chemotactic response in selected patients with recurrent episodes of otitis media and diarrhea. Ichimura (1982) identified defective neutrophil chemotaxis in 20 children who had had recurrent episodes of otitis media (four or more episodes during the preceding year) but were well at the time of examination. These data suggest that recurrent episodes of otitis media in some children may be due to or associated with depressed functions of polymorphonuclear leukocytes.

IMMUNOLOGY OF CHRONIC OTITIS MEDIA WITH EFFUSION

Role of Antibody in Middle Ear Fluid

All the major classes of immunoglobulins, IgA, IgG, IgM, IgD, and IgE have been identified in the middle ear fluids of patients with chronic otitis media with effusion. SIgA, IgA, and IgG are synthesized by the mucosa of the middle ear; synthesis of other immunoglobulins in the middle ear is less certain (Bernstein and Reisman, 1974). Both IgA and IgG are present in middle ear effusions in concentrations higher than those found in simultaneously obtained serum, whereas IgM and IgE are present in equivalent or lower concentrations in effusion than are found in serum. The highest concentrations of each of the major classes of immunoglobulins are present in mucoid effusions; the lowest are found in serous effusions, and intermediate values occur in leukocytic middle ear effusions.

Polymorphonuclear Leukocyte Response

Giebink and colleagues (1980) studied the polymorphonuclear leukocyte response in children with chronic otitis media with effusion at the time of myringotomy or placement of ventilating tubes and, in a few cases, two to eight weeks later. In some children there were transient abnormalities of polymorphonuclear leukocyte motility (depressed chemotactic responsiveness), phagocytosis (depressed polymorphonuclear leukocyte bactericidal activity), or intracellular oxidation (depressed polymorphonuclear leukocyte chemiluminescence). Repeat studies performed after surgery found these indices to be normal in the majority of children, suggesting that leukocyte dysfunction was transient and probably associated with the inflammatory reaction that elicited the middle ear fluid.

Immune Complexes

Some investigators suggest that chronic otitis media with effusion may be an immune complex disease. Antigen (microbial agents or allergens) may combine with antibody (locally produced or derived from serum) to form an immune complex, which activates the complement sequence through the classical or alternate pathways. Polymorphonuclear leukocytes and monocytes are attracted to the site. With the death of these cells, intracellular enzymes are released, producing local tissue damage and stimulating effusion. Maxim and colleagues identified immune complexes in middle ear fluids by use of the fluorescent Raji cell assay (Maxim et al., 1977). Others have not been able to corroborate the results (Bernstein et al., 1981). If immune complexes do occur in middle ear fluid, they may represent microbial antigen-antibody complexes as a part of the normal process of elimination of infectious product through phagocytosis.

CHILDREN WITH DEFECTS OF THE IMMUNE SYSTEM

Most children with recurrent episodes of otitis media with effusion have no apparent systemic or local immune defect. These children have normal concentrations of immunoglobulin in serum, normal systemic cell-mediated responses, and normal phagocytic and bactericidal capacity of neutrophils in peripheral blood (Giebink and Quie, 1978). Available data about the immune system of the middle ear in children with recurrent otitis media with effusion indicate that most have the essential elements for immunological resistance, including T- and B-cell responses that are fully operative, macrophages that are available for engulfing and ingesting antigenic material, and appropriate antibody response by middle ear mucosa (Palva et al., 1980).

Children with congenital or acquired immunodeficiency may have defects of phagocyte function or humoral systems. Infections of the respiratory tract, including otitis media, are associated with defects of chemotaxis, phagocytosis (neutropenia or intrinsic cellular defects), or killing (chronic granulomatous disease); problems with the humoral system include deficiency of circulating antibody (hypo- or agammaglobulinemia), mucosal antibody (IgA deficiency), or complement deficiency. Human immunodeficiency virus (HIV), the organism responsible for the acquired immunodeficiency syndrome (AIDS), is highly tropic for T-lymphocytes. Children with AIDS have abnormalities of T-cell, B-cell and complement functions and phagocytosis. The children are susceptible to local and systemic pyogenic infections, and otitis media is only one of the many bacterial diseases that may occur.

Multiple infections in the same system (respiratory tract, urinary tract, or central nervous system) suggest a local anatomical or physiological defect. The vast majority of children with recurrent episodes of otitis media as the sole form of recurrent infectious disease probably have an underlying defect that is not immunologically mediated, e.g. eustachian tube dysfunction. A few children have recurrent respiratory infections, including recurrent otitis media and pyogenic infections in other systems, as part of an immunodeficiency syndrome (Berdal et al., 1976; Johnston, 1984). Two or more serious pyogenic skin infections (furunculosis, subcutaneous abscess, or cellulitis), accompanied by pneumonia or recurrent otitis media, raises suspicion of neutropenia, defective chemotaxis, or problems with phagocytosis. A pattern of subcutaneous abscesses of furunculosis, accompanied by abscess formation in lymph nodes, liver, or lung, and recurrent acute otitis media suggests chronic granulomatous disease. Meningitis, osteomyelitis, septic arthritis with recurrent acute otitis media, or pneumonia raises concern for a deficiency of antibody or C3. Protracted diarrhea, when accompanied by recurrent episodes of otitis media, sinusitis, or pneumonia, suggests IgA deficiency (although many children with deficiencies of IgA are otherwise normal without undue susceptibility to infection). Children with selective IgG2 or IgG3 subclass deficiency had recurrent sinopulmonary infections and otitis media (more than six episodes per year) (Umetsu et al., 1985).

Patients with defects in splenic function are susceptible to overwhelming infection due to encapsulated organisms such as *S. pneumoniae* or *H. influenzae* type b. Such patients, including those with congenital or acquired asplenia and those with sickle cell disease, have not been identified as groups with unusual susceptibility to infections at local sites, such as the skin and soft tissues or middle ear.

THE ROLE OF ALLERGY IN OTITIS MEDIA WITH EFFUSION

The role of allergy as an etiological factor in otitis media with effusion is uncertain. The role of allergy and eustachian tube function is discussed in Chapter Three, Physiology, Pathophysiology, and Pathogenesis. Few critical studies of appropriate design are available to clarify the relationship of allergy and otitis media with effusion. Available studies are often biased (enrollees include children referred for allergy evaluation) and do not include appropriate control patients. However, the association of reaginic antibody with IgE provides a specific measure for precise definition of allergy and has already provided some significant information about the primary or secondary role of allergy in otitis media with effusion.

The evidence for a role for allergy in recurrent otitis media with effusion in some children was presented by Siegel (1979) and Bernstein (1980):

1. Many patients with recurrent otitis media with effusion have concomitant allergic respiratory disease.

2. A history of one or more major allergic illnesses in parents is usually present.

3. Nasal or peripheral eosinophils are often present in increased numbers.

4. Positive skin tests to allergens or positive radioallergosorbent tests (RAST) are present in many patients.

5. Elevated IgE levels in middle ear effusions and in serum of some children have been identified.

6. Mast cells (some that are degranulating)

are found frequently throughout the middle ear mucosa.

Evidence against a major role for allergy in otitis media with effusion was summarized by Bernstein (1980).

1. In unselected series of cases of otitis media with effusion, fewer than one third of patients are atopic. Allergic airway disease was not a predisposing factor for Arizona Indian children with recurrent otitis media (Todd and Feldman, 1985). These children are likely to have other factors responsible for the susceptibility to middle ear infection.

2. The seasonal incidence of otitis media with effusion (winter to spring) is contrary to the season when grasses, trees, and pollens cause acute nasal allergy (late spring and early fall).

3. Most studies indicate an absence of eosinophils and absence of, or only small numbers of, IgE-producing cells in middle ear fluids and middle ear mucosa.

4. A failure to improve with aggressive allergic treatment, including hyposensitization and use of antihistamines in spite of improvement in nasal symptoms, is seen in most patients.

Thus, many patients may be allergic and many children have recurrent otitis media, but there is no substantive evidence correlating the two conditions. However, it is likely that the allergic response plays a role in some children with otitis media with effusion or in some episodes of otitis media with effusion. The presence of specific IgE on mast cells in middle ear mucosa could result in release of mediators of inflammation, with the mucosa functioning as a shock organ similar to respiratory mucosa in others areas. Alternately, the allergic reaction might be a predisposing factor producing congestion of the mucosa of the nose and eustachian tube, leading to obstruction of the tube with retention of fluid in the middle ear.

BACTERIAL VACCINES AND IMMUNOGLOBULINS FOR PREVENTION OF OTITIS MEDIA

If type-specific serum antibody is correlated with protection from homotypic infection, bacterial vaccines may be an effective mode of prevention of type-specific otitis media. Among bacterial vaccines currently under investigation, the meningococcal vaccines and the *H. influenzae* type b vaccine are of limited interest because of the infrequency of acute otitis media caused by these organisms. A vaccine for nontypable *H. influenzae* is not available, but current investigations focus on use of outer membrane antigens for development of a vaccine (Gnehm et al., 1985). A multitype pneumococcal vaccine is available and is of major interest because of the importance of this organism as a cause of otitis media in all age groups. The clinical and microbiological results of recent trials of pneumococcal vaccine to prevent recurrences of acute otitis media are presented in the section on immunoprophylaxis (Chapter Eight). Usage of immune globulins for prevention of acute otitis media is also discussed in Chapter Eight.

References

Austrian, R., Howie, V. M., and Ploussard, J. H.: The bacteriology of pneumococcal otitis media. Johns Hopkins Med. J. 141:104–111, 1977.

Barenkamp, S. J., Shurin, P. A., Marchant, C. D., Karasic, R. B., Pelton, S. I., Howie, V. M., and Granoff, D. M.: Do children with recurrent *Hemophilus influenzae* otitis media become infected with a new organism or reacquire the original strain? J. Pediatr. 105:533–537, 1984.

Berdal, P., Brandtzaeg, P., Froland, S., Henriksen, S., and Skrede, S.: Immunodeficiency syndromes with otorhinolaryngological manifestations. Acta Otolaryngol. (Stockh.) 82:185–192, 1976.

Berger, G., Hawke, M., Proops, D. W., Ranadive, N. S., and Wong, D.: Histamine levels in middle ear effusions. Acta Otolaryngol. (Stockh.) 98:385–390, 1984.

Bernstein, J. M.: Biological mediators of inflammation in middle ear effusions. Ann. Otol. Rhinol. Laryngol. 85(25):90–96, 1976.

Bernstein, J. M.: Immunological reactivity in otitis media with effusion. *In* Oehling, A., Mathov, E., Glazer, I., and Arbesman, C. (Eds.): *Advances in Allergology and Immunology.* Oxford, Pergamon Press, 1980, pp. 139–146.

Bernstein, J. M.: Observations on immune mechanisms in otitis media with effusion. Int. J. Pediatr. Otorhinolaryngol. 8:125–138, 1984.

Bernstein, J. M., Hayes, E. R., Ishikawa, T., Tomasi, T. B., and Herd, J. K.: Secretory otitis media: A histopathologic and immunochemical report. TAAOO 76:1305–1318, 1972.

Bernstein, J. M., and Reisman, R.: The role of acute hypersensitivity in secretory otitis media. TAAOO 78:ORL 120–ORL 127, 1974.

Bernstein, J. M., Okazaki, T., and Reisman, R. E.: Prostaglandins in middle ear effusions. Arch Otolaryngol. 102:257–258, 1976.

Bernstein, J. M., Schenkein, H. A., Genco, R. J., and Bartholomew, W.: Complement activity in middle ear effusions. Clin. Exp. Immunol. 33:340–346, 1978a.

Bernstein, J. M., Szymanski, C., Albini, B., Sun, M., and Ogra, P. L.: Lymphocyte subpopulations in otitis media with effusion. Pediatr. Res. 12:786–788, 1978b.

Bernstein, J. M., Brentjens, J., and Vladutziu, A.: Immune complex determination in otitis media with effusion. Presented at the ARO Midwinter Meeting, January, 1981, St. Petersburg, Florida.

DeMaria, T. F., McGhee, R. B., Jr., and Lim, D. J.: Rheumatoid factor in otitis media with effusion. Arch. Otolaryngol. 110:279–280, 1984.

Freijd, A., Oxelius V.-A., Rynnel-Dagoo, B.: A prospective study demonstrating an association between plasma IgG2 concentrations and susceptibility to otitis media in children. Scand. J. Infect. Dis. 17:115–120, 1985.

Giebink, G. S., and Quie, P. G.: Otitis media: The spectrum of middle ear inflammation. Ann. Rev. Med. 29:285–306, 1978.

Giebink, G. S., Berzins, I. K., Cates, K. L., Huff, J. S., and Quie, P. G.: Polymorphonuclear leukocyte function during otitis media. Ann. Otol. Rhinol. Laryngol. 89(68):138–142, 1980.

Gnehm, H. E., Pelton, S. I., Gulati, S., and Rice, P. A.: Characterization of antigens from nontypable *Haemophilus influenzae* recognized by human bactericidal antibodies. J. Clin. Invest. 75:1645–1658, 1985.

Granstrom, G., and Holmquist, J., Jarlstedt, J., and Renvall, U.: Collagenase activity in middle ear effusion. Acta Otolaryngol. (Stockh.) 100:405–413, 1985.

Hill, H. R., Book, L. S., Hemming, V. G., and Herbst, J. J.: Defective neutrophil chemotactic responses in patients with recurrent episodes of otitis media and chronic diarrhea. Am. J. Dis. Child. 131:433–436, 1977.

Howie, V. M., Ploussard, J. H., Sloyer, J. L., and Johnston, R.B., Jr.: Immunoglobulins of the middle ear fluid in acute otitis media: Relationship to serum immunoglobulin concentrations and bacterial cultures. Infec. Immun. 7:589–593, 1973.

Ichimura, K.: Neutrophil chemotaxis in children with recurrent otitis media. Int. J. Pediatr. Otorhinolaryngol. 4:47–55, 1982.

Johnston, R. B., Jr.: Recurrent bacterial infections in children. N. Engl. J. Med. 310:1237–1243, 1984.

Koskela, M., Leinonen, M., and Luotonen, J.: Serum antibody response to pneumococcal otitis media. Pediatr. Inf. Dis. 1:245–252, 1982.

Lewis, D. M., Schram, J. L., Lim, D. J., Birck, H. G., and Gleich, G.: Immunoglobulin E in chronic middle ear effusions: Comparison of RIST, PRIST, and RIA techniques. Ann. Otol. Rhinol. Laryngol. 87:197–201, 1978.

Maxim, P. E., Veltri, R. W., Sprinkle, P. M., and Pusateri, R. J.: Chronic serous otitis media: An immune complex disease. TAAOO 84:234–238, 1977.

Meri, S., Lehtinen, T., and Palva, T.: Complement in chronic secretory otitis media: C3 breakdown and C3 splitting activity. Arch. Otolaryngol. 110:774–778, 1984.

Meurman, O. H., Sarkkinen, H. K., Puhakka, H. J., Virolainen, E. S., and Meurman, O. H.: Local IgA-class antibodies against respiratory viruses in middle ear and nasopharyngeal secretions of children with secretory otitis media. Laryngoscope 90:304–311, 1980.

Mogi, G., Yoshida, T., Honjo, S., and Maeda, S.: Middle ear effusions: Quantitative analysis of immunoglobulins. Ann. Otol. Rhinol. Laryngol. 82:196–202, 1973.

Mogi, G., Honjo, S., Maeda, S., Yoshida, T., and Watanabe, N.: Immunoglobulin E (IgE) in middle ear effusions. Ann. Otol. Rhinol. Laryngol. 83:393–398, 1974.

Palva, T., Holopainen, E., and Karma, P.: Protein and cellular protein of glue ear secretions. Ann. Otol. Rhinol. Laryngol. 85(25):103–109, 1976.

Palva, T., Hayry, P., and Ylikoski, J.: Lymphocyte mor-

phology in middle ear effusions. Ann. Otol. Rhinol. Laryngol. 89(68):143–146, 1980.

Phillips, M. J., Knight, N. J., Manning, H., Abbott, A. L., and Tripp, W. G.: IgE and secretory otitis media. Lancet 2:1176–1178, 1974.

Prellner, K., Nilsson, N. I., Johnson, U., and Laurell, A. B.: Complement and C1q binding substances in otitis media. Ann. Otol. Rhinol. Laryngol. 89(68):129–132, 1980.

Qvarnberg, Y., Holopainen, E., and Palva, T.: Aspiration cytology in acute otitis media. Acta Otolaryngol. (Stockh.) 97:443–449, 1984.

Shurin, P. A., Pelton, S. I., Tager, I. B., and Kasper, D. L.: Bactericidal antibody and susceptibility to otitis media caused by nontypable strains of *Haemophilus influenzae*. J. Pediatr. 97:364–369, 1980.

Siegel, S. C.: Allergy as it relates to otitis media. *In* Wiet, R. J., and Coulthard, S. W. (Eds.): *Proceedings of the Second National Conference on Otitis Media.* Columbus, Ohio, Ross Laboratories, 1979, pp. 25–29.

Sipila, P., and Karma, P.: Inflammatory cells in mucoid effusion of secretory otitis media. Acta Otolaryngol. (Stockh.) 94:467–472, 1982.

Sloyer, J. L., Jr., Howie, V. M., Ploussard, J. H., Amman, A. J., Austrian, R., and Johnston, R. B.: Immune response to acute otitis media in children. I. Serotypes isolated in serum and middle ear fluid antibody in pneumococcal otitis media. Infect. Immun. 9:1028–1032, 1974.

Sloyer, J. L., Jr., Cate, C. D., Howie, V. M., Ploussard, J. H., and Johnston, R. B.: The immune response to acute otitis media in children. II. Serum and middle ear antibody in otitis media due to *Haemophilus influenzae*. J. Infect. Dis. 132:685–688, 1975.

Sloyer, J. L., Howie, V. M., Ploussard, J. H., Schiffman, G. D., and Johnston, R. B.: Immune response to acute otitis media: Association between middle ear antibody and the clearing of clinical infection. J. Clin. Microbiol. 4:306–308, 1976.

Sloyer, J. L., Jr., Howie, V. M., Ploussard, J. H., Bradoc, J., Hatercorn, M., and Ogra, P. L.: Immune response to acute otitis media in children. III. Implications of viral antibody in middle ear fluid. J. Immunol. 118:248–250, 1977.

Todd, N. W., and Feldman, C. M.: Allergic airway disease and otitis media in children. Int. J. Pediatr. Otorhinolaryngol. 10:27–35, 1985.

Umetsu, D. T., Ambrosino, D. M., Quinti, I., Siber, E. R., and Geha, R. S.: Recurrent sinopulmonary infection and impaired antibody response to bacterial capsular polysaccharide antigen in children with selective IgG-subclass deficiency. N. Engl. J. Med. 313:1247–1251, 1985.

Veltri, R. W., and Sprinkle, P. M.: Serous otitis media: Immunoglobulin and lysozyme levels in middle ear fluids and serum. Ann. Otol. Rhinol. Laryngol. 82:297–301, 1973.

Ward, P. A., and McClean, R.: Complement activity. *In* Bellanti, J. A. (Ed.): *Immunology II.* Philadelphia, W. B. Saunders Co., 1978, pp. 138–150.

Wong, D. T., and Ogra, P. L.: Immunology of tonsils and adenoids—an update. Int. J. Pediatr. Otorhinolaryngol. 2:181–191, 1980.

Yamaguchi, T., Urasawa, T., and Kataura, A.: Secretory immunoglobulin A antibodies to respiratory viruses in middle ear effusion of chronic otitis media with effusion. Ann. Otol. Rhinol. Laryngol. 93:73–75, 1984.

Yamanaka, T., Bernstein, J. B., Cumella, J., Parker, C., and Ogra, P. L.: Immunologic aspects of otitis media with effusion: Characteristics of lymphocyte and macrophage reactivity. J. Infect. Dis. 145:804–810, 1982.

7

Diagnosis

Of the various methods currently used for diagnosis of otitis media with effusion in children, the medical history and physical examination, including pneumatic otoscopy, are usually sufficient to establish the diagnosis. However, the most significant advance in the identification of middle ear effusion is the use of the electroacoustic impedance bridge, with which a tympanogram can be obtained. Audiometry is of limited value as a diagnostic method for identification of otitis media with effusion, but it can be helpful in evaluation of the effect of middle ear disease on hearing; it is also an aid in selection of management options.

SIGNS AND SYMPTOMS OF OTITIS MEDIA

Children with acute otitis media may have nonspecific signs and symptoms, including fever, irritability, headache, apathy, anorexia, vomiting, and diarrhea. Fever occurs in one third (Schwartz et al., 1981) to two thirds (Mortimer and Watterson, 1956) of children with otitis media, and high fever (over 40° C) is unusual unless accompanied by bacteremia or a significant focus elsewhere.

Eight specific signs and symptoms are associated with otitis media and its complications and sequelae.

Otalgia, or ear pain, is by far the most common complaint in children with acute otitis media. In infants, however, pulling at the ear or irritability, especially when associated with fever, may be the only sign of ear pain. Otalgia may also be the result of inflammation of the external canal or may originate outside the ear (e.g., from the temporomandibular joint, teeth, or pharynx). In most cases, otalgia not associated with otitis media can be identified as referred pain due to discomfort with swallowing (tonsillitis), nasal obstruction, or pain in the throat (pharyngitis), but any lesion in the areas of the trigeminal, facial, glossopharyngeal, vagus, great auricular, or lesser occipital nerve supply can result in earache (Ingvarsson, 1982). On the other hand, earache does not occur in some children with acute otitis media; approximately one fifth of 335 consecutively diagnosed episodes in a pediatric practice were without earache (usually among children older than two years of age) (Hayden and Schwartz, 1985).

Otorrhea is a discharge, either from the middle ear through a defect in the tympanic membrane or from the external auditory canal when inflamed, or from both.

Hearing loss is a frequent symptom associated with otitis media when elicited from older children. In infants and younger children who are not able to verbalize this loss of function, the only sign of disease in the middle ear may be the parents' suspicion of hearing loss.

Vertigo is not a common complaint in children, but otitis media or eustachian tube dysfunction, or both, are the most common causes of this disorder. The vestibular system is more commonly affected by unilateral middle ear effusion than it is by bilateral disease. Vertigo may also be due to labyrinthitis. Older children describe a feeling of spinning or turning, whereas younger children may not be able to describe these symptoms but manifest *dysequilibrium* by falling, stumbling, or "clumsiness."

69

Nystagmus, which is usually associated with vertigo of labyrinthine origin, is of unidirectional, horizontal, jerk type in otitis media.

Tinnitus is another symptom that children describe infrequently but, like vertigo, is commonly due to otitis media and eustachian tube dysfunction.

Swelling about the ear, especially in the postauricular area, may indicate disease of the mastoid (e.g., periostitis or subperiosteal abscess) but must be differentiated from diffuse external otitis, adenopathy, or adenitis.

Facial paralysis in children, when it is due to disease within the temporal bone, most commonly occurs as a complication of acute otitis media or chronic otitis media with perforation and discharge, or as a result of cholesteatoma.

Recent articles cite the frequent occurrence of purulent *conjunctivitis* with acute otitis media. The conjunctivae are injected with pain, there is tearing or purulent discharge and, in some children, concurrent ear pain (Bodor, 1982). Simultaneous cultures of conjunctivae and middle ear exudates reveal nontypable *Haemophilus influenzae* in almost all cases (Bodor et al., 1985).

PHYSICAL EXAMINATION

Aside from the history, the most useful method for diagnosing otitis media is a physical examination that includes pneumatic otoscopy. Adequate examination of the head and neck can lead to identification of a condition that may predispose to, or be associated with, otitis media.

The appearance of the child's face may be an important clue to susceptibility to middle ear disease. Many craniofacial anomalies, such as mandibulofacial dysostosis (Treacher Collins syndrome) or trisomy 21 (Down syndrome), are associated with increased incidence of ear disease.

The character of speech may be altered. Mouth breathing and hyponasality may indicate intranasal or postnasal obstruction, whereas hypernasality is a sign of velopharyngeal insufficiency.

Examination of the oropharyngeal cavity may uncover an overt cleft palate or a submucous cleft (Fig. 7–1), both of which predispose the infant to otitis media with effusion (Paradise et al., 1969; Stool and Randall, 1967). A bifid uvula is also associated with increased incidence of middle ear disease (Taylor, 1972). Posterior nasal or pharyngeal inflammation and discharge may be present.

Pathological conditions of the nose such as polyposis, severe deviation of the nasal septum, or a nasopharyngeal tumor may be associated with otitis media.

Examination of the ear is the most critical part of the clinician's assessment of the patient, but it must be performed systematically. The auricle and external auditory meatus should be examined first; all too frequently these areas are overlooked in the physician's haste to make a diagnosis by otoscopic examination. The presence or absence of signs of infection in these areas may be of aid later in the differential diagnosis or evaluation of complications of otitis media. For instance, eczematoid external otitis may result from acute otitis media with discharge, or inflam-

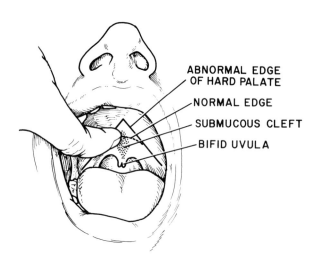

ABNORMAL EDGE OF HARD PALATE

NORMAL EDGE

SUBMUCOUS CLEFT

BIFID UVULA

Figure 7–1. Bifid uvula, widening and attenuation of the median raphe of the soft palate, and a V-shaped midline notch (rather than a smooth curve) are diagnostic of a submucous cleft palate.

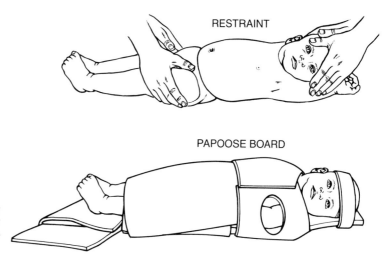

RESTRAINT

PAPOOSE BOARD

Figure 7–2. Methods of restraining an infant for examination and for procedures such as tympanocentesis or myringotomy.

mation of the postauricular area may be indicative of a periostitis or subperiosteal abscess that has extended from the mastoid air cells. Palpation of these areas will determine if tenderness is present: exquisite pain upon palpation of the tragus would indicate the presence of acute, diffuse external otitis.

After examination of the external ear and canal, the clinician may proceed to the most important part of the physical assessment, the otoscopic examination.

OTOSCOPY

Positioning the Patient for Examination

The position of the patient for otoscopy depends upon the patient's age, his or her ability to cooperate, the clinical setting, and the preference of the examiner. Otoscopic evaluation of an infant is best performed on an examining table, and a parent or assistant is necessary to restrain the baby, since undue movement usually prevents an adequate evaluation (Fig. 7–2). Some clinicians prefer to place the infant prone on the table, whereas others prefer the patient to be supine. Use of the examining table is also desirable for older infants who are uncooperative or when a tympanocentesis or myringotomy is performed without general anesthesia. Figure 7–3 shows that infants and young children who are just apprehensive and not struggling actively can be evaluated adequately while sitting on the parent's lap; when necessary, the child may be restrained firmly on an

adult's lap if the parent holds the child's wrists over the abdomen with one hand and holds the patient's head against the adult's chest with the other hand. If necessary, the child's legs can be held between the adult's thighs. Some infants can be examined by placing the child's head on the parent's knee (Fig. 7–4). Cooperative children sitting in a chair or on the edge of an examination table can usually be evaluated successfully. The otoscope should be held with the hand or finger placed firmly against the child's head or face, so that the otoscope will move with the head rather than cause trauma (pain) to the ear canal if the child moves suddenly (Fig. 7–5). Pulling up and out on the pinna will usually straighten the ear canal enough to allow exposure of the tympanic membrane. In the young infant, the tragus must be moved forward and out of the way.

Removal of Cerumen

Before adequate visualization of the external canal and tympanic membrane can be obtained, all obstructing cerumen must be removed from the canal. Many children with acute otitis media have moderate to large accumulations of cerumen in the ear canal. For optimal visualization of the tympanic membrane, mechanical removal was necessary in approximately one third of 279 patients observed by Schwartz and colleagues (1983); cerumen removal was inversely proportional to age with more than half of infants under one year of age. Removal of cerumen can usually be accomplished by use of an otoscope with a surgical head and a

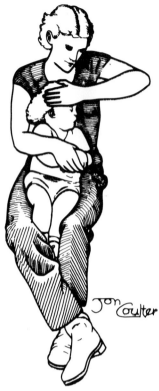

Figure 7–3. Mother assisting in restraining a child for examination of the ear.

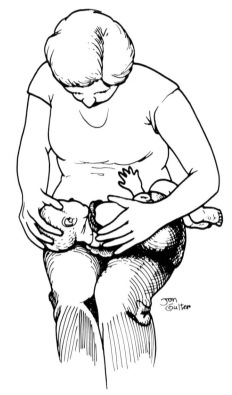

Figure 7–4. Mother using lap position of infant for examination of the infant's ear.

wire loop or a blunt cerumen curette (Fig. 7–6) or by irrigating the ear canal *gently* with warm water delivered through a dental irrigator (Water Pik) (Fig. 7–7).

Carbamide peroxide in glycerol (Debrox) can be used by the patient for a few days prior to irrigation. Reported use of other commercial preparations (e.g., triethanolamine polypeptide oleate-condensate [Cerumenex]) may cause severe eczematoid allergic reactions of the external canal.

The Otoscope

For proper assessment of the tympanic membrane and its mobility, a pneumatic otoscope in which the diagnostic head has an adequate seal should be used. Currently, the quality of the otoscopic examination is limited by deficiencies in the designs of commercially available otoscopes. The speculum employed should have the largest lumen that comfortably can fit in the child' s cartilaginous external auditory meatus. If the speculum is too small, adequate visualization may be im-

paired and the speculum may touch the bony canal, which can be painful. In most models an airtight seal is usually not possible because of a leak of air within the otoscope head or

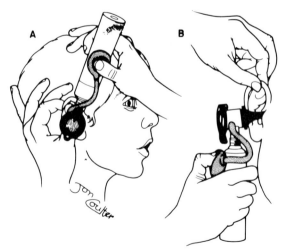

Figure 7–5. Positioning otoscope to enhance visualization and to minimize the chance that head movement will result in trauma to the ear canal. Both of the otoscopist's hands can be used (*A*), or, when the child is cooperative, a finger touching the child's cheek is sufficient (*B*).

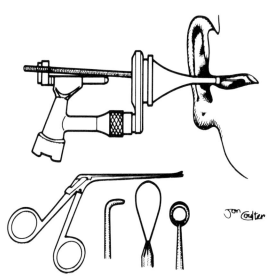

Figure 7–6. Method for removing cerumen from the external ear canal by employing the surgical head attached to the otoscope. Instruments that can be used are also illustrated.

between the stiff ear speculum and the external auditory canal, although leaks at the latter location can be stopped by cutting off a small section of rubber tubing and slipping it over the tip of the ear speculum (Fig. 7–8).

The Examination

Inspection of the tympanic membrane should include evaluation of its (1) position,

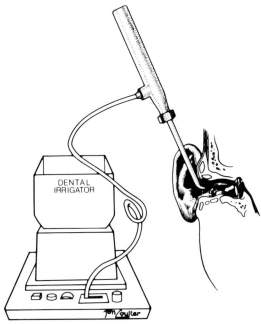

Figure 7–7. Irrigation of the external canal with a dental irrigator to remove cerumen.

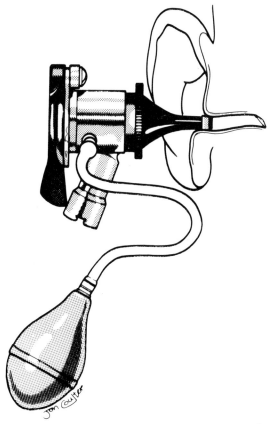

Figure 7–8. Pneumatic otoscope, with rubber tip on the end of the ear speculum to give a better seal in the external auditory canal.

(2) color, (3) degree of translucency, and (4) mobility. Assessment of the light reflex is of limited value because it does not reflect the status of the middle ear in the evaluation of tympanic membrane–middle ear disorders.

Position of the Tympanic Membrane

The positions of the tympanic membrane when the middle ear is aerated and when effusion is present are illustrated in Figure 7–9.

The normal eardrum should be in the neutral position, with the short process of the malleus visible but not prominent through the membrane.

Mild retraction of the tympanic membrane usually indicates the presence of negative middle ear pressure or an effusion, or both. The short process of the malleus and posterior mallear fold are prominent, and the manubrium of the malleus appears to be foreshortened.

Severe retraction of the tympanic membrane is characterized by a very prominent

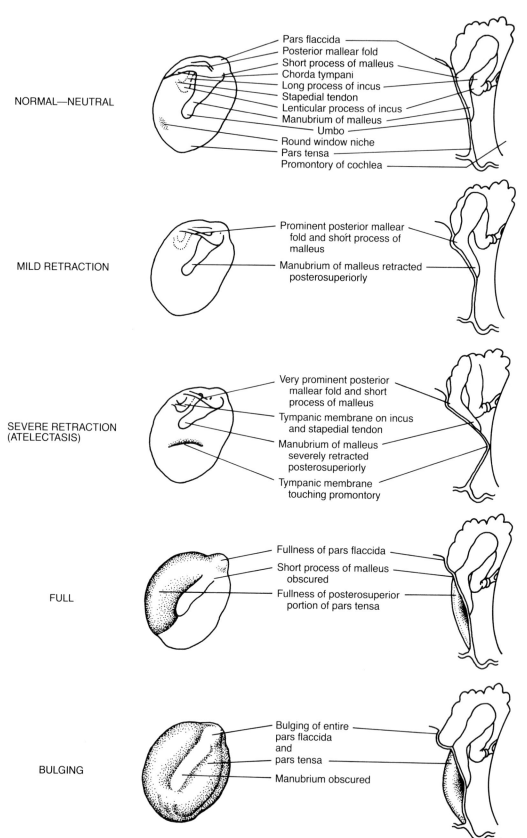

TYMPANIC MEMBRANE POSITION

OTOSCOPIC VIEW

LATERAL SECTION THROUGH TYMPANIC MEMBRANE AND MIDDLE EAR

NORMAL—NEUTRAL

Pars flaccida
Posterior mallear fold
Short process of malleus
Chorda tympani
Long process of incus
Stapedial tendon
Lenticular process of incus
Manubrium of malleus
Umbo
Round window niche
Pars tensa
Promontory of cochlea

MILD RETRACTION

Prominent posterior mallear fold and short process of malleus
Manubrium of malleus retracted posterosuperiorly

SEVERE RETRACTION (ATELECTASIS)

Very prominent posterior mallear fold and short process of malleus
Tympanic membrane on incus and stapedial tendon
Manubrium of malleus severely retracted posterosuperiorly
Tympanic membrane touching promontory

FULL

Fullness of pars flaccida
Short process of malleus obscured
Fullness of posterosuperior portion of pars tensa

BULGING

Bulging of entire pars flaccida and pars tensa
Manubrium obscured

Figure 7–9. Otoscopic views and corresponding lateral sections through the tympanic membrane and middle ear demonstrate the various positions of the drum with their respective anatomic landmarks (see text).

posterior mallear fold and short process of the malleus and a severely foreshortened manubrium. The tympanic membrane may be severely retracted, presumably owing to high negative pressure in association with a middle ear effusion.

Fullness of the tympanic membrane is apparent initially in the posterosuperior portion of the pars tensa and the pars flaccida, since these two areas are the most highly compliant parts of the tympanic membrane. The short process of the malleus is commonly obscured. The fullness is caused by increased air pressure or effusion, or both, within the middle ear. When bulging of the entire tympanic membrane occurs, the malleus is usually obscured, which occurs when the middle ear–mastoid system is filled with an effusion.

Appearance of the Tympanic Membrane

The normal tympanic membrane has a ground-glass appearance; a blue or yellow color usually indicates a middle ear effusion seen through a translucent tympanic membrane. A red tympanic membrane may not alone be indicative of a pathological condition, since the blood vessels of the drum head may be engorged as the result of the patient's crying, sneezing, or nose-blowing. It is critical to distinguish between translucency and opacification of the eardrum in order to identify a middle ear effusion. The normal tympanic membrane should be translucent, and the observer should be able to look through the drum and visualize the middle ear landmarks (the incudostapedial joint, promontory, round window niche, and, frequently, the chorda tympani nerve) (Fig. 7–10). If a middle ear effusion is present medial to a translucent drum, an air-fluid level or bubbles of air admixed with the liquid

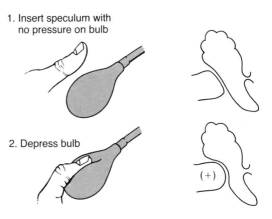

TO OBTAIN POSITIVE PRESSURE:

1. Insert speculum with no pressure on bulb

2. Depress bulb

(+)

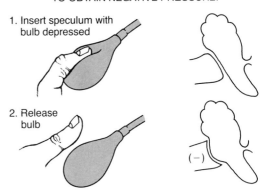

TO OBTAIN NEGATIVE PRESSURE:

1. Insert speculum with bulb depressed

2. Release bulb

(−)

Figure 7–11. Pressure applied to the rubber bulb attached to the pneumatic otoscope will deflect the normal tympanic membrane inward with applied positive pressure and outward with applied negative pressure if the middle ear air pressure is ambient. The movement of the eardrum is proportionate to the degree of pressure exerted on the bulb until the tympanic membrane has reached its limit of compliance.

may be visible. Inability to visualize the middle ear structures indicates opacification of the drum, which is usually the result of thickening of the tympanic membrane or the presence of an effusion, or both.

Mobility of the Tympanic Membrane

Abnormalities of the tympanic membrane and middle ear are reflected in the pattern of tympanic membrane mobility when first positive and then negative pressure is applied to the external auditory canal with the pneumatic otoscope. As shown in Figure 7–11, this is achieved by first applying slight pressure on the rubber bulb (positive pressure) and then, after momentarily breaking the seal, releasing the bulb (negative pressure). The presence of effusion or high negative

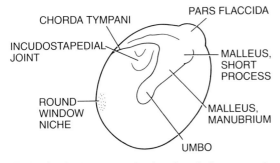

CHORDA TYMPANI
PARS FLACCIDA
INCUDOSTAPEDIAL JOINT
MALLEUS, SHORT PROCESS
ROUND WINDOW NICHE
MALLEUS, MANUBRIUM
UMBO

Figure 7–10. Important landmarks of the tympanic membrane that usually can be visualized with the otoscope.

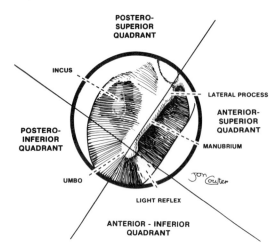

Figure 7–12. The four quadrants of the pars tensa of a right tympanic membrane.

pressure, or both, within the middle ear can markedly dampen the movements of the eardrum. When the middle ear pressure is ambient, the normal tympanic membrane moves inward with slight positive pressure in the ear canal and outward toward the examiner with slight negative pressure. The motion observed is proportionate to the applied pressure and is best visualized in the posterosuperior quadrant of the tympanic membrane (Fig. 7–12). If a two-layered membrane or atrophic scar (secondary to a healed perforation) is present, mobility of the tympanic membrane can also be assessed more readily by observing the movement of the flaccid area.

Figure 7–13 shows the relationship between mobility of the tympanic membrane, as measured by pneumatic otoscopy, and the middle ear contents and pressure. In Figure 7–13, Frame 1 shows the normal tympanic membrane when the middle ear contains only air at ambient pressure. A hypermobile eardrum (Frame 2) is seen most frequently in children whose membranes are atrophic or flaccid. The mobility of the tympanic membrane is greater than normal (the drum is said to be highly compliant) if the drum

			PNEUMATIC OTOSCOPY					MIDDLE EAR	
		EARDRUM POSITION*	EARDRUM MOVEMENT †					CONTENTS	PRESSURE
			POSITIVE ▽ PRESSURE		NEGATIVE PRESSURE				
			LOW	HIGH	LOW	HIGH			
1.	NEUTRAL	EXT. CANAL / MIDDLE EAR	1+	2+	1+	2+		AIR	AMBIENT
2.	NEUTRAL		2+	3+	2+	3+		AIR	AMBIENT
3.	NEUTRAL		0	1+	0	1+		AIR OR AIR AND EFFUSION	AMBIENT
4.	RETRACTED		0	0	1+	2+		AIR OR AIR AND EFFUSION	LOW NEGATIVE
5.	RETRACTED		0	0	0	1+		AIR OR EFFUSION AND AIR	HIGH NEGATIVE
6.	RETRACTED		0	0	0	0		AIR OR EFFUSION OR BOTH	VERY HIGH NEGATIVE OR INDETERMINATE
7.	FULL		0	1+	0	0		AIR AND EFFUSION	POSITIVE OR INDETERMINATE
8.	BULGING		0	0	0	0		EFFUSION	POSITIVE OR INDETERMINATE

* POSITION OF EARDRUM
—— AT REST;--- POSITIVE PRESSURE APPLIED (BULB COMPRESSED);
⋯ NEGATIVE PRESSURE APPLIED (RELEASE BULB)

† DEGREE OF TYMPANIC MEMBRANE MOVEMENT AS VISUALIZED THROUGH THE OTOSCOPE; 0 = NONE, 1+ = SLIGHT, 2+ = MODERATE, 3+ = EXCESSIVE

▽ COMPRESSION OF BULB EXERTS POSITIVE PRESSURE ; RELEASE OF A COMPRESSED BULB INDUCES NEGATIVE PRESSURE

Figure 7–13. Pneumatic otoscopic findings related to middle ear contents and pressure (see text).

moves when even slight positive or negative external canal pressure is applied, and if the drum moves equally well to both applied positive and negative pressures, the middle ear pressure is approximately ambient. However, if the tympanic membrane is hypermobile to applied negative pressure but is immobile when positive pressure is applied, the tympanic membrane is flaccid and negative pressure is present within the middle ear. A middle ear effusion is rarely present when the tympanic membrane is hypermobile, even though high negative middle ear pressure is present. A thickened tympanic membrane (secondary to inflammation or scarring, or both) or a partly effusion-filled middle ear (in which the middle ear air pressure is ambient) shows decreased mobility to applied pressures, both positive and negative (Frame 3).

Normal middle ear pressure is reflected by the neutral position of the tympanic membrane as well as by its response to both positive and negative pressures in each of the previous examples (Frames 1 through 3). In other cases, the eardrum may be retracted—usually because negative middle ear pressure is present (Frames 4 through 6). The compliant membrane is maximally retracted by even moderate negative middle ear pressure and hence cannot visibly be deflected inward further with applied positive pressure in the ear canal. Negative pressure produced by releasing the rubber bulb of the otoscope will, however, cause a return of the eardrum toward the neutral position if a negative pressure equivalent to that in the middle ear can be created by releasing the rubber bulb, a condition (Frame 4) that occurs when air, with or without an effusion, is present in the middle ear. When the middle ear pressure is even lower, there may be only slight outward mobility of the tympanic membrane (Frame 5) because of the limited negative pressure that can be exerted through the otoscopes currently available. If the eardrum is severely retracted with extremely high negative middle ear pressure or in the presence of a middle ear effusion, or both, the examiner is not able to produce significant outward movement (Frame 6).

The tympanic membrane that exhibits fullness (Frame 7) will move to applied positive pressure but not to applied negative pressure if the pressure within the middle ear is positive and air, with or without an effusion, is present. In such an instance, the tympanic membrane is stretched laterally to the point

of maximum compliance and will not visibly move outward any farther to the applied negative pressure but will move inward to applied positive pressure as long as some air is present within the middle ear–mastoid air cell system. When this system is filled with an effusion and little or no air is present, the mobility of the bulging tympanic membrane (Frame 8) is severely decreased or absent to both applied positive and negative pressure.

Figure 7–14 shows examples of common conditions of the middle ear as assessed with the otoscope, in which position, color, degree of translucency, and mobility of the tympanic membrane are diagnostic aids.

Otoscopy in the Newborn Infant

The tympanic membrane of the neonate is in a different position from that of the older infant and child; if this is not kept in mind, the examiner may perceive the eardrum to be smaller and retracted, since in the neonate the tympanic membrane appears to be as wide as it is in older children but not as high (Fig. 7–15). Figure 7–16 shows that this perception is due to the more horizontal position of the neonatal eardrum, which frequently makes it difficult for the examiner to distinguish the pars flaccida of the tympanic membrane from the skin of the wall of the deep superior external canal.

In the first few days of life, the ear canal is filled with vernix caseosa, but this material is readily removed with a small curette or suction tube. The canal walls of the young infant are pliable and tend to expand and collapse with insufflation during pneumatic otoscopy. Because of the pliability of the canal walls, it is necessary to advance the speculum farther into the canal than would be the case for the older child. The tympanic membrane often appears thickened and opaque during the first few days. In many infants the membrane is in an extreme oblique position, with the superior aspect proximal to the observer (Fig. 7–15). The tympanic membrane and the superior canal wall may appear to lie almost in the same plane, so that it is often difficult to distinguish the point where the canal ends and the pars flaccida begins. The inferior canal wall bulges loosely over the inferior position of the tympanic membrane and moves with positive pressure, simulating the movement of the tympanic membrane. The examiner must distinguish the movement of the canal walls

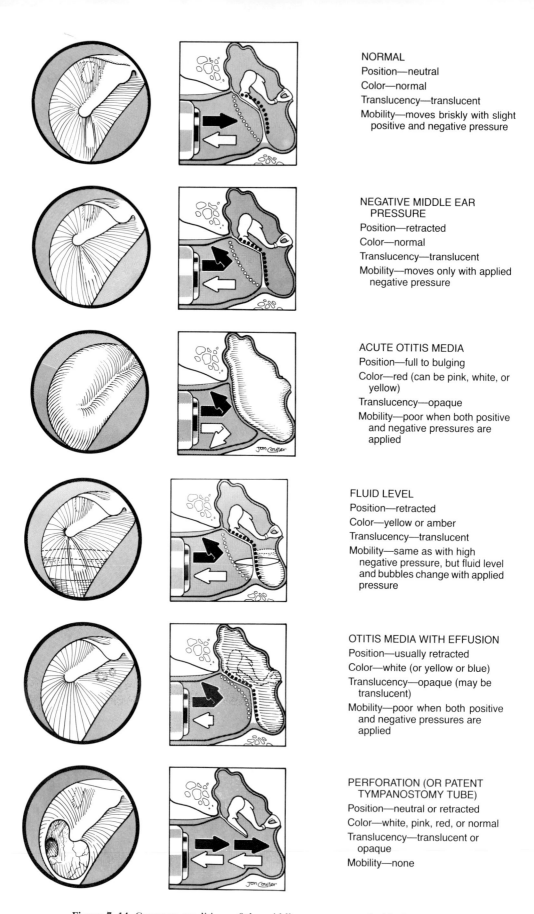

NORMAL
Position—neutral
Color—normal
Translucency—translucent
Mobility—moves briskly with slight positive and negative pressure

NEGATIVE MIDDLE EAR PRESSURE
Position—retracted
Color—normal
Translucency—translucent
Mobility—moves only with applied negative pressure

ACUTE OTITIS MEDIA
Position—full to bulging
Color—red (can be pink, white, or yellow)
Translucency—opaque
Mobility—poor when both positive and negative pressures are applied

FLUID LEVEL
Position—retracted
Color—yellow or amber
Translucency—translucent
Mobility—same as with high negative pressure, but fluid level and bubbles change with applied pressure

OTITIS MEDIA WITH EFFUSION
Position—usually retracted
Color—white (or yellow or blue)
Translucency—opaque (may be translucent)
Mobility—poor when both positive and negative pressures are applied

PERFORATION (OR PATENT TYMPANOSTOMY TUBE)
Position—neutral or retracted
Color—white, pink, red, or normal
Translucency—translucent or opaque
Mobility—none

Figure 7–14. Common conditions of the middle ear, as assessed with the otoscope.

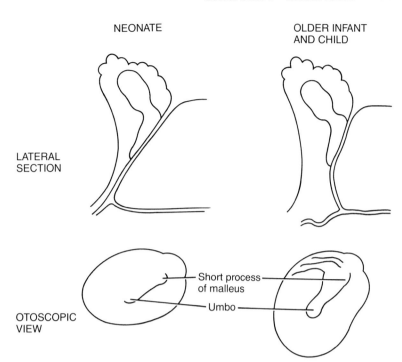

NEONATE

OLDER INFANT
AND CHILD

LATERAL
SECTION

Short process
of malleus

Umbo

OTOSCOPIC
VIEW

Figure 7–15. Otoscopic view of tympanic membrane of neonate, compared with that seen in the older infant and child.

and the movement of the membrane. The following should be considered to distinguish the movement of these structures: vessels are seen within the tympanic membrane but not in the skin of the ear canal, the tympanic membrane moves during crying or respiration, and inferiorly, the wall of the external canal and the tympanic membrane lie at an acute angle. By one month of age, the tympanic membrane has assumed an oblique position, one with which the examiner is familiar in the older child. During the first

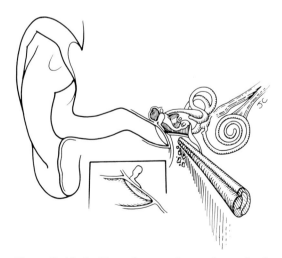

Figure 7–16. Position of tympanic membrane in the child is more vertical than it is in the neonate.

few weeks of life, however, examination of the ear requires patience and careful appraisal of the structures of the external canal and the tympanic membrane.

Accuracy and Validation

Otoscopy is subjective and thus is usually an imprecise method of assessing the condition of the tympanic membrane and middle ear. Many clinicians do not use a pneumatic otoscope, and few have been trained adequately to make a correct diagnosis. The primary reason for this lack of proper education is the method of teaching employed. Since otoscopy is a monocular assessment of the tympanic membrane, the teacher cannot verify that the student actually saw the anatomical features that led to the diagnosis. A new otoscope with a second viewing port is available (Welch-Allyn Co.) (Fig. 7–17). Teacher and student can make observations together, and student errors can be corrected immediately. One of the most effective means of education currently available is the correlation of otoscopic findings with that of the otomicroscope that has an observer tube for the student. In this manner, the instructor can point out critical landmarks and demonstrate tympanic mobility.

Assessment techniques can also be improved by correlating otoscopy findings with

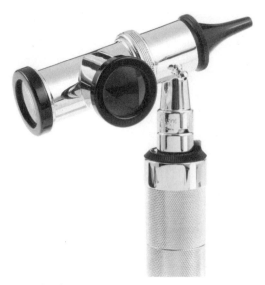

Figure 7–17. Teaching otoscope with sidearm viewer. (From Welch-Allyn and Co., New York.)

a tympanogram taken immediately after the otoscopic examination. Lack of agreement between the otoscopic findings and tympanometry usually results in a second otoscopic examination, since tympanometry is in general very accurate in distinguishing between normal and abnormal tympanic membranes and middle ears (specifically, in the identification of middle ear effusions). The presence or absence (and degree) of negative pressure within the middle ear as measured by pneumatic otoscopy can only be verified by similar results as measured on the tympanogram.

Validation of otoscopic skills is important for education of individuals and for documenting the adequacy of participants in research programs. Validation of the presence or absence of effusion as observed by otoscopy is best achieved by performing a tympanocentesis or myringotomy immediately after the examination. When surgical opening of the tympanic membrane is indicated, preliminary otoscopy by the examiner is a very effective way of validating the otoscopist. This method has been described for research purposes (Bluestone and Cantekin, 1979; Cantekin et al., 1980), but the method should be part of every clinician-otoscopist's method to improve the accuracy of diagnoses of otitis media.

CLINICAL DESCRIPTION

Acute Otitis Media

The usual picture of acute otitis media is seen in a child who has had an upper respiratory tract infection for several days and suddenly develops otalgia, fever, and hearing loss. Examination with the pneumatic otoscope reveals a hyperemic, opaque, bulging tympanic membrane that has poor mobility (Fig. 7–14). Purulent otorrhea is usually also a reliable sign. In addition to fever, other systemic signs and symptoms may include irritability, lethargy, anorexia, vomiting, and diarrhea. However, none of these may be present, and even earache and fever are unreliable guides and may frequently be absent. Likewise, otoscopic findings may consist only of a bulging or full, opaque, poorly mobile eardrum without evidence of erythema. Hearing loss will not be a complaint of the very young and may not even be noted by the parents.

Because of the variability of symptoms, infants and young children presenting with diminished or absent mobility and opacification of the tympanic membrane should be suspected of having acute otitis media.

Otitis Media with Effusion

Most children with otitis media with effusion for prolonged periods of time are asymptomatic. Some may complain of hearing loss and, less commonly, tinnitus and vertigo. In children the attention of an alert parent or teacher may be drawn to a suspected hearing loss. Sometimes, the child presents with a behavioral disorder due to the hearing deficit and consequent inability to communicate adequately. More often, the reason for referral is the detection of a hearing loss during a school hearing screening test or when acute otitis media fails to resolve completely. Occasionally, the first evidence of the disease is discovered during a routine examination or in high-risk cases, such as in children with a cleft palate.

Older children will describe a frank hearing loss or, more commonly, a "plugged" feeling or "popping" in their ears. The symptoms are usually bilateral. Unilateral signs and symptoms of chronic middle ear effusion may uncommonly be secondary to a naso-pharyngeal neoplasm such as an angiofi-broma or even a malignancy.

Pneumatic otoscopy will frequently reveal either a retracted or full tympanic membrane that is usually opaque; however, when the membrane is translucent, an air-fluid level or air bubbles may be visualized, and a blue or amber color is present. The mobility of the eardrum is almost always altered (Fig. 7–14).

It is evident from the preceding clinical description of acute otitis media and otitis media with effusion that there is considerable overlap, and it is often very difficult for the clinician to distinguish between acute and chronic forms unless the child has been observed over a period of time before the onset of disease or there are associated specific (otalgia) or systemic (fever) symptoms. It may not be possible to distinguish between the two even when the middle ear effusion is aspirated (tympanocentesis) since in both acute and chronic otitis the effusion may be either serous, mucoid, or purulent. In approximately half of chronic effusions, bacteria have been cultured that are frequently found in ears of children with classic signs and symptoms of acute otitis media (Riding et al., 1978a).

Atelectasis of the Tympanic Membrane–Middle Ear and High Negative Pressure

Atelectasis of the tympanic membrane may be acute or chronic, generalized or localized, and mild or severe. The tympanic membrane may be retracted or collapsed. High negative pressure may be present or absent (Fig. 7–14). When middle ear effusion is also present, the clinical description is the same as described previously for cases in which an acute or chronic otitis media is present. In such cases, it is not unusual to visualize through the otoscope a severely retracted malleus in association with a tympanic membrane that is full or even bulging in the posterior portion. The malleus is retracted by concurrent high negative middle ear pressure or chronic inflammation of the tensor tympani muscle or the mallear ligaments, or both, whereas the hydrostatic pressure of the effusion (not completely filling the middle ear–mastoid air cell system) results in bulging of the most compliant (floppy) portion of the

pars tensa, the posterosuperior and postero-inferior quadrants. Frequently an effusion is evident by the presence of an air-fluid level or bubbles behind a severely retracted tympanic membrane.

Just as when there is a middle ear effusion present, there may be a lack of specific otological symptoms when atelectasis but no effusion is present. The child may have a severely retracted translucent tympanic membrane with evidence of high negative pressure by pneumatic otoscopy (immobile to applied positive pressure and either decreased or absent mobility to applied negative pressure) or a high negative middle ear pressure tracing on the tympanogram. The otoscopist can look through the tympanic membrane and see that there is no effusion present. Some children with such an otoscopic (and tympanometric) examination may not have any complaint, whereas others may have a feeling of fullness in the ear, otalgia, tinnitus, hearing loss, and even vertigo. The condition may be self-limited and, in some, physiological, owing to temporary eustachian tube obstruction. But in others, especially those with symptoms, the condition is pathological and should be managed in a similar manner as described when an effusion is present.

When there is localized atelectasis or a retraction pocket, especially in the pars flaccida or posterosuperior portion of the pars tensa of the tympanic membrane, then the condition may be more serious than when only generalized atelectasis is present. The child may be totally asymptomatic, but the retraction pocket may be associated with a significant conductive hearing loss, especially if there is erosion of one or more of the ossicles. Erosion of the long process of the incus may be present when a deep posterosuperior retraction pocket is seen (Fig. 7–18). It is extremely important to inspect these areas of the tympanic membrane to determine if a retraction pocket is present and, if present, if there is destruction of one of the ossicles. It is important to distinguish between a retraction pocket and a cholesteatoma. If the otoscopic examination is not adequate to make this differential diagnosis, then referral to an otolaryngologist for examination with the otomicroscope should be considered; the otolaryngologist should not hesitate to perform otomicroscopic examination under general anesthesia when indicated. Cholestea-

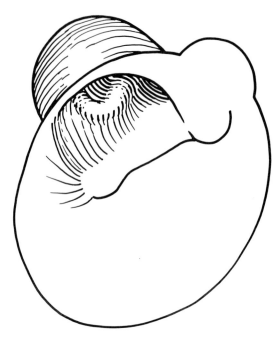

Figure 7–18. An atelectatic membrane that has a severe retraction pocket in the posterosuperior quadrant of the pars tensa.

toma, like its precursor, the deep retraction pocket, may be without signs and symptoms (other than the otoscopic appearance) unless conductive hearing loss or otorrhea is present.

Eustachian Tube Dysfunction

Some children, especially older ones, will complain of a periodic popping or snapping sound in the ear that may be preceded or accompanied by a feeling of fullness in the ear, hearing loss, tinnitus, or vertigo. Otoscopic examination may reveal a normal tympanic membrane or possibly slight retraction of the eardrum, but the middle ear pressure is within normal limits. These children have obstruction of the eustachian tube that is not severe enough to cause atelectasis or a middle ear effusion but nevertheless may be quite disconcerting. When this condition is troublesome, the child should be managed as described for the children who have middle ear effusion.

On occasion, older children may complain of autophony (hearing one's own voice in the ear) and hearing their own breathing. The eustachian tube is most likely patulous (abnormally patent), in which case the tympanic membrane will appear normal when visualized through the otoscope. Middle ear pressure will be normal; however, if the child is asked to breathe forcefully through one nasal cavity while the opposite one is occluded with a finger, the posterosuperior portion of the tympanic membrane will be observed to move in and out with respiration, which will confirm the diagnosis. Tympanometry may also aid in diagnosis.

ACOUSTIC IMPEDANCE MEASUREMENT, INCLUDING TYMPANOMETRY

The function of the electroacoustic impedance bridge depends on the principles of sound in relation to the physiological characteristics of the ear. The most effective transfer of energy occurs when a force flows from one medium to another medium of similar impedance (i.e., with similar mechanical properties of stiffness, mass, and friction). The middle ear facilitates the transfer of sound energy from an air medium with low impedance to a liquid medium with relatively high impedance (cochlea) (Fig. 7–19A). The tympanic membrane and middle ear, therefore, act as an impedance matching transformer. Abnormalities that interfere with this function impair hearing. Three basic observations about acoustic impedance can be made with the electroacoustic impedance bridge: a tympanogram can be obtained, and middle ear muscle reflex and static compliance can be measured. The instrument has become increasingly popular, and it is currently used in a wide variety of clinical settings both for diagnosis and screening. A tympanic membrane–middle ear system that has an increase in one or more of the components of impedance (stiffness, mass, or friction) will not transfer sound energy efficiently to the cochlear fluids. In such an instance, acoustic impedance is increased, or, stated reciprocally, acoustic compliance is reduced. Therefore, a greater amount of sound energy will be reflected from the tympanic membrane–middle ear region and a smaller amount of sound energy will be transmitted to the cochlea. An excellent example of this type is a middle ear that contains an effusion (Fig. 7–19B). Conversely, the tympanic membrane and middle ear may have a decrease in impedance (or increase in compliance), such as may occur with disarticulation of the ossicular

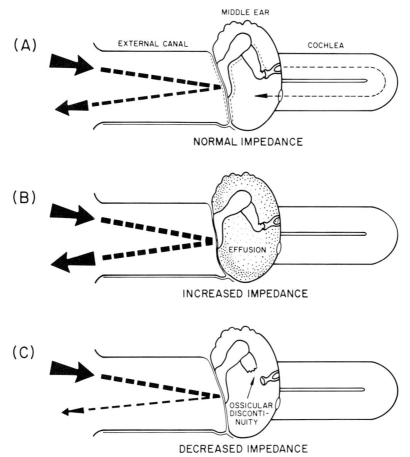

Figure 7–19. Examples of normal, increased, and decreased middle ear impedance. In the normal condition (*A*), some sound is transmitted through the tympanic membrane–middle ear to the cochlea, and some portion is reflected back into the external canal. When there is increased impedance (*B*), such as with an effusion in the middle ear, less sound is transmitted to the cochlea and more sound is reflected back into the ear canal than in the normal condition. When decreased middle ear impedance (*C*) exists, such as with an ossicular chain discontinuity, sound is stored in the middle ear instead of being effectively transferred to the cochlea and reflected back into the ear canal, but at a point in time that is opposite to that when the tympanic membrane–middle ear impedance is increased.

chain, in which case an increased amount of sound energy is received by the middle ear but is not transmitted to the cochlea (Fig. 7–19*C*).

The Electroacoustic Impedance Bridge

Measurements made with the electroacoustic impedance bridge provide an objective assessment of the mobility of the tympanic membrane and the dynamics of the ossicular chain, the intra-aural muscles with their attachments, and the middle ear air cushion. Its design permits the introduction of a signal through one of three small openings in the probe tip, which is hermetically sealed in the external auditory canal (Fig. 7–20). A certain amount of the signal is transmitted into and through the tympanic membrane and middle ear, whereas a certain amount is reflected back into the ear canal. The reflected sound is received by a microphone circuit, connected to a second opening in the probe tip in the ear canal, which has a certain amplitude and phase related to the mechanical properties of the tympanic membrane; the frequency of the signal is determined by the frequency of the probe tip, which is usually 220 Hz. The third aperture of the probe is connected to an air pump that varies the air pressure in the closed ear canal. With this arrangement, impedance can be monitored with a varying air pressure load on the tympanic membrane, or with a static air pressure load. The air pressure can be varied either

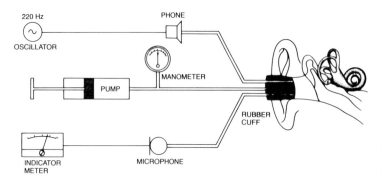

Figure 7–20. Schematic design of electroacoustic impedance bridge (see text).

manually or automatically with most bridges. The measurement of impedance changes at the tympanic membrane with a dynamic air pressure load is called tympanometry, and when there is a static pressure load, static compliance can be measured.

Tympanometry

Tympanometry employing most available instruments involves varying canal air pressure in a single sweep from 200 to −400 mm H_2O (or −600 mm H_2O), thereby altering the stiffness of the tympanic membrane. Changing the stiffness of the tympanic membrane results in an alteration of the relationship between the probe tone and the sound pressure level in the canal; this changing relationship is recorded as tympanic membrane impedance, which can be calculated and displayed graphically as a tympanogram. The abscissa of the tympanogram records air pressure in millimeters of water, and the ordinate records compliance, an arbitrary unit. Figure 7–21 shows an example of a normal tympanogram. Since the tympanic membrane compliance is maximum when the air pressure on both sides of the drum is equal, the peak of the normal tympanogram tracing occurs at approximately 0 mm H_2O. If pressure within the middle ear is negative, the tympanometric peak will be in the negative pressure zone of the tympanogram (Fig. 7–22). Thus, the position of the peak of the trace along the horizontal axis usually is indicative of the middle ear pressure. Also important is the height of the peak. Normally, the height of the peak is between half and full scale on the ordinate. Conditions that increase the impedance of the tympanic membrane–middle ear system (e.g., otitis media with effusion) can result in a tympanogram peak that is less than half scale, showing

low compliance. Conversely, conditions that decrease the impedance of the system (e.g., a flaccid tympanic membrane) elevate the peak to exceed full-scale deflection. Therefore, the position of the peak along both the ordinate and the abscissa provides information regarding middle ear pressure and the acoustic impedance of the system. In addition, the shape of the peak or, more specifically, the gradient (slope) is also important. A peak that has a gradual slope (rounded) rather than a steep one is usually associated with some degree of tympanic membrane–middle ear disorder.

Validation of Tympanometry

By assessing the pressure, compliance, and shape of the tympanometric trace, the normal tympanic membrane–middle ear system can be distinguished from the abnormal one with a reasonable degree of certainty. In addition, the types of abnormality may also be determined. To this end, the tympanometric patterns have been classified and related to various pathological conditions involving the eardrum and middle ear. Bluestone, Beery, and Paradise (1973) attempted to relate these patterns (with the Madsen instrument) to the presence or absence of effusion at myringotomy but found a high percentage of false positive results (i.e., the tympanometric patterns indicated the presence of an effusion but none was found at myringotomy). In a later study from Pittsburgh, Paradise, Smith, and Bluestone (1976) proposed a pattern classification with the same type of instrument for the identification of middle ear effusion based on otoscopy and, in many instances, the myringotomy findings. The accuracy of the diagnosis of effusion was higher with the Paradise, Smith, and Bluestone (1976) classification

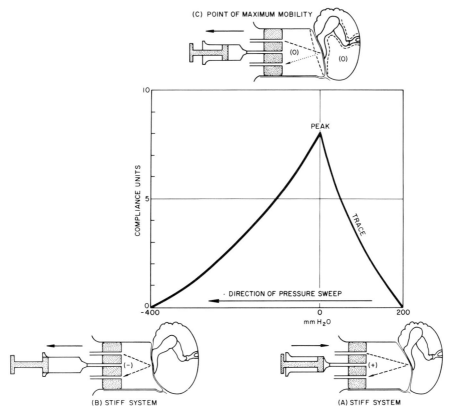

Figure 7–21. Tympanogram showing trace (pressure, compliance, and shape) related diagrammatically to the tympanic membrane position during tympanometry procedure. Initially, 200 mm H_2O is applied to the external canal, which stiffens the tympanic membrane–middle ear system to produce reduced compliance (increased impedance) (A). The pressure in the external canal is then progressively lowered to -400 mm H_2O, which also stiffens the tympanic membrane–middle ear (B). In the normal ear the peak of the trace is recorded on the graph at ambient pressure, which is the point of maximum compliance (lowest impedance) and the pressure within the middle ear (C).

than with the previously proposed patterns. The study also demonstrated that tympanometry in infants less than seven months of age was not valid because of their highly compliant external auditory canals. More recently, a study conducted in San Antonio confirmed the diagnostic accuracy of this pattern classification (Gates et al., 1986). Beery and coworkers (1975a), employing the Grason-Stadler otoadmittance meter, also related myringotomy findings to the tympanometric patterns and proposed a pattern classification for the diagnosis of middle ear effusion. The patterns were 93 percent accurate. Shurin, Pelton, and Finkelstein (1977) also employed the Grason-Stadler instrument and proposed a pattern classification based on measurements with a planimeter. Cantekin, Beery, and Bluestone (1977a) compared the two instruments—the Madsen electroacoustic impedance bridge and the

Grason-Stadler otoadmittance meter—as to their abilities to identify middle ear effusions; the tympanometric findings were validated by myringotomy, and the same number of false-negative and false-positive patterns were recorded for both instruments.

Tympanometric Patterns

From all of these studies, it appears that using the electroacoustic impedance bridge is a very accurate way of identifying middle ear effusions, but it is not perfect. The instrument can be an invaluable aid in diagnosis and, under certain conditions, in screening for middle ear disease. Figure 7–23 shows the types of tympanograms and their common variants that relate to expected conditions of the eardrum and middle ear. This chart is currently employed by the authors,

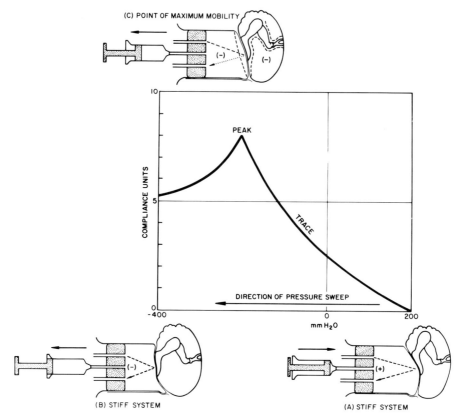

Figure 7–22. Tympanogram showing a trace of an ear with negative middle ear pressure. The procedure is the same as illustrated diagrammatically in Figure 7–21, but in this example, the peak of the trace, or point of maximum compliance, is in the negative pressure zone.

TYMPANOGRAM TYPES AND VARIANTS RELATED TO CLINICAL FINDINGS

	TYMPANOGRAM TYPES	COMMON VARIANTS	PRESUMPTIVE DIAGNOSIS OF TYMPANIC MEMBRANE MIDDLE EAR CONDITION
1.	NORMAL	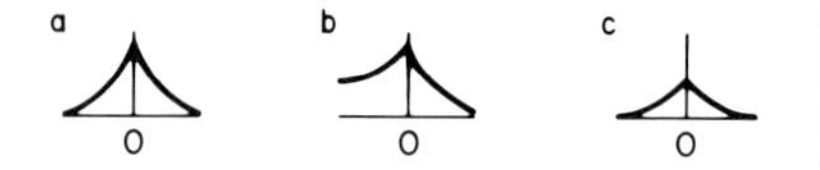	NORMAL
2.	HIGH COMPLIANCE (NORMAL PRESSURE)	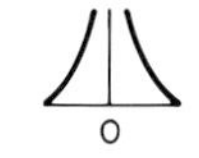	FLACCID TYMPANIC MEMBRANE OR OSSICULAR DISCONTINUITY
3.	NEGATIVE PRESSURE (NORMAL COMPLIANCE)	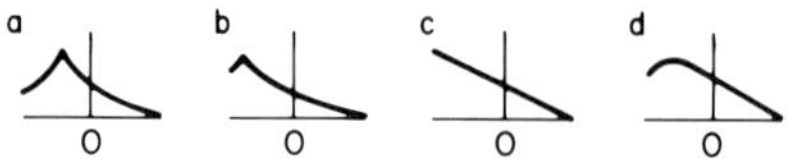	HIGH NEGATIVE PRESSURE WITH OR WITHOUT MIDDLE EAR EFFUSION
4.	HIGH NEGATIVE PRESSURE AND HIGH COMPLIANCE	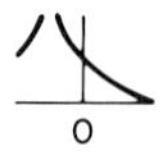	FLACCID TYMPANIC MEMBRANE AND HIGH NEGATIVE PRESSURE (OR OSSICULAR DISCONTINUITY AND HIGH NEGATIVE PRESSURE)
5.	HIGH POSITIVE PRESSURE		HIGH POSITIVE PRESSURE WITH OR WITHOUT MIDDLE EAR EFFUSION
6.	LOW COMPLIANCE	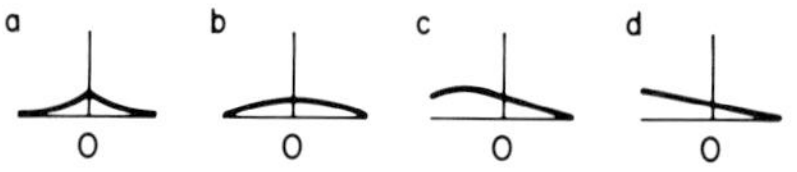	MIDDLE EAR EFFUSION, &/OR THICKENED TYMPANIC MEMBRANE, &/OR OSSICULAR FIXATION &/OR ADHESIVE OTITIS MEDIA

Figure 7–23. Tympanogram types related to presumptive conditions of the middle ear (see text).

and much of this information is based on the myringotomy findings of a study of 425 ears of 238 subjects ranging in age from seven months to 15 years, with a median age of six years (Bluestone and Cantekin, 1979). Tympanograms that are considered normal are those included in the first frame of the figure. Ears that yield tympanograms of variant *a* will on occasion (2 percent) be found to have an effusion, especially a scant, thin, serous effusion usually seen as an air-fluid level or bubbles behind a translucent eardrum. Variant *b*, even though it has a somewhat low compliance, is usually not obtained when an effusion is present. The tympanogram type that has an open end (peak off graph) at or near the normal pressure zone (Frame 2) is the result of very high compliance and is most commonly associated with a flaccid tympanic membrane that is secondary to wide fluctuations in middle ear pressure and loss of drum elasticity resulting from eustachian tube dysfunction. However, an effusion is not present. When this type of tympanogram is associated with a significant conductive hearing loss (usually between 40 and 60 dB), then an ossicular discontinuity should be suspected.

The negative pressure type of tympanogram (Frame 3) has many variants, of which the four most common are shown. Unfortunately, at present there is no totally reliable way of predicting the presence or absence of effusion by the variant, as all may be associated with a middle ear effusion. However, the probability that an ear yielding a tympanogram of variant *a* has an effusion is less than the probability of effusion in ears giving the other three variants, and an ear from which a tympanogram of variant *d* (with a rounded peak) is recorded has the highest probability of having an effusion present. When the tympanogram trace is open without a peak and is in the negative pressure zone (Frame 4), the tympanic membrane is flaccid and only rarely will an effusion be present within the middle ear. The explanation for the floppy tympanic membrane is the same as that described for the type of tympanogram in Frame 2, but in this type, negative pressure is evident at the time of testing. Again, as described previously (Frame 2), if a significant air-bone audiometric gap is found, an ossicular chain discontinuity should be suspected. The tympanogram type that shows a high positive pressure (Frame 5) may be associated with an effusion, usually an acute otitis media with effusion,

particularly with variant *b*. All of the variants shown for the types of tympanograms that have low compliance (Frame 6) are usually associated with a middle ear effusion; ears from which tympanograms of variants *a* and *b* are recorded may or may not have an effusion, whereas 90 percent of ears with tympanograms of variants *c* and *d* will have an effusion. Other pathological conditions that can result in this type of pattern are conditions that can increase the acoustic impedance of the system (e.g., thickening of the tympanic membrane, ossicular chain fixation, or adhesive otitis media).

The problem in attempting to diagnose either a fixation or a discontinuity of the ossicular chain by the tympanogram pattern is that other parts of the tympanic membrane–middle ear system may be abnormal and mask the condition. An example of this would be a middle ear in which one of the ossicles is fixed (e.g., stapes, with adhesive otitis media) but the tympanogram is either normal or reveals high compliance because the tympanic membrane is flaccid. Therefore, making a definitive diagnosis of an ossicular pathological disorder usually must depend on the audiogram or, ultimately, an exploratory tympanotomy.

The Acoustic Middle Ear Muscle Reflex

Acoustic impedance instrumentation can also be used to detect the contraction of the middle ear muscles, the stapedius and tensor tympani, to intense sound stimulation. This contraction is called the acoustic middle ear muscle reflex, or, simply, the acoustic reflex.

The anatomy of the acoustic reflex arc is depicted in Figure 7–24. The afferent portion of the arc, up to and including the superior olivary complex, is shared with the hearing mechanism. The efferent fibers of the acoustic reflex arc arise from neuronal connections in the brain stem between the olivary and the facial nerve nucleus for the stapedius muscle and the trigeminal nerve nucleus for the tensor tympani muscle.

The acoustic impedance bridge indicates the status of the acoustic reflex in two ways: first, the reflex results in a stiffening of the ossicular chain and a concomitant increase in impedance; second, because the reflex is bilateral to a unilateral stimulus (the muscles of both sides contract when one ear is stimulated), an earphone can be placed on one

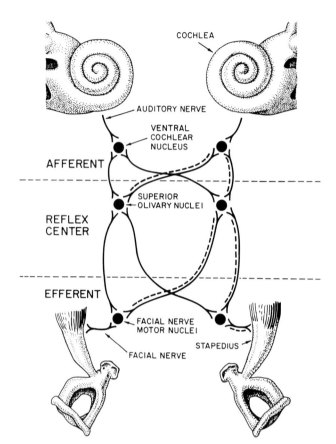

Figure 7–24. Diagrammatic representation of the acoustic reflex arc (see text).

ear to deliver an intense stimulus, and the probe tip of the impedance bridge, inserted in the opposite ear, can detect the impedance change caused by the reflex.

When the impedance bridge is used to detect an acoustic reflex elicited by stimulating the opposite ear, the response is commonly called the "contralateral" or "crossed" acoustic reflex. Many acoustic impedance bridges marketed today have probe tips designed both to stimulate and to detect the acoustic reflex in the same ear; the reflex is elicited and its effect on impedance is detected in the same ear. Under these conditions, the response is called the "ipsilateral" or "uncrossed" acoustic reflex.

The threshold of the acoustic reflex is operationally defined as the minimum stimulus intensity required to produce an observable change in monitored impedance. This minimum intensity, or acoustic reflex threshold is typically specified as a certain number of decibels (dB), referenced to either "sensation level" or "hearing level." Sensation level (SL) refers to the individual's behavioral hearing threshold for a given stimulus, and hearing level (HL) refers to normal hearing

for a group of young adults (i.e., 0 dB on the audiogram). For example, a reflex threshold of 85 dB HL, for a 1000-Hz pure tone, can also be expressed as 85 dB SL if the individual's hearing threshold for that stimulus is 0 dB HL. If the individual's hearing threshold for the same 1000-Hz pure tone is 30 dB HL, then the reflex threshold of 85 dB HL can also be expressed as 55 dB SL. These relationships between sensation level and hearing level are important to an understanding of the acoustic reflex parameters.

In adults with normal hearing, the contralateral acoustic reflex threshold for pure tones of different frequencies is approximately 85 dB poorer than behavioral hearing thresholds (i.e., 85 dB SL). Approximately 20 dB less intensity is required to elicit a reflex with a broad-band noise stimulus. Ipsilateral reflex thresholds are approximately 10 dB better than contralateral thresholds.

The influence of a middle ear effusion and attendant conductive hearing loss on the reflex is not simply a result of the mode of reflex stimulation. Ipsilateral acoustic reflex tests stimulate and detect the response in the same ear through the impedance bridge probe tip. In the middle ear with an effusion, the impedance is already abnormally altered, and further changes in impedance, due to middle ear muscle contraction, may not be observable; to be detectable, these changes may require elevated stimulus intensity levels.

It follows that ipsilateral acoustic reflex testing in a middle ear with an effusion will most probably yield no response; if the response is present, the threshold of the response will tend to be elevated.

The influence of a middle ear effusion on the contralateral acoustic reflex may be somewhat harder to understand. The contralateral reflex will probably be absent if the middle ear having the probe tip has an effusion or if the effusion-filled middle ear having the stimulus earphone has a moderate to moderately severe conductive hearing loss. The reason for the first situation was described above. In the second situation, the conductive hearing loss necessitates reflex stimulus levels that may be beyond the instrument's output capabilities. For these reasons, the contralateral acoustic reflex is generally absent in cases of bilateral otitis media with effusion. When the effusion is unilateral, the contralateral reflex will probably be absent for both ears, if the impaired ear has a moderate to moderately severe conductive hearing loss.

Static Compliance (Physical Volume Test)

Compliance, or the mobility of the tympanic membrane–middle ear system, can be measured by the amplitude of the tympanogram trace and can also be measured separately—it is usually expressed in absolute units of volume (cubic centimeters). However, the measurement has limited clinical value except for determining the volume of the system, which can be used to determine whether the tympanic membrane is intact or perforated or if a functioning tympanostomy tube is present. Clinically, a microscopic perforation can be detected with the measurement, even when the tympanic membrane appears to be mobile when positive or negative pressure is applied by the pneumatic otoscope (assuming that the perforation is small enough and the magnitude of the pressure exerted by the otoscope is sufficient to move the eardrum). A similar condition frequently exists when a tympanostomy tube is in the tympanic membrane but the patency of the tube is questionable. The volume meas-

ured by all of the currently available bridges is probably not accurate, but the technique is still useful for determination of an intact or nonintact tympanic membrane.

The volume of the middle ear is measured by applying 200 mm H_2O pressure to the external canal with the impedance bridge. If the tympanic membrane is intact, the measurement should be approximately 0.6 to 0.8 cc in a younger child and between 1.0 and 1.5 cc in the older child and adult. If the eardrum is not intact, then greater values are found: more than 2 cc in the child and 2.5 cc in the adult. However, some children have rather large ear canal volumes that may exceed 2 cc when the tympanic membrane is intact. Therefore, in such a case an additional method should be attempted to determine if a nonintact tympanic membrane is present. The external canal pressure should be raised to 400 mm H_2O, and, if the eardrum has an opening, the eustachian tube will be forced open in most children and rapid drops in pressure will be noted on the bridge manometer. All infants and children from whom a tympanogram is obtained should have static compliance (volume) recorded also, since a flat or rounded tympanogram apparently indicating an effusion may be found in a child who actually has a nonintact eardrum.

Screening for Ear Disease with Acoustic Impedance Measurements

Emphasis has been placed here on interpreting the three acoustic impedance measurements—tympanometry, static compliance, and the acoustic reflex—as a whole. This approach provides the best opportunity for accurate diagnostic assessment. There have been numerous attempts, however, to separate certain impedance measurements as screening tools, particularly for the detection of middle ear disease in children.

Several published investigations have evaluated the screening effectiveness of tympanometry, the acoustic reflex, or both (Brooks, 1973, 1976, 1977; Cooper et al., 1974; Ferrer, 1974; Harker and Van Wagoner, 1974; Lewis et al., 1974; McCandless and Thomas, 1974; McCurdy et al., 1976; Orchik and Herdman, 1974; Renvall et al., 1973; Roberts, 1976). Brooks (1978) supported the utility of the acoustic reflex alone as a screening tool for detection of middle ear disease in children. These investigators commonly agree that impedance measurements are easy to perform, noninvasive, reliable, and highly sensitive to the presence of middle ear disease. These factors would favor the use of tympanometry and the acoustic reflex as screening measurements for the detection of disease. However, definitive data supporting the validity of using impedance measurements for screening are still lacking. Although the measurements are sensitive to disease, when it is present, they are considerably less accurate in sorting out children without disease, and the percentage of false-positive errors obtained is uncomfortably high (Fria et al., 1978; Paradise and Smith, 1978). The resulting over-referral rate argues against the cost-effectiveness of *mass* screening for middle ear disease with acoustic impedance measurements. A review of the state-of-the-art and suggested guidelines for impedance screening for middle ear disease in children was presented at a workshop on screening by Bluestone and coworkers (1986).

Tympanometric Screening for Otitis Media with Effusion

Screening for otitis media with effusion is a process that is intended to identify children who may have the disease but in whom it would otherwise go undetected. Otitis media is a disease that appears to be important to screen since it is highly prevalent, is associated with varying degrees of conductive hearing loss, and may lead to other, more serious complications and sequelae. Otoscopy performed by an expert is an excellent method to identify otitis media and should be employed by professionals who care for children as a routine part of the examination. This is especially important in infants and young children. However, for mass screening, otoscopy is not feasible. Audiometry, employing the routine audiological screening criteria, has been shown to identify only half of a group of children with middle ear effusion (Bluestone et al., 1973). In addition, audiometry, employing standard methods, cannot be obtained on young infants in whom the prevalence of the disease is the highest. However, impedance screening employing tympanometry and possibly the acoustic reflex is a highly sensitive method to screen for otitis media with effusion. Impedance testing is acceptable to both the child and the health care provider because it is safe, noninvasive, and simply executed. Studies have shown

impedance measurements to be reliable, but these studies have not involved subjects of all age groups or all instruments that are available, many of which have been designed specifically for screening purposes.

The validity of criteria for referral for specific diagnostic criteria based on impedance measurements (i.e., their association, singly or in combination, with the presence or absence of middle ear effusion) has not been established completely, and further studies are required. In addition, neither the epidemiology nor the natural history of the disease have been adequately studied in the various age groups affected, which makes most of the methods of management currently employed difficult to evaluate. Otitis media with effusion in many instances spontaneously disappears. Because of these problems, the referral criteria for children who are identified with a middle ear effusion remain controversial.

Current Recommendations

A task force convened in 1977 addressed the use of tympanometry for screening for ear disease and advised against mass screening on a routine basis for the detection of middle ear disorders in children of any age group (Harford et al., 1978). Although not recommending mass screening, the task force did advise screening methods that employed impedance measurements in small, carefully controlled programs in order to determine the best method for larger screening programs. More recently, the workshop on screening for otitis media again advised against mass screening (Bluestone et al., 1986).

The following is a summary of the 1977 task force's recommendations. Middle ear effusion has its highest prevalence and incidence in the age group beween six and 36 months. Following episodes of acute infection, asymptomatic otitis media with effusion continues for extended periods in a large number of infants, and there is concern about the possible effects of undetected effusions on a child's function and development. In children younger than seven months of age, the relations between tympanometric findings currently employed and middle ear disease are not well understood, although the limited data now available indicate that the sensitivity of tympanometry as usually performed is relatively low. There are also feasibility problems associated with impedance screening of infants. Logistically, it may be difficult to gather infants for testing after they leave their place of birth. Moreover, impedance testing in infants may sometimes be difficult and time-consuming. However, if these difficulties can be overcome, impedance testing of infants should be attempted, if feasible.

Even though mass screening of preschool and school-age children by impedance measurements is not recommended at present, it should be carried out in a planned manner in a smaller program. The following procedures and criteria have been judged to be minimal:

1. A combination of tympanometry and acoustic reflex measurement should be used.

2. For eliciting the acoustic reflex, a signal of 105 dB HTL (hearing threshold level) should be used in the contralateral mode, or a signal of 105 dB SPL (sound pressure level) in the ipsilateral mode, or both.

3. Whether broad-band noise or pure tone is preferable as an eliciting stimulus for the acoustic reflex remains to be established. A pure tone between 1000 and 3000 Hz would be acceptable for this purpose. The stimulus should be specified or described, or both.

4. Acoustic reflex measurements can be obtained either with the ear canal air pressure that results in minimum acoustic impedance or with ear canal air pressure equal to ambient pressure. The condition used should be specified.

5. For tympanometry, a 220-Hz probe tone is preferred.

6. For tympanometry, an air pressure range of -400 to $+100$ mm H_2O is preferred. However, a range of -300 to $+100$ mm H_2O is acceptable. Automatic recording should be used whenever possible, and the rate of air pressure change should be specified.

7. Failure on the initial screening test is denoted by either an absent acoustic reflex or an abnormal tympanogram. An abnormal tympanogram is defined as one that either (a) is flat or rounded (i.e., without a definite peak) or (b) has a peak at, or more negative than, -200 mm H_2O. Flat or rounded tympanograms appear to be more highly correlated with middle ear effusions than are tympanograms with peaks at negative pressure readings.

8. Any child failing the initial screening should be retested in four to six weeks. Parents or guardians should be advised accordingly. Any child who has an acoustic reflex and a normal tympanogram result on the initial screening passes and is "cleared."

9. The schema on Table 7–1 is recommended for various screening findings. Classifications I and II should constitute the majority of children in a given population. Referral, when indicated after confirmatory retest, should be made to an appropriate health care provider in the community. Classification III constitutes a group of children that requires special monitoring by the agency responsible for the screening program. These "at risk" children should be retested periodically to determine the best possible need for future medical referral.

10. An optimal time and frequency for screening or referring particular populations could not be advised because of lack of adequate information. Future research is needed.

11. The agency responsible for a testing program must have facilities available for referral that include expert management. Prior to the initiation of a screening program, referral and management procedures must be defined.

12. Impedance testing should be supervised by professionals who are qualified by training and experience to perform and interpret impedance measurements.

13. Programs should be designed to gather information of value in defining the role of impedance measurement in screening children for middle ear disease.

Impedance Instrumentation

During the last 15 years, an increasing number of instrument companies have introduced electroacoustic impedance bridges to the market. This has been primarily due to the widespread acceptance of this technique of assessment, which is related to the ever-growing number of studies that have shown that impedance testing improves the accuracy of diagnosing otitis media and related conditions. Tympanometry is a reliable, simple procedure that is easily carried out in a short time by nonprofessional personnel. For all of these reasons, the instruments have become enormously popular, and with this has come a technological explosion in instrumentation that has resulted in confusion among professionals who wish to purchase new instruments and concern by those who find their relatively new instruments outdated in only

Table 7–1. **SCHEMA FOR TYMPANOMETRIC SCREENING**

Classification	Initial Screen	Retest	Subject Outcome
I	Acoustic reflex present and Tympanogram normal	Not required	Cleared
II	Acoustic reflex absent and/or Typanogram normal	Acoustic reflex absent and/or Tympanogram normal	Referred
III	Acoustic reflex absent and/or Tympanogram abnormal	Acoustic reflex present and Tympanogram normal	At risk—Recheck at later date

a few years. In addition, most of the new or modified instruments are not field tested and validated prior to their introduction to the market; this presents a distinct hazard to the clinician who wishes to use a validated, reliable instrument. However, some of the instruments have been validated and are reliable, as demonstrated over many years of use by both clinicians and investigators.

The first commercially available instrument to measure acoustic impedance was developed in Denmark during the 1950s by Terkildsen and Nielson (1960), and in 1958 it was manufactured by Madsen Electronics as their model ZO61. In 1963, Madsen introduced model ZO70, which rapidly became the prototype for all of the impedance bridges that followed and has provided the latest information on the invaluable diagnostic capabilities of electroacoustic impedance measurements. In 1971, Madsen introduced the ZO72, which incorporated an audiometer so that a contralateral acoustic reflex could be measured, and a later model added the ability to measure the ipsilateral acoustic reflex. In 1970, the Grason-Stadler Company introduced the otoadmittance meter, which measures the complex components of acoustic impedance. The measurement as described by the developers is termed acoustic admittance, which is divided into acoustic susceptance (compliance) and acoustic conductance (resistance) and is expressed in acoustic milliohms (Grason, 1972). Subsequent to the popularity of the Madsen model ZO70, many other companies have entered into manufacturing impedance bridges. Some are designed for diagnostic use, others are purely for screening, and still others can be used for both diagnostic and screening purposes. The clinician should make a decision regarding which instrument to purchase based on the need; however, availability of repair services should also be a consideration.

The only instruments that have been validated by comparing the patterns obtained with a bridge and the findings at myringotomy are: (1) Madsen model ZO70 (Bluestone et al., 1973; Cantekin et al., 1977a; Paradise et al., 1976), (2) Grason-Stadler model 1720 (Beery et al., 1975a; Cantekin et al., 1977a; Shurin et al., 1977), and (3) Grason-Stadler model 1722 (Fria et al., 1980).

ACOUSTIC REFLECTOMETRY

The acoustic otoscope, or reflectometer (Endeco Medical, Marion, MA), is a hand-held instrument that is placed next to the opening of the child's external ear canal; it uses an 80-dB sound source that varies from 2000 to 4500 Hz over a 100-ms period (Fig. 7–25; Teele and Teele, 1984). A microphone located in the probe tip measures the total level of transmitted and reflected sound (Fig. 7–26). Since no pressurization of the external canal is required, no seal with the canal is needed. Acoustic energy is reflected back toward the probe tip from the ear canal and eardrum. The operating principle is based on the fact that a sound wave in a closed tube will be reflected when it strikes the end of the tube. Reflected sound waves from the middle ear cancel the transmitted sound one quarter of a wavelength from the eardrum, thus providing information related to the presence or absence of a middle ear effusion, as will an estimate of ear canal length; the more sound reflected, the greater the likelihood of an effusion being present. Sound reflectivity is measured in units ranging from zero through nine; a vertical scale indicates status of the middle ear by the sound reflected, and a horizontal score indicates canal length.

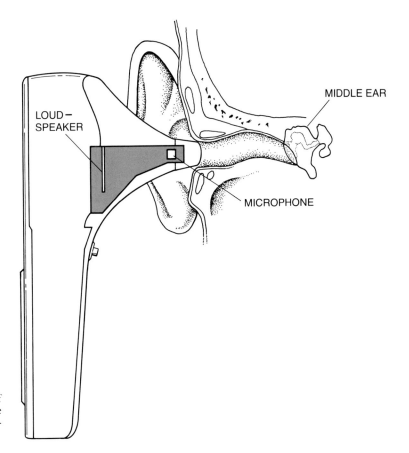

Figure 7–25. Cutaway view of probe assembly, showing relative position of microphone and loudspeaker.

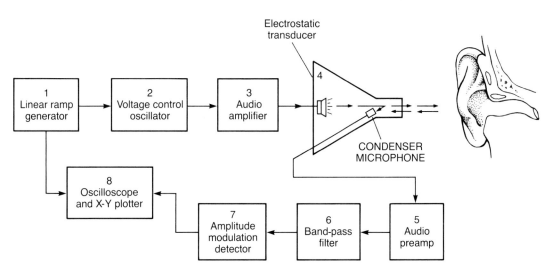

Figure 7–26. Block diagram of acoustic reflectometer.

ASSESSMENT OF HEARING

The assessment of hearing in infants and children is not an accurate method for identifying the presence of a middle ear effusion but can be valuable in determining the effect of middle ear disease on hearing function and is important in decision-making regarding management.

Hearing loss is by far the most prevalent complication and morbid outcome of otitis media, and it may be caused by one or more of the intra-aural complications or sequelae. To a varying degree, fluctuating or persistent loss of hearing is almost always associated with otitis media. The audiogram usually reveals a mild to moderate conductive loss; when otitis media is present the average loss is 27 dB (Fria et al., 1985). However, there may be a sensorineural component, generally attributed to the effect of increased tension and stiffness of the round window membrane. This hearing loss is usually reversible with resolution of the effusion, but permanent conductive hearing loss can result from irreversible changes secondary to recurrent acute or chronic inflammation (e.g., adhesive otitis, tympanosclerosis, or ossicular discontinuity). Irreparable sensorineural loss may also occur, presumably as the result of spread of infection through the round or oval window membrane (Paparella et al., 1972) or a labyrinthitis due to perilymphatic fistulae (Supance and Bluestone, 1983). Audiometry can be reliably performed in children as young as six months. Children under two years are the group at highest risk for effusions and associated hearing loss, and in these patients standard audiometric assessment may be difficult to perform reliably. Therefore, infants and young children may require nonbehavioral tests of hearing.

All infants and children should have their hearing evaluated, if possible, when a chronic middle ear effusion is present since the type (i.e., conductive or sensorineural, or both) and the degree of hearing loss will have a bearing on the selection and timing of the various management options available to the clinician.

Methods

In general, there are two methods to evaluate hearing in children: behavioral and nonbehavioral. The age and the ability of the child to cooperate usually dictates the tests that are selected (Northern and Downs, 1978).

Behavioral Tests

The neonatal reactions to sudden, intense sound are predominantly reflexive and include the Moro reflex, the aural palpebral reflex, and the arousal and cessation responses.

The *Moro reflex* is a generalized motor response that is commonly known as the "startle reflex." Classically, the neonate (also, most infants) will thrust the head backward and suddenly move the arms and legs up and outward when a stimulus of 80 to 85 dB SPL (Sound Pressure Level) is presented. The *aural palpebral reflex,* or "eyeblink" reflex, consists of a contraction of the orbicularis oculi muscles and, frequently, closing of the eyelids. A stimulus of 105 to 115 dB SPL will usually be required. The *arousal* and *cessation reflexes* involve clear contrasts in the neonate's pre- and poststimulus activity. A stimulus of 90 dB SPL should awaken or arouse the sleeping or drowsy neonate, and in the cessation reflex, a decrease or inhibition of activity in the restless or crying baby is observed. However, these reactions are primarily reflexive, require rather intense stimuli, and are qualitative rather than quantitative.

Behavioral observation audiometry (BOA) is a technique used for neonates and young infants in which the examiner presents a stimulus sound and observes the child's associated behavioral response, which does not require conditioning. Simple noise-makers, such as rattles, squeak toys, and bells, are common stimulus devices used in the office setting, but calibrated stimuli are used in a test booth in audiology centers.

Visual reinforcement audiometry (VRA) also involves the presentation of a stimulus sound and the observation of the child's conditioned head-turn response (Fig. 7–27). The response, however, is rewarded with a visual reinforcement, such as a blinking light, an illuminated picture or toy, or an animated toy that is located above the loudspeaker through which the stimulus is presented. The test is most successful for assessing infants age 6 months to two years.

Tangible reinforcement audiometry, or *tangible reinforcement operant conditioning audiometry* (TROCA), uses candy or sugar-coated cereal to reward the child for pressing a bar when

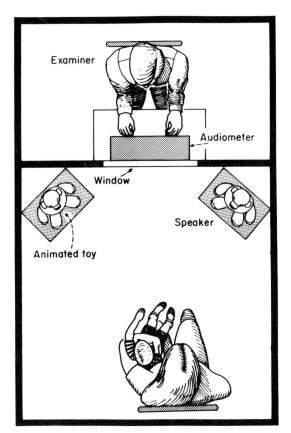

Figure 7–27. Visual reinforcement audiometry (VRA). Infant sits on mother's lap and is observed by examiner, who presents a sound stimulus through speaker to right or left of child. The infant response, a head-turn toward the sound stimulus, is rewarded by activation and illumination of the animated toy.

the sound stimulus is presented (Fig. 7–28). It is a test appropriate for assessment of difficult-to-test children, such as the mentally retarded, as well as infants.

These tests will provide some indication of the degree of hearing loss present but not the type (conductive or sensorineural). However, in some children, the VRA and TROCA tests may be able to determine the hearing level in the individual ear. They are appropriate for children younger than three years of age.

Play audiometry is similar to conventional tests given to older children and adults and can be used to assess the hearing of children two years of age and older. Conventional audiometric techniques can be used, but they must be modified to be more interesting for the young child, which usually is in the form of "play." The assessment can provide information regarding both speech and pure-tone stimuli and can determine the degree of loss for the individual ear. In addition, play au-

diometry can provide threshold information on both air and bone conduction and, therefore, can determine whether a loss is conductive or sensorineural, or both.

Conventional audiometry is usually reserved for the child five years of age and older but can be used for certain younger children, depending on the examiner and the cooperation of the child. The assessment should include pure-tone and speech audiometry to determine air and bone conduction thresholds on children with chronic otitis media with effusion to determine the type and degree of hearing loss for each ear.

Nonbehavioral Tests

The nonbehavioral techniques to assess hearing include acoustic impedance measurements, auditory brain stem–response record-

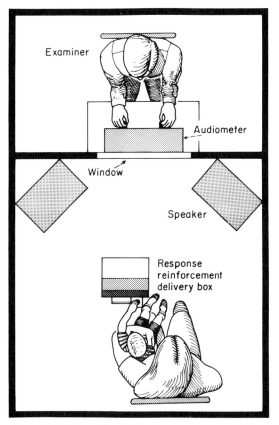

Figure 7–28. Tangible reinforcement operant conditioning audiometry (TROCA). Infant or young child sits on mother's lap and is observed by audiologist, who presents sound stimulus through speakers to right or left of child. The infant or child responds by pressing the bar on the TROCA device. Correct responses are rewarded by delivery of a tangible object, such as cereal, candy, or small toys.

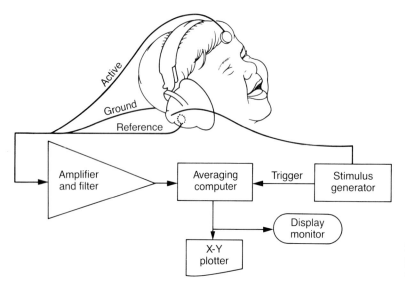

Figure 7–29. A schematic diagram of the equipment used for ABR audiometry (see text).

ings, cardiac audiometry, and respiratory audiometry. However, of all of these tests, the *auditory brain stem response* (ABR) is currently the best available and most widely used method. It is a test that is relatively independent of the child's behavioral response and is ordinarily used to evaluate infants and children for whom information on behavioral hearing tests is either unobtainable or unreliable. Figure 7–29 shows a diagram of the equipment used for the test procedure. Three miniature electrodes placed on the scalp are used to record the responses. The

NORMAL ADULT

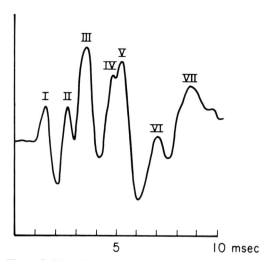

Figure 7–30. ABR to a 60 dB normal hearing level click stimulus in patient with normal hearing. Major wave components are labeled with Roman numerals I through VII.

ABR consists of five to seven vertex-positive waves labeled I to VII, occurring in the first 10 msec following the onset of the stimulus (Fig. 7–30). Waves I through III presumably reflect activity of the eighth cranial nerve fibers (wave I) and auditory centers in the pons (waves II and III). Waves IV and V apparently reflect activity of the auditory centers in the mid to rostral pons and the caudal midbrain, respectively, whereas the neural generators for waves VI and VII are less certain.

The electrical configuration for the ABR includes the active electrode on the vertex of the skull, or midforehead at the hairline, and the reference and ground electrodes, respectively, on the ipsilateral and contralateral mastoid processes, or earlobes. The responses to 2000 to 4000 Hz clicks, filtered clicks, or brief, pure-tone bursts are typically averaged for each stimulus intensity employed. The stimuli are presented at a rapid rate (10 to 30 per second) and a complete run, at a given stimulus intensity, requires 1.5 minutes; the entire procedure for both ears, in most cases, at several stimulus intensities, average less than an hour.

Since excessive muscle activity can interfere with the test, the child must be completely relaxed or, preferably, asleep. Natural sleep can be facilitated by feeding babies, up to about six months of age, immediately prior to the test. Children seven years of age or older can lie quietly for the procedure; however, infants and children between these ages require sedation or even a general anesthesia.

The test can be very sensitive in identifying a conductive hearing loss associated with a

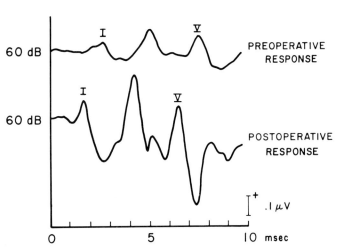

AGE 6 MONTHS

Figure 7–31. The ABR in a six-month-old infant with otitis media with effusion, showing an example of latency delay. The top trace was recorded immediately prior to myringotomy and the bottom trace, immediately thereafter. (From Fria, T. J., and Sabo, D. L.: Auditory brainstem responses in children with otitis media and effusion. Ann. Otol. Rhinol. Laryngol. 89(68):200–206, 1980.)

chronic middle ear effusion, and it is especially valuable in the young infant. However, the technique does not assess the perceptual event called "hearing." The ABR reflects auditory neural electric responses that are adequately correlated to behavioral hearing thresholds, but a normal result on the ABR only suggests that the auditory system up to midbrain level is responsive to the stimulus employed—it does not guarantee normal "hearing."

In cases of middle ear impairment, the entire series of ABR waves is delayed in time by an amount commensurate with the degree of attendant conductive hearing loss (Fria and Sabo, 1980). Latency of wave I provides a better index of middle ear impairment (Fig. 7–31). The consistent nature of the ABR in young infants makes it particularly useful in the evaluation of hearing when a chronic middle ear effusion is present.

Indications

Infants and children who have frequently recurrent otitis media or chronic otitis media with effusion, or both, should have their hearing assessed. It is important to know the degree of hearing loss and if that loss is conductive, sensorineural, or both. If the loss is only conductive and mild, management may consist of watchful waiting in hopes that the natural history of the effusion is in favor of spontaneous resolution. On the other hand, if there is significant bilateral conductive loss, such as greater than 30 dB, surgical intervention (e.g., tympanostomy tubes) may

be an appropriate option, since the hearing loss may interfere with the child's development. The degree of conductive loss present in each ear would be more desirable information, since there may be a sequela or chronic middle ear effusion present in one ear and not in the other. An ossicular chain disarticulation secondary to rarefying osteitis, or ossicular fixation resulting from adhesive otitis media, may cause a maximum conductive hearing loss (i.e., 50 to 60 dB). In addition, a cholesteatoma may also be present even though there is no apparent defect in the tympanic membrane, and this may cause ossicular damage and a conductive loss. When the hearing loss (conductive) appears to be out of proportion to that expected with chronic otitis media with effusion, an examination employing the otomicroscope is necessary to exclude the possibility of a retraction pocket or cholesteatoma, or both, in either the pars flaccida or the posterosuperior quadrant of the pars tensa. If the awake child cannot be examined adequately, then general anesthesia will be required. At this time, a myringotomy and aspiration can be performed and a tympanostomy tube can be inserted. In addition, if the patient is either too young for assessment of hearing with behavioral methods, difficult to assess, or not cooperative, then an ABR can be performed at the time of general anesthesia. The test should be performed after the aspiration of the effusion to determine if a residual conductive hearing loss is present that might be indicative of the presence of an ossicular abnormality.

When a conductive hearing loss is present

in association with a middle ear effusion and the effusion either spontaneously resolves in response to medical treatment or is removed by myringotomy, another audiogram should be obtained to verify that hearing has returned to normal limits. An audiogram should be obtained on every child approximately two weeks following the insertion of tympanostomy tubes (as long as there is no otorrhea present). A persistent, marked conductive hearing loss in the absence of an effusion would be presumptive evidence of an acquired ossicular defect or a concurrent congenital anomaly. The presence of both a chronic otitis media with effusion and a congenital ossicular deformity occurs quite frequently in the child with Down syndrome.

When a mixed hearing loss (conductive and sensorineural) is identified after the assessment, the clinician must be suspect of a middle ear effusion that may be causing a serous ("toxic") labyrinthitis resulting from penetration of the round window or, possibly, a congenital or acquired defect in either the oval or round window, or both; in these cases the infection spreads directly into the labyrinth. Progressive or fluctuating sensorineural hearing loss with or without vertigo may be present, and, if documented, the patient should have further assessment (e.g., vestibular testing, computed tomography of the temporal bone), and possible exploration (tympanotomy) of the middle ear in search for a perilymphatic fistula (Supance and Bluestone, 1983).

If the sensorineural hearing loss is not due to a condition that can be corrected, as described previously, but to a known cause of sensorineural hearing loss in children (such as neonatal asphyxia or meningitis), then more aggressive management of chronic otitis media with effusion may be required than is needed for a child who does not have a sensorineural hearing loss. The added conductive hearing loss to a permanent sensorineural hearing loss may be quite handicapping for the child. This is especially true for the patient who has a moderate to severe sensorineural hearing loss and is "mainstreamed" or is in a school for the deaf. Myringotomy and tympanostomy tubes are early treatment options for such children, rather than prolonged observation. Again, if a mixed hearing loss is suspected because the degree of loss appears to be greater than would be expected due to otitis media with effusion, then an accurate assessment of

hearing is mandatory, regardless of the child's age. High-risk infants and children, in whom there is a family history of sensorineural hearing loss, would be of greatest concern. For such an infant, a procedure including an examination under anesthesia, a myringotomy, and insertion of tubes, followed by an ABR, is the best method to establish a definitive diagnosis as well as treat the chronic otitis media with effusion.

Screening for Hearing Loss

The identification of hearing loss is an important part of screening programs for preschool and school children, since identification of significant hearing problems must be followed by more definitive testing, evaluation, and, possibly, habilitation or rehabilitation of the child. However, audiometric screening to identify a middle ear effusion does not have a high enough sensitivity and specificity to warrant its use. Bluestone and coworkers (1973) found that only half of a group of children (58 ears) with chronic middle ear effusion would have been identified by using an auditory screening test if 25 dB had been used as the criterion for failure (Fig. 7–32). However, audiometric screening is still necessary to identify those children with sensorineural hearing loss.

Recommended Audiometers

A hand-held screening instrument that provides audiometric testing at 500, 1000, 2000, and 4000 Hz at a 25-dB hearing level has been developed by the Welch-Allyn Co. (Audioscope). Gershel and colleagues compared the Audioscope with traditional audiological screening and pure-tone and speech audiometry (Gershel et al., 1985). There was general agreement between traditional hearing screening results and those obtained from the Audioscope. More experience in use of the Audioscope under office conditions is required to determine its value for screening children for hearing loss.

Every otolaryngologist and pediatrician should have an audiometer available to test children. For the pediatrician, a soundproof room and a sophisticated instrument is not necessary, but a screening audiometer should be part of pediatric ambulatory clinical facilities. Those children found to have a hearing

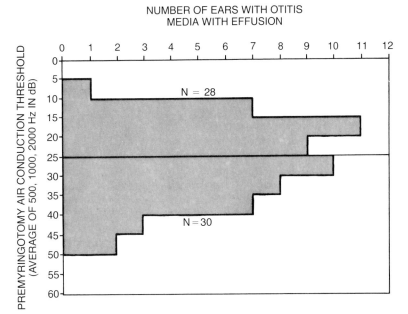

NUMBER OF EARS WITH OTITIS
MEDIA WITH EFFUSION

Figure 7–32. Audiometric findings in 58 ears with middle ear effusion (see text).

loss that is out of proportion to the disease under management (e.g., otitis media) or those infants and children who are difficult to treat should be referred to an otolaryngologist or diagnostic hearing center, or both.

Special Populations

Because of high risk, serious consequences, or known high prevalence of middle ear disease, certain populations of children warrant special consideration, beginning soon after birth, for early detection of and surveillance for this disorder. These populations include children with known sensorineural hearing loss, developmentally delayed and mentally impaired children, children with cleft palate or other craniofacial anomalies, and native American children (Indian and Eskimo).

VESTIBULAR TESTING

Otitis media with effusion and eustachian tube dysfunction are the most common causes of dysequilibrium (e.g., vertigo, falling, and "clumsiness") in infants and children. The dysequilibrium almost invariably is resolved when the middle ear effusion is absent or the child no longer has fluctuating middle ear pressures. Frequently, the parents will report a dramatic disappearance of dysequilibrium immediately following insertion of tympanostomy tubes for recurrent acute or chronic otitis media with effusion or eustachian tube obstruction (fluctuating high negative pressure).

For most infants and children with otitis media and signs and symptoms of dysequilibrium, sophisticated vestibular testing is not indicated, since nonsurgical or surgical management of the eustachian tube–middle ear disorder will resolve the problem. In addition, the tests that are currently available are usually not feasible in children, especially infants. However, when the dysequilibrium persists despite the resolution of the middle ear effusion and the presence of normal middle ear pressures, then the child should be referred to an otolaryngologist for assessment of vestibular function to rule out the possibility of another cause of imbalance (Busis, 1983). Also, children who have frequent attacks of vertigo, with or without fluctuating or progressive sensorineural hearing loss, in association with otitis should be suspect of having a labyrinthine fistula.

The tests that can access vestibular function in infants and children have been described by Eviatar and Eviatar (1983). Rotational tests and gross caloric testing can be performed in the infant and young child, and electronystagmography is feasible in the older child.

HIGH–RISK POPULATIONS

Cleft Palate

In patients with cleft palate, ear disease and hearing loss have long been recognized as common problems. This association was first reported by Alt in 1878, who noted hearing improvement following treatment of otorrhea associated with cleft palate. Thorington, in 1892, reported increased hearing in a patient following artificial correction of a destroyed palate. In 1893, Gutzmann noted hearing loss in one half of his patients with cleft palate. In 1906, the need for otological examination of patients with cleft palate was stressed by Brunck. Since these early descriptions, many reports have appeared in the literature related to the incidence, nature, and degree of hearing loss in patients with cleft palate.

Hearing Loss

The prevalence of hearing loss in the cleft palate population, as reported in the literature, varies considerably. Of all studies, the average prevalence is approximately 50 percent. Even though the criteria of hearing loss have not been generally agreed upon, it has been identified as conductive and usually bilateral. Halfond and Ballenger (1956) found that, of the 69 patients tested, 37 (54 percent) had a hearing loss of 20 dB or greater. Miller (1956) reported that 19 (54 percent) of 35 children with cleft palate had a hearing loss greater than 30 dB. That the prevalence may be even greater is suggested by Walton (1973), who studied 93 school-age children with cleft palate: one half of those who would have passed conventional audiometric screening at the 20-dB level were found to have air-bone gaps indicative of conductive hearing loss. This contention is supported by the study of Bluestone, Beery, and Paradise (1973), who found high-viscosity middle ear effusions in children, including those with cleft palate, who would have passed a 25-dB screening audiogram. Even though a conductive hearing impairment would be expected, Bennett, Ward, and Tait (1968) reported 30 percent of 100 adults with cleft palate had either sensorineural or mixed hearing loss. This finding might be explained by the work of Paparella and coworkers (1972), who found sensorineural hearing loss in some patients with otitis media and ascribed this to directly associated pathological changes in the inner ear, presumably mediated via the round window. Unfortunately, no information is available in the literature concerning hearing in the infant with cleft palate.

Aural Pathology

Infants. Variot, in 1904, was the first to report ear disease in an infant with cleft palate. Sataloff and Fraser, in 1952, reported that, in their experience, "examination of the ears of very young children with cleft palate reveals a high incidence of pathologic changes, despite the absence of subjective symptoms of otitis media." In 1958, Skolnick reported that only 6 percent of cleft palate patients below the age of one, and only 27 percent of those between the ages of one and four years, had aural disorders. However, Linthicum, Body, and Keaster in 1959 discovered pathological ear changes in 77 percent of a group of 100 infants and children with cleft palate. In 1967, Stool and Randall reported that middle ear effusion was present at myringotomy in 94 percent of 25 infants with cleft palate. In 1969, Paradise, Bluestone, and Felder, employing standard office otoscopy, diagnosed middle ear disease in 49 of 50 infants with cleft palate. Most had full or bulging, opaque, immobile tympanic membranes, although spontaneous perforations and otorrhea were observed. Subsequent studies by the same team indicate that throughout the first two years of life in infants with unrepaired cleft palate, otitis media is a virtually constant complication (Bluestone, 1971; Paradise and Bluestone, 1974).

Older Children and Adults. Although the criteria for aural disorders in older children and adults with cleft palate varies considerably, its prevalence appears to be quite high. Meissner (1939) examined 213 such patients between the ages of 10 and 35 years and found that 83 percent had abnormal tympanic membranes. Skolnick (1958) found that the prevalence of aural pathological change was 67 percent in patients above the age of five. Graham and Lierle (1962) found ear disorders in 44 percent of 29 patients with cleft palate and in 55 percent of 146 with a cleft of both palate and lip. In a group of 82 patients, Aschan (1966) found 78 percent had aural disorders. In a retrospective, longitudinal study of 191 patients with cleft palate between five and 27 years of age, Severeid (1972) reported that 83 percent had a middle ear effusion confirmed by myringotomy. In Bennett's study (1972) of 100 adults with cleft palate, 30 percent had aural pathological signs consisting of eustachian tube obstruction (13 percent), chronic suppurative otitis media with or without mastoiditis (8 percent), dry tympanic membrane perforation (6 percent), and chronic adhesive otitis media (3 percent).

Other High-Risk Populations

Infants and children who have parents or siblings, or both, with otitis media with effusion appear to have an increased risk of also developing the disorder than do those whose parents or siblings have no evidence of the disease. Teele, Klein, and Rosner (1980) studied 2565 infants from birth to their third birthdays. They found that children who had single or recurrent episodes of otitis media were more likely to have parents or siblings with histories of significant middle ear infections than were children who had no episodes of otitis media. Therefore, children whose siblings have had otitis media are at higher risk and should have more frequent otological examinations than children whose siblings have not had the disease.

Upper respiratory allergy is thought to be involved in the development of otitis media and therefore requires close surveillance. Even though there is no proof that children who have an upper respiratory allergy have a higher incidence of otitis media than do children without such an allergy, they should be examined frequently for possible occurrence of otitis media.

Any child with a craniofacial malformation should be suspected of having a middle ear effusion. Children with Down syndrome have a very high prevalence and incidence of otitis media with effusion.

Certain racial groups such as American natives (Indians and Eskimos), Maoris of New Zealand, and aborigines of Australia are known to have a high prevalence of otitis media, which in the past has been characterized as chronic suppurative otitis media with perforation and discharge; however, as these groups obtain improved health care, otitis media with effusion has become increasingly more prevalent.

Other possible risk factors such as prematurity or other reasons for being in a neonatal intensive care unit (Berman et al., 1978), first episode of otitis media during early infancy (Howie et al., 1975), malnutrition, and child abuse (Downs, 1980) are not proved but warrant consideration for close surveillance until these factors are disproved by further studies.

The Deaf

Severely deaf to profoundly deaf children (primarily those whose hearing loss is sensorineural), whether enrolled in a special class in a regular school ("mainstreamed") or in a residential school for the deaf, are of particular concern when middle ear effusion is present. Should a conductive hearing loss secondary to chronic or recurrent otitis media with effusion or high negative pressure, or both, be superimposed on the pre-existing hearing loss, auditory input may be severely affected. This may critically interfere with the education of such children (Ruben and Math, 1978).

The incidence of middle ear problems in deaf children has not been studied systematically, but the few studies that have been reported indicate the incidence to be equal to or possibly higher than that in nondeaf children. Porter (1974) found that 25 percent of 79 deaf children aged six to 10 years had abnormal tympanograms. Brooks (1974) reported that five-year-old children in a residential school for the deaf in England had a higher incidence of abnormal tympanograms than did nondeaf children. Mehta and Erlich (1978) found a high incidence of otitis media with effusion in children in a school for the deaf. Rubin (1978) reported the incidence of middle ear effusion in children three to six years of age to be 30 percent. Over a period of one year, Stool, Craig, and Laird (1980) conducted otoscopic, tympanometric, and audiometric evaluations on 446 students at the Western Pennsylvania School for the Deaf and reported that the incidence of middle ear effusions was 8 percent, whereas that of high negative middle ear pressure was 21 percent. However, the incidence of otitis media with effusion in this study was 26 percent in the two- to five-year age group. In addition, they found that 79 percent of the students who initially were identified as having high negative middle ear pressure consistently had abnormal negative pressures during the one-year observation period.

Table 7–2. **SUGGESTED SCREENING FOR MIDDLE EAR DISEASE
IN PROGRAMS AND SCHOOLS FOR DEAF CHILDREN**

	Population Groups				
	Infants and Young Children (also multiply handicapped children of all ages)		Older Children and Adolescents		
First Year Upon Entry					
Frequency of examination	Monthly*		Every Three Months*		
Experience at the end of the first year	No disease or infrequent disease of short duration	Frequently recurrent or chronic disease	No disease	Infrequent disease of short duration	Frequently recurrent or chronic disease
Second Year (and each succeeding year until experience changes)	Every two to three months*	Monthly*	Yearly	Every three months*	Monthly

*And with every upper respiratory tract infection or the appearance of otological signs and symptoms (e.g., otalgia, otorrhea).

From these few studies, it is apparent that continuous surveillance for middle ear disease and early treatment should be part of every program or school for deaf children. This is especially critical for those children with some residual hearing who benefit from amplification, since even the slightest conductive hearing loss may decrease or eliminate the efficacy of amplification. It is recommended that every school for deaf children be afforded appropriate health care professionals who are competent in otoscopy, tympanometry, audiometry, and treatment of otological disorders to carry out this program. Most schools for the deaf do not have sufficient provisions for such care.

Because the external canals of deaf children are frequently obstructed with cerumen, frequent examination and removal of the cerumen may be extremely beneficial, especially for those who wear a hearing aid (Riding et al., 1978b). This finding alone is reason enough for frequent periodic otological examination; however, a schedule for screening for otitis media with effusion and high negative pressure should be established. Until a formal long-term study has been completed in order to offer recommendations for a screening program in schools for the deaf, we propose the following schedule of examinations of such children, based on the findings of Findlay, Stool, and Svitko (1977); Riding and coworkers (1978b); Craig, Stool, and Laird (1979); and Stool, Craig, and Laird (1980): all children should have an otoscopic, tympanometric, and audiometric examination upon entering the school and periodically during the first school year (Table 7–2). Since infants and young children are at highest risk, they should be examined once a month by otoscopy (and tympanometry when indicated) during this first year. Older children and adolescents probably can be evaluated upon entry and every three months during the first year, since the incidence of middle ear disease in this age group is less than in the younger age group. All students should be examined during periods of an upper respiratory tract infection and whenever there are signs or symptoms related to the ear, such as otalgia or otorrhea. In addition, a child should be examined if the teacher or parent suspects a middle ear problem, owing to a noticeable lack of attention, sudden or gradual failure to benefit from the amplification, or overt, progressive loss of hearing. After the first year of follow-up the children will usually separate into one of four groups, based on the occurrence of otitis media with effusion or high negative pressure or both: (1) no disease; (2) infrequent disease and, when present, of short duration; (3) frequently recurrent disease; and (4) chronic disease. Infants and young children who fit into either of the first two categories, based on the examination of the first year, may be examined at less frequent intervals, such as every two to three months during the second year. Older children who have no evidence of disease during the first year probably can be examined once a year, either upon entering in the fall or, more ideally, during the winter months. Older children with infrequent problems during the first year should probably be examined every three months during the second year. All infants and children who have frequently recurrent or chronic middle ear disease during the first year must be examined every month and with each upper respiratory tract infection until they, too, have a year without significant problems. Screening during the succeeding years should be related to the occurrence of middle ear disease in the preceding year. Children who have multiple handicaps in addition to deafness are considered to be at high risk for middle ear disease, which can significantly compound their handicap due to the attendant conductive hearing loss. Therefore, screening for all such students during the first year should be the program recommended for infants and young children.

Ideally, every examination should be conducted by a physician who is expert in the diseases of the middle ear, but this is not always feasible. Therefore, a nurse should be trained to perform routine otoscopy, examination of the nose and throat, and removal of cerumen from the external canal when present. Tympanometry can be performed by the nurse, a technician, or, if available, an audiologist. Even though an otologist cannot examine every child with the frequency recommended, every school for the deaf must have a physician, preferably an otologist, assigned to the school for diagnosis and treatment of those children found to have middle ear disease.

It is important that all children with severe or profound deafness be considered to be at risk for developing middle ear disease. Therefore, they should have regular periodic examinations of the ear by competent health care professionals and appropriate early management instituted so that their educational handicap is not further compromised by a condition that is amenable to medical or surgical management.

MICROBIOLOGICAL DIAGNOSIS

The correlation between bacterial cultures of the nasopharynx or the oropharynx and cultures of middle ear fluids is poor. The poor correlation occurs because of the frequency of colonization of the upper respiratory tract with organisms of known pathogenicity for the middle ear and, less commonly, because of absence in cultures of the oro- or nasopharynx of the pathogen responsible for infection of the middle ear. Thus, cultures of the upper respiratory tract are of limited value in specific bacteriological diagnosis of otitis media. The consistent results of microbiological studies of middle ear fluid of children with acute otitis media provide an accurate guide to the most likely pathogens. Thus, initial therapy in the uncomplicated case does not require obtaining specimens for bacterial diagnosis.

Specific microbiological diagnosis is achieved by culture of middle ear fluid, obtained by needle aspiration through the intact tympanic membrane (tympanocentesis). If the patient has toxic symptoms or a localized infection elsewhere, culture of the blood or the focus of infection should be performed.

Tympanocentesis

When the diagnosis of acute otitis media is in doubt or when determination of the etiological agent is desirable, aspiration of the middle ear should be performed. Indications for tympanocentesis or myringotomy (Fig. 7–33) include the following:

1. Otitis media in patients who are seriously ill or appear toxic.
2. Unsatisfactory response to antimicrobial therapy.
3. Onset of otitis media in a patient who is receiving antimicrobial agents.
4. Presence of suppurative complications.
5. Otitis media in the newborn infant, or in the immunologically deficient patient, in each of whom an unusual organism may be present.

Both tympanocentesis and myringotomy can usually be performed without general anesthesia. In certain instances, premedication with a combination of a short-acting barbiturate and either morphine or meperidine, or even a general anesthetic, is advisable. The procedures can be carried out using an otoscope with a surgical head or with the otomicroscope. Adequate immobilization of the patient is essential when a general anesthetic is not used.

Diagnostic aspiration may be performed through the inferior portion of the tympanic membrane by an 18-gauge spinal needle attached to a syringe or collection trap (Fig. 7–34). Culture of the ear canal and cleansing of the canal with alcohol should precede the procedure (Fig. 7–35). The canal culture is helpful in determining whether organisms cultured are contaminants from the exterior

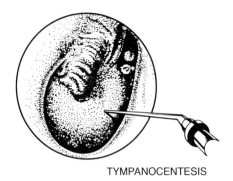

TYMPANOCENTESIS

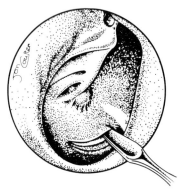

MYRINGOTOMY

Figure 7–33. Tympanocentesis, a needle aspiration of a middle ear effusion, is used primarily for diagnosis of the presence or absence of an effusion and for microbiologic study (*upper*). Myringotomy is an incision in the tympanic membrane used primarily for therapeutic drainage (*lower*).

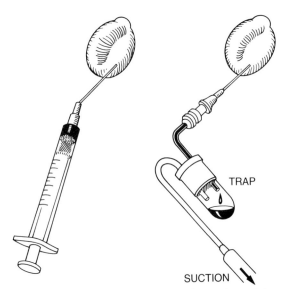

TRAP

SUCTION

Figure 7–34. Tympanocentesis can be performed by employing a needle attached to a tuberculin syringe (*left*) or by using an Alden-Senturia trap (Storz Instrument Co., St. Louis, Mo.).

canal or pathogens from the middle ear. When therapeutic drainage is required, a myringotomy knife should be employed and the incision should be large enough to allow for adequate drainage and aeration of the middle ear.

Following tympanocentesis, the effusion caught in the syringe or collection trap is sent to the laboratory for culture. A gram-stained smear may provide immediate information about the bacterial pathogens. The smear is of particular value if cultures are negative because antibiotics have been administered prior to culture or if infection is due to fastidious organisms such as anaerobic bacteria.

The external ear swab and the fluids aspirated from the middle ear are inoculated onto appropriate solid media and into broth to isolate the likely organisms. Sensitivities of organisms isolated should be tested by the standard method described by Bauer and coworkers (1966). If available, techniques for assay of pneumococcal antigens may yield useful information. Future studies may utilize rapid diagnosis of the virus.

When spontaneous perforation has occurred, the exudate will generally be contaminated with a mixed flora. The ear canal should be carefully cleaned and cultures taken from the area of the perforation or, preferably, by needle aspiration from within the middle ear.

Nasopharyngeal Culture

In an attempt to identify the causative organism in a child with acute otitis media, the results of a nasopharyngeal culture would be less traumatic than a tympanocentesis or myringotomy. The concept is an attractive one, since the bacteria found in middle ear aspirates are the same type found in the nasopharynx of children with acute otitis media. However, the correlation between the organisms found in the middle ear and nasopharynx as reported in the past has not proved to be high enough to warrant the procedure in the usual clinical setting to justify its routine use. A possible exception would be when an ampicillin-resistant strain of *H. influenzae* is suspected. Schwartz and coworkers (1979) and Long and associates (1984) reported a technique that improved the correlation of organisms isolated by the nasopharyngeal culture with bacteria identi-

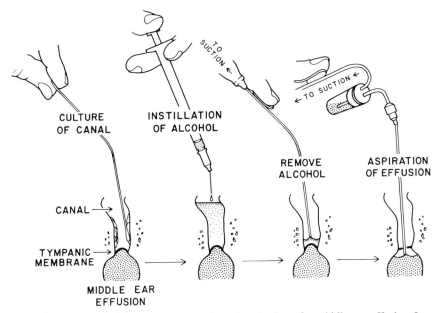

Figure 7–35. Method recommended for tympanocentesis and aspiration of a middle ear effusion for microbiologic assessment. A culture of the external auditory canal is obtained with a Calgiswab (Falton, Oxford, Ca.), which has been moistened with trypticase soy broth. The canal is then filled with 70 percent ethyl alcohol for one minute, after which as much as possible of the alcohol is removed from the ear canal by aspiration. Tympanocentesis is performed in the inferior portion of the tympanic membrane with an Alden-Senturia trap (Storz Instrument Co., St. Louis, Mo.), with a needle attached. Care is taken not to close the suction hole in the trap before entering the middle ear.

fied by culture of middle ear fluid. The method used involved immediate plating of the nasopharyngeal swab on solid media and a semiquantitative estimation of colonies growing on culture plates.

Blood Culture

Bacteremia is rarely associated with otitis media due to nontypable strains of *H. influenzae,* uncommonly associated with otitis media due to *S. pneumoniae,* and frequently associated with otitis media due to type b strains of *H. influenzae* (Harding et al., 1973).

House officers at Boston City Hospital obtained blood for culture from 600 consecutive children one to 24 months of age coming to the walk-in clinic with fever. One hundred and sixty-six children had a diagnosis of otitis; only two (1.2 percent) had concomitant bacteremia (Teele et al., 1975). Studies of young infants include information that is selected because those who had cultures taken of blood showed toxic symptoms or were hospitalized. In four series of infants eight weeks of age or younger (Crain and Shelov, 1982; Greene et al., 1981; Roberts and Borzy, 1977; Shurin et al., 1978) and in two series of patients three months of age or younger (Schlesinger, 1982; Tetzlaff et al.,

1977) five of 136 infants (3.7 percent) with otitis media had positive results of blood cultures (two group B streptococcus, one *S. pneumoniae,* one *P. aeruginosa,* and one enterococcus). The yield of cultures of blood is low in children with uncomplicated otitis media, but it is likely to be higher in children who have toxic symptoms, high fever, or concurrent infection at other foci (pneumonia, meningitis).

White Blood Cell Count

Although white blood cell counts are too variable to be helpful in distinguishing the child with otitis media due to a bacterial pathogen from the child with otitis media and a sterile effusion, there are data that suggest mean white blood cell counts of children with bacterial otitis media are higher than those of children with sterile middle ear effusions. Lahikainen (1953) noted that the mean white blood cell counts (per mm^3) of children with otitis due to *S. pyogenes* was 13,400, due to *S. pneumoniae* was 10,500, and due to *H. influenzae* was 11,500; of children with sterile middle ear effusion, the mean count was 8700. Mortimer and Watterson (1956) found similar results in children who had a bacterial pathogen in the middle ear effusion in whom the mean white blood cell count (per mm^3) was 10,300; the mean white blood cell count was 6700 in children with sterile effusions. Feingold and colleagues (1966) found an association of higher white blood cell counts with isolation of bacterial pathogen from the middle ear effusion; of 35 children with white blood cell counts of 15,000 or more, 27 (77 percent) had a bacterial pathogen grown from the middle ear effusion, whereas of children with a white blood cell count of 9000 or less, eight of 20 (40 percent) had a bacterial pathogen grown from the middle ear effusion.

Sedimentation Rate

Lahikainen (1953) found increases in sedimentation rate in children with otitis media and differences among the bacterial pathogens isolated from the middle ear effusion. The mean sedimentation rate for 104 children with otitis media due to *S. pyogenes* was 43.7; for 171 children with otitis media due to *S. pneumoniae*, 30.2; for 43 with otitis media due to *H. influenzae*, 17.3; and for 85 children with sterile effusion, 21.3.

Radiological Imaging

For the uncomplicated case of acute or chronic otitis media with effusion, radiographs of the temporal bone are not indicated. However, when recurrent acute or chronic otitis media with effusion is present, roentgenographic evaluation of the paranasal sinuses may be helpful in identifying sinusitis that may be related causally to the otitis media. When there are signs and symptoms of sinusitis present (e.g., purulent nasal discharge, cough, and fetor oris), conventional radiographic examination of the paranasal sinuses is the simplest, least expensive, and most practical examination. The occipitomental (Waters), frontal (Caldwell), basal (submentovertical), and lateral erect views should be obtained. In addition, the lateral view is beneficial in assessing the adenoid size in relation to the nasopharynx. The submentovertical view is helpful in evaluation of the ethmoid and sphenoid sinuses, and both views can be diagnostic of a nasopharyngeal tumor, which can mechanically obstruct the eustachian tube and cause otitis media with effusion. Chronic nasal obstruction, with or without epistaxis or cervical lymphadenopa-

thy, in association with otitis media should prompt the clinician to suspect a nasopharyngeal tumor. The A-mode ultrasound can also be useful in determining the presence of an effusion in the maxillary sinuses (Edell and Isaacson, 1978; Revonta, 1979).

When certain complications or sequelae of otitis media are suspect or present, then radiological evaluation of the temporal bone is indicated. Plain radiographs (Towne, Laws, Stenvers) can be helpful in the diagnosis of osteitis of the mastoid or a cholesteatoma, but polydirectional tomography or computerized tomography is more precise and should be obtained if a suppurative intratemporal or intracranial complication is suspected (see Chapters Nine and Ten on intracranial and intratemporal complications and sequelae).

EUSTACHIAN TUBE FUNCTION IN THE CLINICAL SETTING

The roentgenographic tests developed to assess the protective and clearance system of the eustachian tube–middle ear system have been helpful in understanding these functions but are not feasible in the usual clinical setting. However, methods to assess the ventilatory function of the system are readily available to the clinician and should be performed when indicated (described later). The ventilatory function is the most important of the three functions, since adequate hearing depends upon the maintenance of equal air pressure on both sides of the tympanic membrane. In addition, impairment of the ventilatory function can result not only in hearing loss but also in otitis media.

Prior to the examination of the patient, the presence of certain signs and symptoms may be helpful in determining if eustachian tube dysfunction is present. Conductive hearing loss, otalgia, otorrhea, tinnitus, or vertigo may be present with this disorder.

Otoscopy

Visual inspection of the tympanic membrane is one of the simplest (and oldest) ways to assess the functioning of the eustachian tube. The appearance of a middle ear effusion or the presence of high negative middle ear pressure, or both, as determined by the *pneumatic* otoscope (Bluestone and Shurin, 1974), is presumptive evidence of eustachian tube dysfunction, but the type of impairment, such as functional or mechanical obstruction, as well as the degree of abnormality, cannot be determined by this method. Moreover, a normal-appearing tympanic membrane cannot be considered to be evidence of normal functioning of the eustachian tube: for instance, a patulous or semipatulous eustachian tube may be present when the tympanic membrane appears to be normal. In addition, the presence of one or more of the complications or sequelae of otitis media (such as a perforation or atelectasis, as observed through the otoscope) may not correlate with dysfunction of the eustachian tube at the time of the examination, since eustachian tube function may improve with growth and development.

Nasopharyngoscopy

Indirect mirror examination of the nasopharyngeal end of the eustachian tube is also an old but still important part of the clinical assessment of a patient with middle ear disease. For instance, a neoplasm in the fossa of Rosenmüller may be diagnosed by this simple technique. The development of endoscopic instruments has greatly improved the accuracy of this type of examination, but the function of the eustachian tube cannot be determined with the aid of currently available instruments.

Tympanometry

The use of an electroacoustic impedance instrument to obtain a tympanogram is an excellent way of determining the status of the tympanic membrane–middle ear system, and it can be helpful in the assessment of eustachian tube function (Bluestone, 1980) (see Fig. 7–23). The presence of a middle ear effusion or high negative middle ear pressure as determined by this method usually indicates impaired eustachian tube function; however, unlike the otoscopic evaluation, the tympanogram is an objective way of determining the degree of negative pressure present in the middle ear. Unfortunately, assessing the abnormality of values of negative pressure is not so simple: high negative pressure may be present in some patients, especially children, who are asymptomatic and who have relatively good hearing, whereas in others, symptoms such as hearing

loss, otalgia, vertigo, and tinnitus may be associated with modest degrees of negative pressure or even with normal middle ear pressures. The middle ear air pressure may depend upon the time of day, season of the year, or condition of the other parts of the system, such as the presence of an upper respiratory tract infection. For instance, a young child with a common cold may have transitory high negative pressure within the middle ear while he has the cold but may be otherwise otologically normal (Casselbrant et al., 1985). The decision as to whether or not high negative pressure is abnormal or is only a physiological variation should be made taking into consideration the presence or absence of signs and symptoms of middle ear disease. If severe atelectasis or adhesive otitis of the tympanic membrane–middle ear system is present, the tympanogram may not be a reliable indicator of the actual pressure within the middle ear.

Therefore, a resting pressure that is highly negative is associated with some degree of eustachian tube obstruction, but the presence of normal middle ear pressure does not necessarily indicate normal eustachian tube function; a normal tympanogram is obtained when the eustachian tube is patulous.

Manometry

The pump-manometer system of the electroacoustic impedance bridge is usually adequate to assess eustachian tube function clinically when the tympanic membrane is not intact. However, due to the limitations of the manometric systems of all of the commercially available instruments, a controlled syringe and manometer (a water manometer will suffice) should be available when these limitations are exceeded (e.g., when eustachian tube opening pressure is in excess of $+400$ to $+600$ mm H_2O.

Methods of Assessing Eustachian Tube Function in the Clinical Setting

Classical Tests of Tubal Patency

Valsalva (see Fig. 8–6) and Politzer (Fig. 8–7) have developed methods to assess patency of the eustachian tube. When the tympanic membrane is intact and the middle ear inflates following one of these tests, then the tube is not totally mechanically obstructed.

Likewise, if the tympanic membrane is not intact, passage of air into the middle ear would indicate patency of the tube. The assessment is more objective with a tympanogram obtained when the tympanic membrane is intact, and with a manometric observation on the impedance instrument when the tympanic membrane is not intact. However, inflation of the eustachian tube and middle ear from the nasopharynx end of the system by one of these classical methods only is an assessment of tubal patency and *not function,* and failure to inflate the middle ear does not necessarily indicate a lack of patency of the eustachian tube. Elner and coworkers (1971) reported that 86 percent of 100 otologically normal adults could perform the Valsalva test. In young children, the Valsalva test is usually more difficult to perform than the Politzer test. However, in a recent study by Bluestone and coworkers (1981), six of seven children who had a traumatic perforation but who were otherwise otologically "normal" could perform the Valsalva test, but only 11 of 28 children who had a retraction pocket or a cholesteatoma could do so. The Valsalva and Politzer maneuvers are more beneficial as management options in selected patients than they are as methods to assess tubal function.

Toynbee Test

One of the oldest and still one of the best tests of eustachian tube function is the Toynbee test (Fig. 7–36). Test results are usually considered positive when an alteration in middle ear pressure results. More specifically, if negative pressure (even transitory in the absence of a patulous tube) develops in the middle ear during closed-nose swallowing, the eustachian tube function can be considered most likely to be normal. When the tympanic membrane is intact, the presence of negative middle ear pressure must be determined by pneumatic otoscopy or, more accurately, by obtaining a tympanogram before and immediately following the test (Fig. 7–37). When the tympanic membrane is not intact, the manometer of the impedance bridge can be observed to determine middle ear pressure. In the study by Elner and coworkers (1971), results of the Toynbee test were positive in 79 percent of normal adults. Cantekin and colleagues (1976) reported that only seven of 106 ears (6.6 percent) of subjects (mostly children) who had had tympanostomy tubes inserted for otitis media could

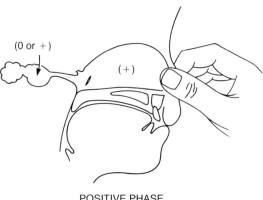

POSITIVE PHASE

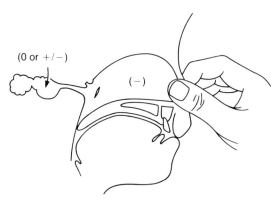

NEGATIVE PHASE

Figure 7–36. The Toynbee test of eustachian tube function. Closed-nose swallowing results in, first, positive pressure in the nose and nasopharynx, followed by a negative pressure phase. When positive pressure is in the nasopharynx, air may enter the middle ear, creating positive pressure. During or after the negative pressure phase, negative pressure may develop in the middle ear, or positive pressure may still be in the middle ear (no change in middle ear pressure during negative phase), or positive pressure may be followed by negative middle ear pressure, or ambient pressure will be present if equilibration takes place before the tube closes. If the tube does not open during either the positive or negative phase, no change in middle ear pressure will occur.

show positive results when given a modification of the Toynbee test (closed-nose equilibration attempt with applied negative middle ear pressure of 100 or 200 mm H_2O). Likewise, in a series of patients, most of whom were older children and adults with chronic perforations of the tympanic membrane, only three of 21 (14.3 percent) passed the test. However, in children with a traumatic perforation of the tympanic membrane but who otherwise had a negative otological history, three of 10 (30 percent) could pass the test. In the study by Bluestone and coworkers (1981) of "normal" children with traumatic perforations, six of seven children could change the middle ear pressure, but *none* of

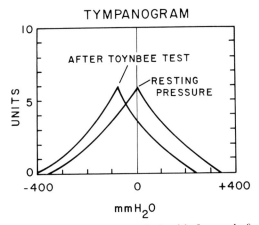

Figure 7–37. Tympanogram obtained before and after Toynbee test. Negative middle ear pressure is objectively demonstrated in the middle ear; this is considered to be associated with good eustachian tube function.

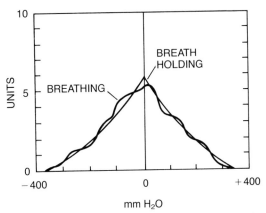

Figure 7–38. Diagnosis of a patulous eustachian tube by employing the tympanogram.

the 21 ears of children who had a retraction pocket or a cholesteatoma showed pressure change. The test is of greater value in determining normal or abnormal eustachian tube function in adults than it is in children. The test is still of considerable value since, regardless of age, if negative pressure develops in the middle ear during or following the test, the eustachian tube function is most likely normal, since the eustachian tube actively opens and is sufficiently stiff to withstand nasopharyngeal negative pressure (i.e., it does not "lock"). If positive pressure is noted or no change in pressure occurs, the function of the eustachian tube still may be normal, and other tests of eustachian tube function should be performed.

Patulous Eustachian Tube Test

If a patulous eustachian tube is suspected, the diagnosis can be confirmed by otoscopy or objectively by tympanometry when the tympanic membrane is intact (Bluestone, 1980). One tympanogram is obtained while the patient is breathing normally, and a second is obtained while the patient holds his breath. Fluctuation of the tympanometric trace that coincides with breathing confirms the diagnosis of a patulous tube (Fig. 7–38). Fluctuation can be exaggerated by asking the patient to occlude one nostril with the mouth closed during forced inspiration and expiration or by performing the Toynbee maneuver. When the tympanic membrane is not intact, a patulous eustachian tube can be identified by the free flow of air into and out of the eustachian tube by using the pump-manometer portion of the electroacoustic

impedance bridge. These tests should not be performed while the patient is in a reclining position, since the patulous eustachian tube will close.

Nine-Step Inflation-Deflation Tympanometric Test

Another method of assessing the function of the eustachian tube when the tympanic membrane is intact, developed by Bluestone (1975), is called the nine-step inflation-deflation tympanometric test, although the applied middle ear pressures are very limited in magnitude. The middle ear must be free of effusion. The nine-step tympanometry procedure may be summarized as follows (Fig. 7–39):

1. The tympanogram records resting middle ear pressure.
2. Ear canal pressure is increased to $+200$ mm H_2O with medial deflection of the tympanic membrane and a corresponding increase in middle ear pressure. The subject swallows to equilibrate middle ear overpressure.
3. While the subject refrains from swallowing, ear canal pressure is returned to normal, thus establishing a slight negative middle ear pressure (as the tympanic membrane moves outward). The tympanogram documents the established middle ear underpressure.
4. The subject swallows in an attempt to equilibrate negative middle ear pressure. If equilibration is successful, airflow is from nasopharynx to middle ear.
5. The tympanogram records the extent of equilibration.
6. Ear canal pressure is decreased to -200 mm H_2O, causing a lateral deflection of the tympanic membrane and a corresponding

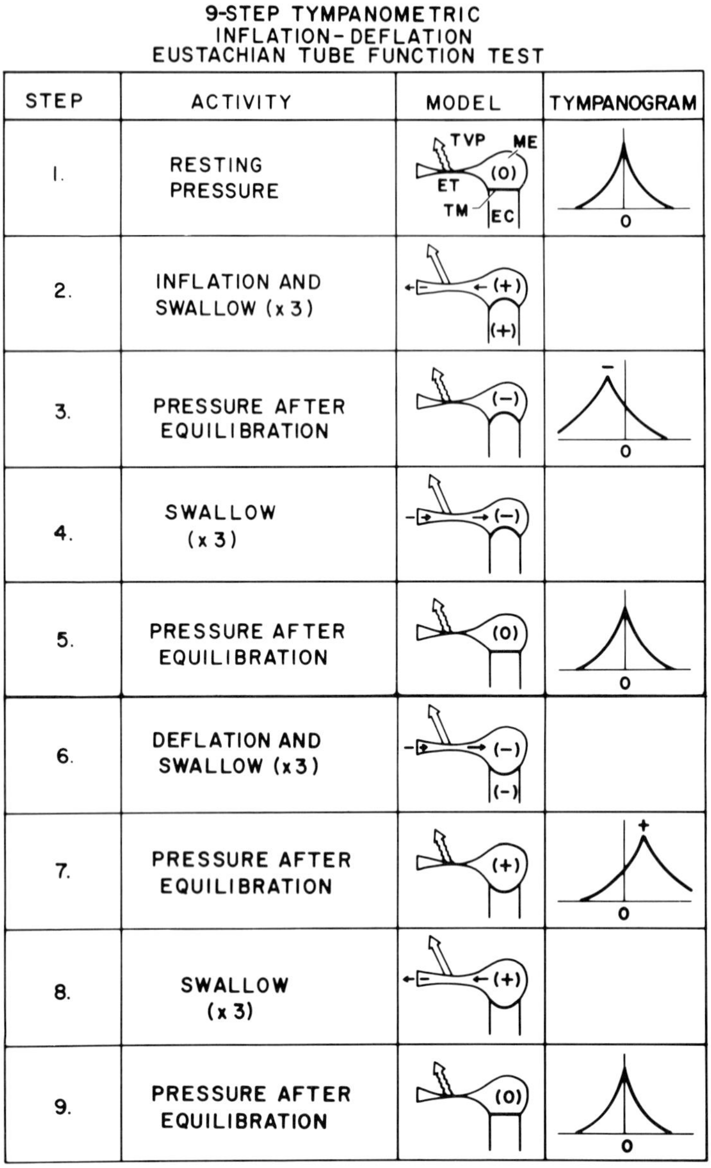

9-STEP TYMPANOMETRIC INFLATION-DEFLATION EUSTACHIAN TUBE FUNCTION TEST

STEP	ACTIVITY	MODEL	TYMPANOGRAM
1.	RESTING PRESSURE	TVP ME ET (0) TM EC	0
2.	INFLATION AND SWALLOW (x 3)	←(+) (+)	
3.	PRESSURE AFTER EQUILIBRATION	(−)	− 0
4.	SWALLOW (x 3)	→(−)	
5.	PRESSURE AFTER EQUILIBRATION	(0)	0
6.	DEFLATION AND SWALLOW (x3)	→(−) (−)	
7.	PRESSURE AFTER EQUILIBRATION	(+)	+ 0
8.	SWALLOW (x 3)	←(+)	
9.	PRESSURE AFTER EQUILIBRATION	(0)	0

Figure 7–39. Nine-step inflation-deflation tympanometric test. *TVP,* tensor veli palatini muscle; *ET,* eustachian tube; *ME,* middle ear; *TM,* tympanic membrane; *EC,* ear canal.

decrease in middle ear pressure. The subject swallows to equilibrate negative middle ear pressure; airflow is from the nasopharynx to the middle ear.

7. The subject refrains from swallowing while external ear canal pressure is returned to normal, thus establishing a slight positive pressure in the middle ear as the tympanic membrane moves medially. The tympanogram records the overpressure established.

8. The subject swallows to reduce overpressure. If equilibration is successful, airflow is from the middle ear to the nasopharynx.

9. The final tympanogram documents the extent of equilibration.

The test is simple to perform, can give useful information regarding eustachian tube function, and should be part of the clinical evaluation of patients with suspected eustachian tube dysfunction. In general, most normal adults can perform all or some parts of this test, but even normal children have difficulty in performing it. However, if a child can pass some or all of the steps, eustachian tube function is considered good.

Modified Inflation-Deflation Test (Nonintact Tympanic Membrane)

When the tympanic membrane is not intact, the pump-manometer system of the electroacoustic impedance bridge can be used to perform the modified inflation-deflation eustachian tube function test (Fig. 7–20), which assesses passive as well as active functioning of the eustachian tube (Cantekin et al., 1976; Ingelstedt and Ortegren, 1963). The middle ear should be free of any drainage for an accurate assessment of eustachian tube function using this test. The middle ear is inflated (i.e., positive pressure is applied) until the eustachian tube spontaneously opens (Fig. 7–40). At this time, the pump is manually stopped and air is discharged through the eustachian tube until the tube closes passively. The pressure at which the eustachian

tube is passively forced open is called the opening pressure, and the pressure at which it closes passively is called the closing pressure. The patient is then instructed to equilibrate the middle ear pressure actively by swallowing. The residual pressure remaining in the middle ear after swallowing is recorded. The active function is also recorded by applying over- and underpressure to the middle ear, which the patient then attempts to equilibrate by swallowing. The residual negative pressure that remains in the middle

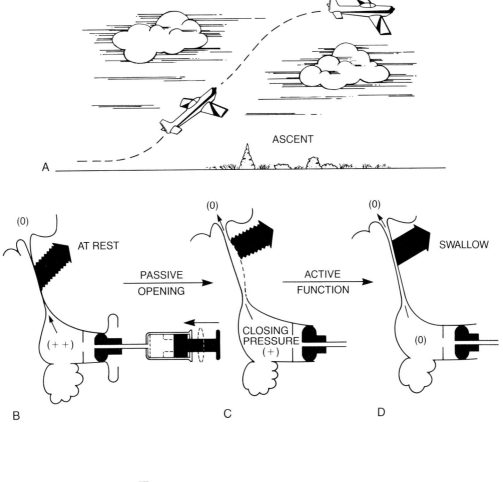

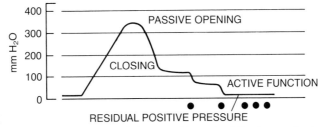

Figure 7–40. Test of passive and active function of the eustachian tube following application of positive middle ear pressure. *A*, Analogous ascent in an airplane. *B*, Assessment of passive function. *C*, Closing pressure. *D*, Assessment of active function (swallowing). *E*, Strip chart recording showing an example of normal pressure tracing. Black circles represent swallows.

ear after the attempt to equilibrate applied negative pressure of −200 mm H_2O is also noted (Fig. 7–41). This procedure is not performed in patients who cannot equilibrate applied overpressure. If the eustachian tube does not open following application of positive pressure using the electroacoustic impedance bridge, and if no reduction in positive pressure occurs during swallowing, then the eustachian tube must be assessed using a manometric system other than that available with the electroacoustic impedance bridge. The opening pressure may be higher than 400 to 600 mm H_2O pressure or not present at all (severe mechanical obstruction). Example A in Figure 7–42 shows that, following

passive opening and closing of the eustachian tube during the inflation phase of the study, the patient was able to equilibrate completely the remaining positive pressure. Active swallowing also completely equilibrated applied negative pressure (deflation). This is considered to be characteristic of normal eustachian tube function. Example B shows the eustachian tube passively opened and closed following inflation, but subsequent swallowing failed to equilibrate the residual positive pressure. In the deflation phase of the study, the patient was unable to equilibrate negative pressure. Inflation to a pressure below the opening pressure but above the closing pressure could not be equilibrated by active swal-

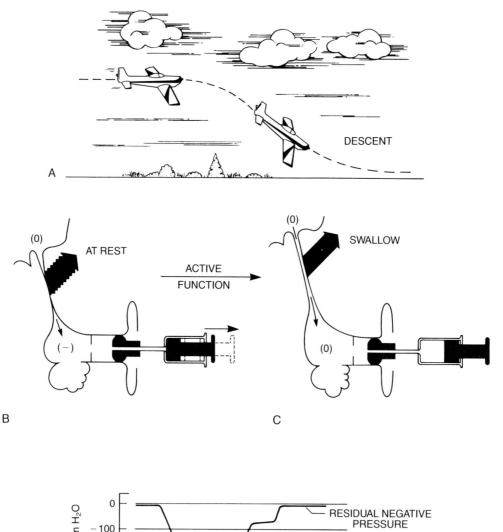

Figure 7–41. Deflation phase of eustachian tube testing. *A,* Analogous descent in an airplane. *B,* Application of low negative pressure to the middle ear. *C,* Equilibration by active tubal opening. *D,* Strip chart recording showing an example of a normal tracing. Black circles represent swallows.

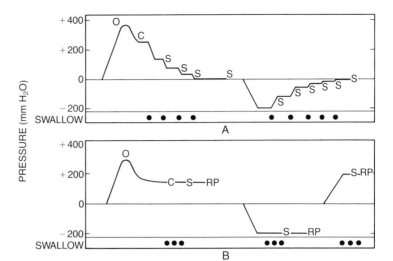

Figure 7–42. Examples of results of inflation-deflation ventilation studies that employed a strip chart recorder. *A,* Normal adult with a traumatic perforation. *B,* Four-year-old boy with a functioning tympanostomy tube who had a persistent otitis media with effusion. *RP,* Residual pressure; *O,* opening pressure; *C,* closing pressure; *S,* pressure after swallow. Black circles represent swallows.

lowing. This type of result is considered to be abnormal but may be found in a few subjects who do not have any obvious otological disease.

Failure to equilibrate the applied negative pressure may indicate locking of the eustachian tube during the test. This type of tube is considered to have increased compliance or to be "floppy" in comparison to a tube with perfect function. The tensor veli palatini muscle is unable to open (dilate) the tube.

Even though the inflation-deflation test of eustachian tube function does not strictly duplicate physiological functions of the tube, the results are helpful in differentiating normal from abnormal function. The mean opening pressure for apparently normal subjects with a traumatic perforation and negative otological history reported by Cantekin and coworkers (1977b) was 330 mm H_2O ($\pm$ 70 mm H_2O). If the test results reveal passive opening and closing within the normal range, if residual positive pressure can be equilibrated by swallowing, and if applied negative pressure can also be equilibrated completely, then the eustachian tube can be considered to have normal function. However, if the tube does not open to a pressure of 1000 mm H_2O, one can assume that total mechanical obstruction is present. This pressure is not hazardous to the middle ear or inner ear windows if the pressure is applied slowly. An extremely high opening pressure (e.g., greater than 500 to 600 mm H_2O) may indicate partial obstruction, whereas a very low opening pressure (e.g., less than 100 mm H_2O) would indicate a semipatulous eustachian tube. Inability to maintain even a modest positive pressure within the middle ear would be consistent with a patulous tube (i.e.,

one that is open at rest). Complete equilibration by swallowing of applied negative pressure is usually associated with normal function, but partial equilibration or even failure to reduce any applied negative pressure may or may not be considered abnormal, since even a normal eustachian tube will lock when negative pressure is rapidly applied. Therefore, inability to equilibrate applied negative pressure may not indicate poor eustachian tube function, especially when it is the only abnormal result of testing.

Other Methods Available for Laboratory Use

There are other available methods to test the functioning of the eustachian tube, but they are currently limited to use in the laboratory for investigational purposes. When the tympanic membrane is intact, the microflow technique (Ingelstedt et al., 1967) or an impedance method (Bylander, 1980), both of which require a pressure chamber, or sonometry (Murti et al., 1980; Virtanen, 1978) may be used. When the tympanic membrane is not intact, the forced-response test (Cantekin et al., 1979) may be used. Sonometry and the forced-response test show great promise for future use in the clinical setting.

CLINICAL INDICATIONS FOR TESTING EUSTACHIAN TUBE FUNCTION

Diagnosis

One of the most important reasons for assessing eustachian tube function is the need to make a differential diagnosis in a patient who has an intact tympanic membrane without evidence of otitis media but who has symptoms that might be related to eustachian tube dysfunction (such as otalgia, snapping or popping in the ear, fluctuating hearing loss, tinnitus, or vertigo). An example of such a case would be a child or adolescent who has a complaint of fullness in the ear without hearing loss at the time of the examination, a symptom that could be related to abnormal functioning of the eustachian tube or could be due to an inner ear disorder. A tympanogram that reveals high negative pressure (-50 mm H_2O or less) is presumptive evidence of tubal obstruction, whereas normal resting middle ear pressure is not diagnostically significant. However, when the resting intratympanic pressure is within normal limits and the patient can develop negative middle ear pressure following Toynbee's test or can perform all or some of the functions in the nine-step inflation-deflation tympanometric test, the eustachian tube is probably functioning normally. Unfortunately, failure to develop negative middle ear pressure during the Toynbee test or inability to pass the nine-step test does not necessarily indicate poor eustachian tube function, since many children who are otologically normal cannot actively open their tubes during these tests. Tympanometry is not only of value in determining if eustachian tube obstruction is present; it can also identify abnormality at the other end of the spectrum of eustachian tube dysfunction, and the presence of an abnormally patent eustachian tube can be confirmed by the results of the tympanometric patulous tube test.

Screening for the presence of high negative pressure in certain high-risk populations (i.e., children with known sensorineural hearing losses, developmentally delayed and mentally impaired children, children with cleft palates or other craniofacial anomalies, American Indian and Eskimo children, and children with Down syndrome) appears to be helpful in identifying those individuals who may need to be monitored closely for the occurrence of otitis media (Harford et al., 1978).

Tympanometry appears to be a reliable method for detecting the presence of high negative pressure as well as of otitis media with effusion in children (Beery et al., 1975b; Brooks, 1968). The identification of high negative pressure without effusion in children is indicative of some degree of eustachian tube obstruction. These children as well as those with middle ear effusions should have follow-up serial tympanograms, since they may be at risk of developing otitis media with effusion.

However, the best methods available to the clinician today for testing eustachian tube function are the nine-step test, when the eardrum is intact, or, when not intact, the inflation-deflation test. A perforation of the tympanic membrane or a tympanostomy tube must be present in order to perform the latter test. The test uses the simple apparatus described earlier, with or without the electroacoustic impedance bridge pump-manometer system. This test will aid in determining the presence or absence of a dysfunction, and the type of dysfunction (obstruction vs. abnormal patency) and its severity when one is present. No other test procedures may be needed if the patient has either functional obstruction of the eustachian tube or an abnormally patent tube. However, if there is a mechanical obstruction, especially if the tube appears to be totally blocked anatomically, then further testing may be indicated. In such instances, computed tomography of the nasopharynx–eustachian tube–middle ear region can be performed to determine the site and cause of the blockage, such as by cholesteatoma or tumor. In most cases in which mechanical obstruction of the tube is found, inflammation is present at the middle ear end of the eustachian tube (osseous portion), and this usually resolves with medical management or middle ear surgery, or both. Serial inflation-deflation studies should show resolution of the mechanical obstruction. However, if no middle ear cause is obvious, other studies should be performed to rule out the possibility of neoplasm in the nasopharynx.

Eustachian Tube Function Tests Related to Management

Ideally, patients with recurrent acute otitis media or chronic otitis media with effusion, or both, should have eustachian tube function studies as part of their otolaryngological workup, but for most children, one can assume eustachian tube function to be poor. However, patients in whom tympanostomy tubes have been inserted may benefit from serial eustachian tube function studies. Improvement in function as indicated by inflation-deflation tests might aid the clinician in determining the proper time to remove the tubes. Cleft palate repair (Bluestone et al., 1972a; Paradise and Bluestone, 1974), adenoidectomy (Bluestone et al., 1972b, 1975), elimination of nasal and nasopharyngeal inflammation (Bluestone et al., 1977), treatment of a nasopharyngeal tumor, or growth and development of a child (Holborow, 1970) may be associated with improvement in eustachian tube function.

Studies of the eustachian tube function of the patient with a chronic perforation of the tympanic membrane may be helpful in determining preoperatively the potential results of tympanoplastic surgery. Holmquist (1968) studied eustachian tube function in adults before and after tympanoplasty and reported that the operation had a high rate of success in patients with good eustachian tube function (i.e., those who could equilibrate applied negative pressure) but that in patients without good tubal function, surgery frequently failed to close the perforation. These results were corroborated (Miller and Bilodeau, 1967; Siedentop, 1972), but other investigators (Cohn et al., 1979; Ekvall, 1970; Lee and Schuknecht, 1971; Virtanen et al., 1980) found no correlation between the results of the inflation-deflation tests and success or failure of tympanoplasty. Most of these studies failed to define the criteria for "success," and the postoperative follow-up period was too short. Bluestone and coworkers (1979) assessed children prior to tympanoplasty and found that of 51 ears of 45 children, eight ears could equilibrate an applied negative pressure (-200 mm H_2O) to some degree; in seven of these ears, the graft took, no middle ear effusion occurred, and no recurrence of the perforation developed during a follow-up period of between one and two years. However, as in the studies in adults, failure to equilibrate an applied negative pressure did not predict failure of the tympanoplasty.

The conclusion to be drawn from these studies is that if the patient is able to equilibrate an applied negative pressure, regardless of age, the success of tympanoplasty is likely, but failure to perform this difficult test will not help the clinician in deciding not to operate. However, the value of testing a patient's ability to equilibrate negative pressure lies in the possibility of determining from the test results if a young child is a candidate for tympanoplasty, when one might decide on the basis of other findings alone to withhold surgery until the child is older.

In children who have unilateral perforation of the tympanic membrane or tympanostomy tube in place and a contralateral tympanic membrane that is intact, the status of the intact side, observed for at least one year, can aid in determining whether tympanoplasty should be performed or a tube should be removed. Repair of the eardrum or removal of the tube is usually successful if the contralateral intact side has remained normal (i.e., no middle ear effusion or high negative pressure). Conversely, if the opposite ear has developed middle ear disease during the previous year, tympanoplasty should be postponed, or, if a tympanostomy tube is in place, it should not be removed.

References

Alt, A.: Heilunger taubstummheit erzielte durch beseitigung einer otorrhea und einer angebornen gaumenspalate. Arch. fur Augen. U. Ohrenh., 7:211, and Schmidt's Jahrbuecher, 183:277.

Aschan, G.: Hearing and nasal function correlated to postoperative speech in cleft palate patients with velopharyngoplasty. Acta. Otolaryngol. (Stockh.) 61:371–379, 1966.

Bauer, A. W., Kirby, W. M., Sherris, J. C., and Turck, M.: Antibiotic susceptibility testing by a standardized single disk method. Am. J. Clin. Pathol. 45:493–496, 1966.

Beery, Q. C., Bluestone, C. D., Andrus, W. S., and Cantekin, E. I.: Tympanometric pattern classification in relation to middle ear effusions. Ann. Otol. Rhinol. Laryngol. 84:56–64, 1975a.

Beery, Q. C., Bluestone C. D., and Cantekin, E. I.: Otologic history, audiometry and tympanometry as a case finding procedure for school screening. Laryngoscope 84:1976–1985, 1975b.

Bennett, M.: The older cleft palate patient: A clinical otologic-audiologic study. Laryngoscope 82:1217–1225, 1972.

Bennett, M., Ward, R. H., and Tait, C. A.: Otologic-audiologic study of cleft palate children. Laryngoscope 78:1011–1019, 1968.

Bergstrom, L.: Congenital and acquired deafness in clefting and craniofacial syndromes. Cleft Palate J. 15(3):254–261, 1978.

Berman, S. A., Balkany, T. J., and Simmons, M. A.: Otitis media in the neonatal intensive care unit. Pediatrics 62:198–201, 1978.

Berry, M. F., and Eisenson, J.: *Speech Disorders: Principles and Practices of Therapy.* New York, Appleton-Century-Crofts, Inc., 1956.

Bess, F. H., Lewis, H. D., and Cieliczka, B. T.: Acoustic impedance measurements in cleft palate children. J. Speech Hear. Res. 40(1):13–24, 1975.

Bluestone, C. D.: Eustachian tube obstruction in the infant with cleft palate. Ann. Otol. Rhinol. Laryngol. 80(2):1–30, 1971.

Bluestone, C. D., Paradise, J. L., Beery, Q. C., and Wittel, R.: Certain effects of cleft palate repair on eustachian tube function. Cleft Palate J. 9:183–193, 1972a.

Bluestone, C. D., Wittel, R., Paradise, J. L., and Felder,

H.: Eustachian tube function as related to adenoidectomy for otitis media. Trans. Am. Acad. Ophthalmol. Otolaryngol. 76:1325–1339, 1972b.

Bluestone, C. D., Beery, Q. C., and Paradise, J. L.: Audiometry and tympanometry in relation to middle ear effusions in children. Laryngoscope 85:594–604, 1973.

Bluestone, C. D., and Shurin, P.: Middle ear diseases in children: Pathogenesis, diagnosis, and management. Ped. Clin. North Am. 21:379–400, 1974.

Bluestone, C. D.: Assessment of eustachian tube function. In Jerger J. (Ed.): Handbook of Clinical Impedance Audiometry. New York, American Electromedics Corp., 1975, pp. 127–148.

Bluestone, C. D., Cantekin, E. I., and Beery, Q. C.: Certain effects of adenoidectomy on eustachian tube ventilatory function. Laryngoscope 85:113–127, 1975.

Bluestone, C. D., Cantekin, E. I., and Beery, Q. C.: Effect of inflammation on the ventilatory function of the eustachian tube. Laryngoscope 87:493–507, 1977.

Bluestone, C. D., and Cantekin, E. I.: Design factors in the characterization and identification of otitis media and certain related conditions. Ann. Otol. Rhinol. Laryngol. 88(60):13–27, 1979.

Bluestone, C. D., Cantekin, E. I., and Douglas, G. S.: Eustachian tube function related to the outcome of tympanoplasty in children. Laryngoscope 89:450–458, 1979.

Bluestone, C. D.: Assessment of eustachian tube function. In Jerger, J., and Northern, J. (Eds.): Clinical Impedance Audiometry. New York, American Electromedics Corp., 1980, pp. 83–108.

Bluestone, C. D., Casselbrant, M. L., and Cantekin, E. I.: Functional Obstruction of the Eustachian Tube in the Pathogenesis of Acquired Cholesteatoma in Children. The Netherlands, Kugler Publications BV, 1981, pp. 211–224.

Bluestone, C. D., Fria, T. J., Arjona, S. K., Casselbrant, M. L., Schwartz, D. M., Ruben, R. J., Gates, G. A., Downs, M. P., Northern, J. L., Jerger, J. F., Paradise, J. L., Bess, F. H., Kenworthy, O. T., and Rogers, K. D.: Controversies in screening for middle ear disease and hearing loss in children. Pediatrics 77(1):57–60, 1986.

Bodor, F. F.: Conjunctivitis-otitis syndrome. Pediatrics 69:695–698, 1982.

Bodor, F. F., Marchant, C. D., Shurin, P. A., and Barenkamp, S. J.: Bacterial etiology of conjunctivitis-otitis media syndrome. Pediatrics 76:26–28, 1985.

Brooks, D. N.: An objective method of detecting fluid in the middle ear. J. Int. Audiol. 7:280–286, 1968.

Brooks, D. N.: A comparative study of an impedance method and pure tone screening. Scand. Audiol. 2:67–72, 1973.

Brooks, D. N.: Impedance bridge studies on normal and hearing impaired children. Acta Otorhinolaryngol. Belg. 28:140–145, 1974.

Brooks, D. N.: School screening for middle ear effusions. Ann. Otol. Rhinol. Laryngol. 25(85):223–228, 1976.

Brooks, D. N.: Mass screening with acoustic impedance. In Proceedings of the Third International Symposium on Impedance Audiometry. New York, American Electromedics Co., 1977.

Brooks, D. N.: Impedance screening for school children—state of the art. In Harford, E. R., Bess, F. H., Bluestone, C. D., and Klein, J. O. (Eds.): Impedance Screening for Middle Ear Disease in Children. New York, Grune and Stratton, 1978, pp. 173–180.

Brunck, W.: Die systematische untersuchung des sprach-

organes bei angeborenen gaumendefekte in ihrer beziehung zur prognose und therapie. B. Leipziz, 1906.

Busis, S.: Vertigo. In Bluestone, C. D. and Stool, S. E. (Eds.): Pediatric Otolaryngology. Philadelphia, W.B. Saunders Co., 1983, pp. 261–270.

Bylander, A.: Comparison of eustachian tube function in children and adults with normal ears. Ann. Otol. Rhinol. Laryngol. 89(Suppl. 68):20–24, 1980.

Cantekin, E. I., Bluestone, C. D., and Parkin, L. P.: Eustachian tube ventilatory function in children. Ann. Otol. Rhinol. Laryngol. 85(Suppl. 25):171–177, 1976.

Cantekin, E. I., Beery, Q. C., and Bluestone, C. D.: Tympanometric patterns found in middle ear effusions. Ann Otol. Rhinol. Laryngol. 86(41):16–20, 1977a.

Cantekin, E. I., Bluestone, C. D., Saez, C., Doyle, W. J., and Philips, D.: Normal and abnormal middle ear ventilation. Ann. Otol. Rhinol. Laryngol. 86(Suppl. 41):1–15, 1977b.

Cantekin, E. I., Saez, C. A., Bluestone, C. D., and Bern, S. A.: Airflow through the eustachian tube. Ann. Otol. Rhinol. Laryngol. 88:603–612, 1979.

Cantekin, E. I., Bluestone, C. D., Fria, T. J., Stool, S. E., Beery, Q. C., and Sabo, D. L.: Identification of otitis media with effusion. Ann. Otol. Rhinol. Laryngol. 89(68):190–195, 1980.

Casselbrant M. L., Brostoff, L. M., Cantekin, E. I., Flaherty, M. R., Doyle, W. J., Bluestone, C. D., and Fria, T. J.: Otitis media with effusion in preschool children. Laryngoscope 95:428–436, 1985.

Chaudhuri, P. K., and Bowen-Jones, E.: An otorhinolaryngological study of children with cleft palates. J. Laryngol. Otol. 92(1):29–40, 1978.

Cohn, A. M., Schwaber, M. K., Anthony, L. S., and Jerger, J. F.: Eustachian tube function and tympanoplasty. Ann. Otol. Rhinol. Laryngol. 88:339–347, 1979.

Cooper, J. C., Gates, G., Owen, J., and Dickson, H.: An abbreviated impedance bridge technique for school screening. J. Speech Hear. Dis. 40:260–269, 1974.

Craig, H. B., Stool, S. E., and Laird, M. A.: Project "ears": Otologic maintenance in a school for the deaf. Am. Ann. Deaf 124:458–467, 1979.

Crain, E. F., and Shelov, S. P.: Febrile infants: Predictors of bacteremia. J. Pediatr. 101:686–689, 1982.

Crysdale, W. S.: Rational management of middle ear effusions in cleft palate patients. J. Otolaryngol. 5(6):463–467, 1976.

Downs, M. P.: Identification of children at risk for middle ear effusion problems. Ann. Otol. Rhinol. Laryngol. 89(68):168–171, 1980.

Drettner, B.: The nasal airway and hearing in patients with cleft palate. Acta Otolaryngol. (Stockh.) 52:131–142, 1960.

Edell, S. L., and Isaacson, S.: A-mode ultrasound evaluation of the maxillary sinus. Otolaryngol. Clin. North Am. 11(2):531–540, 1978.

Ekvall, L.: Eustachian tube function in tympanoplasty. Acta Otolaryngol. (Stockh.) Suppl. 263:33–42, 1970.

Elner, A., Ingelstedt, S., and Ivarsson A.: The normal function of the eustachian tube. Acta Otolaryngol. (Stockh.) 72:320–328, 1971.

Eviatar, L., and Eviatar, A.: The neurovestibular testing of infants and children. In Bluestone, C. D., and Stool, S. E. (Eds.): Pediatric Otolaryngology. Philadelphia, W.B. Saunders Co., 1983, pp. 199–212.

Feingold, M., Klein, J. O., Haslam, G. E., Tilles, J. G., Finland, M., and Gellis, S. S.: Acute otitis media in children: Bacteriological findings in middle ear fluid obtained by needle aspiration. Am. J. Dis. Child. 111:361–365, 1966.

Ferrer, H.: Use of impedance audiometry in school screening. Public Health 88:153–163, 1974.

Findlay, R. C., Stool, S. E., and Svitko, C. A.: Tympanometric and otoscopic evaluations of a school-age deaf population: A longitudinal study. Am. Ann. Deaf 122:407–413, 1977.

Fria, T. J., Sabo, D., and Beery, Q. C.: The acoustic reflex in the identification of otitis media with effusion. Presented at the American Speech and Hearing Association National Convention, 1978.

Fria, T. J., Cantekin, E. I., and Probst, G.: Validation of an automatic otoadmittance middle ear analyzer. Ann. Otol. Rhinol. Laryngol. 89:253–256, 1980.

Fria, T. J., and Sabo, D. L.: Auditory brainstem responses in children with otitis media with effusion. Ann. Otol. Rhinol. Laryngol. 89(68):200–206, 1980.

Fria, T. J., Cantekin, E. I., and Eichler, J. A.: Hearing acuity of children with otitis media with effusion. Arch. Otolaryngol. 111:10–16, 1985.

Gates, G. A., Avery, C., Cooper, J. C., Hearne, E. M., and Holt, G. R.: Predictive value of tympanometry in middle ear effusion. Ann. Otol. Rhinol. Laryngol. 95(1):46–50, 1986.

Gershel, J., Kruger, B., Giraudi-Perry, D., Chobot, J., et al.: Accuracy of the Welch Allyn audioscope and traditional hearing screening for children with known hearing loss. J. Pediatr. 106(1):15–20, 1985.

Goetzinger, C. O., Embrey, J. E., Brooks, R., and Proud, G. O.: Auditory assessment of cleft palate adults. Acta Otolaryngol. (Stockh.) 52:551–557, 1960.

Graham, M. D.: A longitudinal study of ear disease and hearing loss in patients with cleft lips and palates. TAAOO 67:213–222, 1963.

Graham, M. D., and Lierle, D. M.: Posterior pharyngeal flap palatoplasty and its relation to ear disease and hearing loss: A preliminary report. Laryngoscope 72:1750–1755, 1962.

Grason, R. L.: Otoadmittance meters. *In Proceedings of Impedance Symposium*, Rochester, Mn., 1972.

Greene, J. W., Hara, C., O'Connor, S., and Altemeier, W. A., III: Management of febrile outpatient neonates. Clin. Pediatr. 20:375–380, 1981.

Gutzman, H.: Zur prognose und behandlung der angeborenen gaumendefekte. Mschr. Sprachheilk., 1893.

Halfond, M. M., and Ballenger, J. J.: An audiologic and otorhinologic study of cleft lip and cleft palate cases. Arch. Otolaryngol. 64:58–62, 1956.

Harding, A. L., Anderson, P., Howie, V. M., Ploussard, J. H., and Smith, D. H.: *Haemophilus influenzae* isolated from children with otitis media. *In Sell, S. H. W., and Kargon, D. T. (Eds.): Haemophilus influenzae.* Nashville, Vanderbilt University Press, 1973, pp. 21–28.

Harford, E. R., Bess, F. H., Bluestone, C. D., and Klein, J. O.: *Impedance Screening for Middle Ear Disease in Children.* New York, Grune & Stratton, 1978.

Harker, L. A., and Van Wagoner, R.: Application of impedance audiometry as a screening instrument. Acta Otolaryngol. (Stockh.) 77:198–201, 1974.

Harrison, R. J., and Phillips, B. J.: Observations on hearing losses of preschool cleft palate children. J. Speech Hear. Dis. 36(2):252–256, 1971.

Hayden, G. F., and Schwartz, R. H.: Characteristics of earache among children with acute otitis media. Am. J. Dis. Child. 139:721–723, 1985.

Heller, J. C., Hochberg, L., and Milano, G.: Audiologic and otologic evaluation of cleft palate children. Cleft Palate J. 7:774–783, 1970.

Holborow, C.: Eustachian tube function. Arch. Otolaryngol. 92:624–626, 1970.

Holmes, E. M., and Reed, G. F.: Hearing and deafness in cleft palate patients. Arch. Otolaryngol. 62:620–624, 1955.

Holmquist, J.: The role of the eustachian tube in myringoplasty. Acta Otolaryngol. (Stockh.) 66:289–295, 1968.

Howie, V. M., Ploussard, J. H., and Sloyer, J: The "otitis prone" condition. Am. J. Dis. Child. 129:676–678, 1975.

Ingelstedt S., and Ortegren, U.: Qualitative testing of the eustachian tube function. Acta Otolaryngol. (Stockh.) Suppl. 182:7–23, 1963.

Ingelstedt, S., Ivarsson, A., and Jonson, A.: Mechanics of the human middle ear: Pressure regulation in aviation and diving, a nontraumatic method. Acta Otolaryngol. (Stockh.) Suppl. 228:1–57, 1967.

Ingvarsson, L.: Acute otalgia in children—findings and diagnosis. Acta Pediatr. Scand. 71:705–710, 1982.

Kaufman, R. S.: Hearing loss in children with cleft palates. N.Y. State J. Med. 70(20):2555–2558, 1970.

Korsan-Bergsten, M., and Nylen, O.: A follow-up study of cleft children treated with primary bone grafting. Scand. J. Plast. Recon. Surg. 8:161–163, 1974.

Lahikainen, E. A.: Clinico-bacteriologic studies on acute otitis media: Aspiration of tympanum as diagnostic and therapeutic method. Acta Otolaryngol. (Stockh.) Suppl. 107:1–82, 1953.

Lampe, R. M., Weir, M. R., Spier, J., and Rhodes, M. F.: Acoustic reflectometry in the detection of middle ear effusion. Pediatrics 76:75–78, 1985.

Lee, K., and Schuknecht, H. F.: Results of tympanoplasty and mastoidectomy at the Massachusetts Eye and Ear Infirmary. Laryngoscope 81:529–543, 1971.

Lewis, A. N., Barry, M., and Stuart, J.: Screening procedures for the identification of hearing and ear disorders in Australian aboriginal children. J. Laryngol. Otol. 88:335–347, 1974.

Lindsay, W. K., LeMeusurier, A. B., and Farmer, A. W.: A study of the speech results of a large series of cleft palate patients. Plast. Reconstr. Surg. 29:273–288, 1962.

Linthicum, F. H., Body, H., and Keaster, J.: Incidence of middle ear disease in children with cleft palate. Cleft Palate Bull. 9:23–25, 1959.

Loeb, W. J.: Speech, hearing and the cleft palate. Arch. Otolaryngol. 79:4–14, 1964.

Long, S. S., Henretig, F. M., Teter, M. J., and McGowan, K. L.: Nasopharyngeal flora and acute otitis media. Infect. Immunol. 41:987–991, 1984.

Masters, F. W., Bingham, H. G., and Robinson, D. W.: The prevention and treatment of hearing loss in the cleft palate child. Plast. Reconstr. Surg 25:503–509, 1960.

McCandless, G. A., and Thomas, G. K.: Impedance audiometry as a screening procedure for middle ear disease. TAAOO, 78:98–102, 1974.

McCurdy, J. A., Goldstein, J. L., and Gorski, D.: Auditory screening of preschool children with impedance audiometry—a comparison with pure tone audiometry. Clin. Pediatr. 15:436–441, 1976.

Means, B. J., and Irwin, J. V.: An analysis of certain measures of intelligence and hearing loss in a sample of Wisconsin cleft palate population. Cleft Palate Bull. 4:4, 1954.

Mehta, D., and Erlich, M.: Serous otitis media in a school for the deaf. Volta Rev. 80:75–80, 1978.

Meissner, K.: Ohrenerkrankungen bei gaumenspalten. Hals-Nasen-und Ohrenarzt 30:6–20, 1939.

Miller, M. H.: Hearing losses in cleft palate cases: The incidence, type and significance. Laryngoscope 66:1492–1496, 1956.

Miller, G. F., and Bilodeau, R.: Preoperative evaluation of eustachian tubal function in tympanoplasty. South Med. J. 60:868, 1967.

Mortimer, E. A., Jr., and Watterson, R. L., Jr.: A bacteriologic investigation of otitis media in infancy. Pediatrics 17:359–366, 1956.

Murti, K., Stern, R., Catekin, E. I., and Bluestone, C. D.: Sonometric evaluation of eustachian tube function using broadband stimuli. Ann. Otol. Rhinol. Laryngol. 89(Suppl. 68):178–184, 1980.

Noone, R. B., Randall, P., Stool, S. E., Hamilton, R., and Winchester, R. A.: The effect on middle ear disease of fracture of the pterygoid hamulus during palatoplasty. Cleft Palate J. 10:23–33, 1973.

Northern, J.,.L., and Downs, M. P. (Eds.): *Hearing in Children.* 2nd Ed. Baltimore, The Williams and Wilkins, Co., 1978.

Orchik, D. J., and Herdman, S.: Impedance audiometry as a screening device with school-age children. J. Aud. Res. 14:283–286, 1974.

Pannbacker, M.: Hearing loss and cleft palate. Cleft Palate J. 6:50–56, 1969.

Paparella, M. M., Oda, M., Hiraide, F., and Brady, D.: Pathology of sensorineural hearing loss in otitis media. Ann. Otol. Rhinol. Laryngol. 81:632–647, 1972.

Paradise, J. L.: Otitis media in infants and children. Pediatrics 65:917–943, 1980.

Paradise, J. L., Bluestone, C. D., and Felder, H.: The universality of otitis media in fifty infants with cleft palate. Pediatrics 44:35–42, 1969.

Paradise, J. L., and Bluestone, C. D.: Early treatment of the universal otitis media of infants with cleft palate. Pediatrics 53:48–54, 1974.

Paradise, J. L., Smith, C. G., and Bluestone, C. D.: Tympanometric detection of middle ear effusion in infants and young children. Pediatrics 58:198–210, 1976.

Paradise, J. L., and Smith, C. G.: Impedance screening for preschool children—state of the art. *In* Harford, E. R., Bess, F. H., Bluestone, C. D., and Klein, J. O. (Eds.): *Impedance Screening for Middle Ear Disease in Children.* New York, Grune & Stratton, 1978, pp. 113–124.

Pfisterer, H.: Recent knowledge concerning impairment of hearing in patients with palatal fissure. HNO (Berl.) 6:307–309, 1958.

Porter, T. A.: Otoadmittance measurements in a residential deaf population. Am. Ann. Deaf 119:47–52, 1974.

Potsic, W. P., Cohen, M., Randall, P., and Winchester, R.: A retrospective study of hearing impairment in three groups of cleft palate patients. Cleft Palate J. 16(1):56–58, 1979.

Renvall, U., Liden, G., Jungert, S., and Nilsson, E.: Impedance audiometry as a screening method in schoolchildren. Scand. Audiol. 2:133–137, 1973.

Revonta, M.: A-mode ultrasound of maxillary sinusitis in children (Letter). Lancet 1:320, 1979.

Riding, K. H., Bluestone, C. D., Michaels, R. H., Cantekin, E. I., Doyle, W. J., and Poziviak, C.: Microbiology of recurrent and chronic otitis media with effusion. J. Pediatr. 93:739–743, 1978a.

Riding, K. H., Reichert, T. J., Findlay, R. C., and Stool, S. E.: Tympanometric and otologic evaluation of students in a school for the deaf. *In* Harford, E. R., Bess, F. H., Bluestone, C. D., and Klein, J. O. (Eds.): *Impedance Screening for Middle Ear Disease in Children.* New York, Grune & Stratton, 1978b, pp. 279–291.

Roberts, M. E.: Comparative study of pure tone, impedance, and otoscopic hearing screening methods. Arch. Otolaryngol. 102:690–694, 1976.

Roberts, K. B., and Borzy, M. S.: Fever in the first eight weeks of life. Johns Hopkins Med. J. 11:9–13, 1977.

Ruben, R. J., and Math, R.: Serous otitis media associated with sensorineural hearing loss in children. Laryngoscope 88:1139–1154, 1978.

Rubin, M.: Serous otitis media in severely to profoundly hearing impaired children, ages 0 to 6. Volta Rev. 80:81–85, 1978.

Sataloff, J., and Fraser, M.: Hearing loss in children with cleft palates. Arch. Otolaryngol. 55:61–64, 1952.

Schlesinger, P. C.: The significance of fever in infants less than three months old: A retrospective review of one year's experience at Boston City Hospital's pediatric walk-in clinic. Thesis submitted to the Yale University School of Medicine, 1982.

Schwartz, R., Rodriguez, W. J., Mann, R., Khan, W., and Ross, S.: The nasopharyngeal culture in acute otitis media: A reappraisal of its usefulness. JAMA 241:2170–2173, 1979.

Schwartz, R. H., Rodriguez, W. J., Brook, I., and Grundfast, K. M.: The febrile response in acute otitis media. JAMA 245:2057–2058, 1981.

Schwartz, R. H., Rodriguez, W. J., McAveney, W., and Grundfast, K. M.: Cerumen removal: How necessary is it to diagnose acute otitis media? Am. J. Dis. Child. 137:1064–1065, 1983.

Severeid, L. R.: A longitudinal study of the efficacy of adenoidectomy in children with cleft palate and secondary otitis media. TAAOO 76:1319–1324, 1972.

Shurin, P. A., Pelton, S. I., and Finkelstein, B. A.: Tympanometry in the diagnosis of middle ear effusions. N. Engl. J. Med. 296:412–417, 1977.

Shurin, P. A., Howie, V. M., Pelton, S. I., Ploussard, J. H., and Klein, J. O.: Bacteriology of otitis media during the first six weeks of life. J. Pediatr. 92:893–896, 1978.

Siedentop, K. H.: Eustachian tube dynamics, size of the mastoid air cell system, and results with tympanoplasty. Otolaryngol. Clin. North Am. 5:33–44, 1972.

Skolnick, E. M.: Otologic evaluation in cleft palate patients. Laryngoscope 68:1908–1949, 1958.

Spriesterbach, D. C., Lierle, D. M., Moll, K. L., Prather, W. F.: Hearing loss in children with cleft palates. Plast. Reconstr. Surg. 30:336–347, 1962.

Stool, S. E., and Randall, P.: Unexpected ear disease in infants with cleft palate. Cleft Palate J. 4:99–103, 1967.

Stool, S. E., Craig, H. B., and Laird, M. A.: Screening for middle ear disease in a school for the deaf. Ann. Otol. Rhinol. Laryngol. 89(68):172–177, 1980.

Supance, J. S., and Bluestone, C. D.: Perilymph fistulas in infants and children. Otolaryngol. Head Neck Surg. 91:663–671, 1983.

Taylor, G. D.: The bifid uvula. Laryngoscope 82:771–778, 1972.

Teele, D. W., Pelton, S. I., Grant, M. J. A., Herskowitz, J., Rosen, D. J., Allen, C. E., Wimmer, R. S., and Klein, J. O.: Bacteremia in febrile children under 2 years of age: Results of cultures of blood of 600 consecutive febrile children seen in a walk-in clinic. J. Pediatr. 87:227–230, 1975.

Teele, D. W., Klein, J. O., and Rosner, B. A.: Epidemiology of otitis media in children. Ann. Otol. Rhinol. Laryngol. 89(68):5–6, 1980.

Teele, D. W., and Teele, J.: Detection of middle ear effusion by acoustic reflectometry. J. Pediatr. 104:832–838, 1984.

Terkildsen, K., and Nielsen, S. S.: An electroacoustic impedance measuring bridge for clinical use. Arch. Otolaryngol. 72:339–346, 1960.

Tetzlaff, T. F., Ashworth, C., and Nelson, J. D.: Otitis media in children less than 12 weeks of age. Pediatrics 59:827–832, 1977.

Thorington, J.: Almost total destruction of the velum palati corrected by an artificial soft palate, producing not only greatly improved speech, but an immediate increase of audition. Med. News Phila., 61:269–272, 1892.

Variot, G.: Ecoulement de lait par l'oreille d'un nourrisson atteint de devision congenitale du voile du palais. Bull. Soc. de Ped. de Paris 6:387, 1904.

Virtanen H.: Sonotubometry: An acoustical method for objective measurement of auditory tubal opening. Acta Otolaryngol. (Stockh.) 96:93–103, 1978.

Virtanen, H., Palva, T., and Jauhiainen, T.: The prognostic value of eustachian tube function measurements in tympanoplastic surgery. Acta Otolaryngol. (Stockh.) 90:317–323, 1980.

Walton, W. K.: Audiometrically "normal" conductive hearing losses among the cleft palate. Cleft Palate J. 10:99–103, 1973.

Webster, J. C.: Middle ear function in the cleft palate patient. J. Laryngol. Otol. 94(1):31–37, 1980.

Whaley, J. B.: Otolaryngologist's role in the care of cleft palate patients. J. Can. Dent. Assist. 23:574–575, 1957.

Yules, R. B.: Hearing in cleft palate patients. Arch. Otolaryngol. 91:319–323, 1970.

8

Management

The different stages of otitis media and atelectasis are most frequently a continuum, and it is often difficult for the clinician to diagnose the precise stage of a patient's illness accurately. Before the detailed methods of management are presented, an initial overall management plan for each clinical type and the treatment options available will be described (Table 8–1).

OVERVIEW

Acute Otitis Media

Figure 8–1 is a diagram of a recommended management plan for children with acute otitis media. Infants and children who have signs and symptoms of acute otitis media should receive antimicrobial therapy; however, several investigators have questioned

Table 8–1. **OPTIONS FOR MANAGING VARIOUS STAGES OF OTITIS MEDIA**

Antimicrobials
Decongestants
Antihistamines
Corticosteroids
Immunization
Hyposensitization (allergy control)
Inflation of eustachian tube and
  middle ear
Myringotomy with or without
  tympanostomy tube
Adenoidectomy with or without
  tonsillectomy
Tympanoplasty
Tympanomastoidectomy
Watchful waiting
Hearing aid

the need for antimicrobial agents in all cases (Diamant and Diamant, 1974; Laxdal et al., 1970; Mygind et al., 1981; van Buchem et al., 1981). Because the rate of suppurative complications has decreased in the antibiotic era (Sorenson, 1977), antimicrobial therapy is still the treatment of choice.

Since the same bacteria found in acute middle ear effusions have been isolated from the ears not only of children who lack the classic signs and symptoms of acute otitis media but also of those who have chronic effusions, all children who have otitis media, regardless of the stage, should receive an antimicrobial agent if one has not been given during the recent past.

Choice of Antimicrobial Agent

Amoxicillin or ampicillin is the currently preferred drug for initial empiric treatment of otitis media, since both are active both *in vitro* and *in vivo* against *Streptococcus pneumoniae* and *Haemophilus influenzae*. Other regimens that are satisfactory include amoxicillin-clavulanate, trimethoprim-sulfamethoxazole, cefaclor, cefuroxime axetil, cefixime, and combinations of a sulfonamide with benzathine penicillin G (administered by the intramuscular route as a single injection), oral penicillin G or V, or erythromycin. For the child who is allergic to penicillins, trimethoprim-sulfamethoxazole and erythromycin or clindamycin combined with a sulfonamide provide equivalent antimicrobial coverage. If the child has acute otitis media with otorrhea or tympanocentesis was initially performed, Gram's stain, culture, and susceptibility studies of the causative organism will provide

121

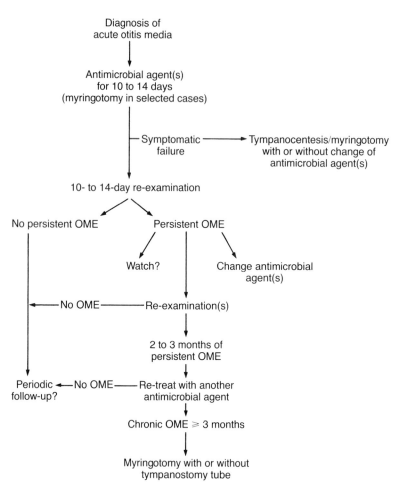

Figure 8–1. Recommended management plan for children with acute otitis media (see text).

more precise selection of an antimicrobial agent (Table 8–2).

Dosage Schedules

Dosage schedules have been determined on the basis of studies of clinical pharmacology and results of clinical trials. Oral ampicillin, 50 to 100 mg/kg/24 hr, in four divided doses for 10 days, is recommended. Amoxicillin, 40 mg/kg/24 hr, is equally effective, can be given in three divided doses, and has fewer side effects such as diarrhea. If the child is allergic to the penicillins, then a

Table 8–2. **EFFICACY OF SELECTED ANTIMICROBIAL AGENTS FOR THE COMMON PATHOGENS IN ACUTE OTITIS MEDIA***

Antimicrobial Agents	S. pneumoniae	H. influenzae Non-beta-lactamase	H. influenzae Beta-lactamase	B. catarrhalis Non-beta-lactamase	B. catarrhalis Beta-lactamase	S. pyogenes
Ampicillin or amoxicillin	+	+	−	+	−	+
Amoxicillin-clavulanate	+	+	+	+	+	+
Penicillin V	+	−	−	+	−	+
Erythromycin	+	−	−	+	+	+
Sulfonamides	−	+	+	+	+	−
Erythromycin-sulfisoxazole	+	+	+	+	+	+
Trimethoprim-sulfamethoxazole	+	+	+	+	+	−
Cefaclor	+	+	+	+	±	+
Cefixime	+	+	+	+	+	+

*Based on available data from clinical trials and *in vitro* studies. Key: + = effective; − = not effective; ± = variable effectiveness.

combination of oral erythromycin, 40 mg/kg/24 hr, and sulfisoxazole, 120 mg/kg/24 hr, in four divided doses is a suitable alternative. Availability of a fixed combination of these two antimicrobial agents is an attractive choice, since patient compliance is improved when only one medication need be given instead of two. If beta-lactamase–producing *H. influenzae* or *B. catarrhalis* is suspected or documented by tympanocentesis, then appropriate choices would be amoxicillin-clavulanate (dosage based on amoxicillin content), trimethoprim-sulfamethoxazole (8 mg trimethoprim and 40 mg sulfamethoxazole per kg/24 hr), cefaclor, 40 mg/kg/24 hr, in three divided doses, or cefixime, 8 mg/kg given in one dose. Intramuscular benzathine penicillin G is an alternative choice if the child is vomiting, there is difficulty in oral administration, or there is doubt concerning patient compliance with the prescribed regimen. This agent is effective against *S. pneumoniae* and *Streptococcus pyogenes,* but it must be combined with a sulfonamide for coverage of *H. influenzae.*

Duration of Therapy

Physicians must rely on empirically derived schedules of therapy to plan drug regimens that lead to rapid and complete resolution of disease but minimal risk in terms of clinical or microbiological failure or drug toxicity. The dosage schedules presented in Table 8–3 are appropriate for a 10-day course on the basis of currently available data.

Other dosage schedules, longer or shorter than the traditional 10- to 14-day course, may be as good, if not better. Studies compared the results of 3- and 10-day courses of amoxicillin (Chaput de Saintonge et al., 1982), treatment with penicillin V for two or seven days (Meistrup-Larsen et al., 1983), and penicillin V administered for five or 10 days (Ingvarsson and Lundgren, 1982). In each study, the shorter course was similar in clinical results to the longer course. Methodological problems, including absence of microbiological diagnosis, limit the validity of the results.

Clinical Course

With appropriate antimicrobial therapy, most children with acute bacterial otitis media are significantly improved within 48 to 72 hours. The physician should be in contact with the patient to ascertain that improvement has occurred; children whose course has become worse should be re-examined by the clinician, since a suppurative complication may have developed. At this stage a tympanocentesis for microbiological diagnosis and possibly myringotomy for drainage is the most effective management option. Complications of otitis media are described in chapters 9 and 10.

If there is persistence or recurrence of otalgia or fever, or both, then the child should also be re-examined before the completion of the antibiotic course. For certain

Table 8–3. DAILY DOSAGE SCHEDULE FOR ANTIMICROBIAL AGENTS USEFUL IN OTITIS MEDIA

Agent	Dosage/24 Hr
Penicillin G	50,000 units/kg in 4 doses*
Penicillin G	600,000 units in 1 dose for ≤30-kg child
(benzathine salt)†	1,200,000 units in 1 dose for >30-kg child
Penicillin V	50 mg/kg in 4 doses
Amoxicillin	40 mg/kg in 3 doses.
Ampicillin	50–100 mg/kg in 4 doses*
Amoxicillin-clavulanate	40 mg/kg in 3 doses
Bacampicillin	25–50 mg/kg in 2 doses
Cyclacillin	50–100 mg/kg in 3 doses
Oxacillin	50 mg/kg in 4 doses*
Cloxacillin	50 mg/kg in 4 doses*
Dicloxacillin	25 mg/kg in 4 doses*
Nafcillin	50 mg/kg in 4 doses*
Cephalexin	100 mg/kg in 4 doses*
Cefaclor	40 mg/kg in 3 doses
Cefixime	8 mg/kg in 1 dose
Erythromycin	40 mg/kg in 4 doses
Clindamycin	25 mg/kg in 4 doses
Sulfisoxazole	120 mg/kg in 4 doses
Trisulfapyrimidine	120 mg/kg in 4 doses
Trimethoprim-sulfamethoxazole (TMP-SMZ)	8 mg TMP and 40 mg SMZ in 2 doses

*Schedule at least one hour before or two hours after meals.
†Intramuscular route; all others are oral dosages.

children in whom severe signs and symptoms of acute infection are present, or for social considerations (e.g., poor home environment), it may be more advantageous to re-examine the child 48 to 72 hours after therapy is initiated. However, at this time the appearance of the tympanic membrane alone should not determine a change in the treatment. Almost all children will have a persistent middle ear effusion, and even erythema and bulging of the tympanic membrane may still be present. Persistent pain or fever, or both, would signal the need either for surgical intervention or for selection of another antimicrobial agent, or for both. Tympanocentesis with or without a myringotomy should be offered as a logical management option in such cases, since culture of the middle ear effusion may reveal the presence of an unusual organism. Further antimicrobial treatment should be based on the results of the culture. If surgery is not feasible (the parents or child might refuse surgery, or the physician is not accustomed to performing this type of surgery, in which case an otolaryngologist should be consulted), then a new antibiotic should be administered. This antibiotic should be chosen to be effective against any unusual bacteria that have been found to be in the community and that have been associated with the treatment failures during the first 10 days. Examples of this situation would be the presence of *H. influenzae* or *B. catarrhalis* that are resistant to ampicillin.

The current incidence of strains of ampicillin-resistant *H. influenzae* and *B. catarrhalis* is low in most communities, and does not require a change in recommendations for initial therapy. However, if the patient does not respond to initial therapy with ampicillin or amoxicillin, infection with a resistant strain of *H. influenzae* or *B. catarrhalis* should be considered. Toxicity with persistent or recurrent fever or otalgia, or both, should prompt the clinician to recommend tympanocentesis or myringotomy, or both, to identify the causative organism; a specific antimicrobial agent may then be chosen on the basis of the results of the culture of the middle ear effusion and sensitivity testing. However, if signs persist but the child shows no toxic symptoms and aspiration to culture the middle ear effusion is not performed, the initial antimicrobial agent should be changed to a regimen to which beta-lactamase–producing *H. influenzae* or *B. catarrhalis* would be sensitive. If ampicillin or amoxicillin was initially

given, then the combination of erythromycin-sulfisoxazole or amoxicillin-clavulanate or trimethoprim-sulfamethoxazole should be administered. Trimethoprim-sulfamethoxazole is not effective when *S. pyogenes* is the causative organism and therefore should not be the drug of choice for initial treatment of otitis media.

In patients with unusually severe earache or toxic symptoms, tympanocentesis and myringotomy may be performed initially in order to provide immediate relief. Tympanocentesis (and possibly myringotomy) should also be performed if the child develops acute otitis media while taking for another condition an antimicrobial agent that should have been effective against the common pathogens that cause otitis. When therapeutic drainage is required for the indications that will be outlined, a myringotomy knife should be used and the incision should be large enough to allow for adequate drainage of the middle ear.

Children may be re-examined at the end of the course of antibiotic therapy, after 10 to 14 days. At this time, some children will have a persistent middle ear effusion: Table 4–3 in Chapter Four, Epidemiology, shows this proportion to be approximately half of those treated with antibiotics. Since the presence of a persistent middle ear effusion after a 10-day trial of an antimicrobial agent is common, this finding alone is not sufficient grounds for performing surgery such as myringotomy and tympanostomy tube insertion.

Although some children who fail clinically at the conclusion of a course of therapy do so because of a bacterial pathogen resistant to initial therapy, many children have bacteria that are susceptible to the drug, and some have negative bacterial cultures and presumably have either a nonbacterial micro-organism as the cause of otitis media or some other reason for the persistent fever.

Neonates and Immunocompromised Children

The method of management of acute otitis media may vary with the age of the patient. Acute otitis media during the neonatal period may warrant more aggressive management than such a condition in an older child. Bland (1972) reported that otitis media in neonates was frequently caused by a more unusual organism than those that usually cause such problems in older infants and in children (i.e., gram-negative bacilli or *S. aureus*). Following this report, many authorities advocated treating these babies in the hospital according to protocols for neonatal sepsis, since the infection could be life-threatening. However, since then other investigators (Schwartz et al., 1978; Shurin et al., 1976, 1978; Tetzlaff et al., 1977) have shown that the incidence of these unusual organisms is relatively low, especially in neonates who were apparently well when discharged from the hospital following birth and then developed an acute otitis media while at home. For these neonates, the acute otitis media should be treated as described above for older infants and children. However, if the neonate appears to be severely ill with toxic symptoms, hospitalization and a tympanocentesis and, possibly, myringotomy is indicated. If the baby is still hospitalized following delivery and develops otitis media, tympanocentesis and myringotomy are indicated, since infection at this time can be life-threatening. Culture of the middle ear aspirate may reveal an unusual organism that would require treatment with an antimicrobial agent different from the antibiotics recommended for treatment of acute otitis media in older children.

The management of acute otitis media may be different in certain infants and children whose underlying condition is known to be associated with otitis caused by an unusual organism. Such children would be primarily those who are immunologically compromised. Tympanocentesis possibly followed by myringotomy would be indicated in an effort to identify the causative organisms and to promote drainage.

Adjunctive Therapies

Additional supportive therapy, including analgesics, antipyretics, and local heat, will usually be helpful. An oral decongestant, such as pseudoephedrine hydrochloride, may relieve nasal congestion, and antihistamines may help patients with known or suspected nasal allergy. However, the efficacy of antihistamines and decongestants in the treatment of acute otitis media has not been proved.

Complete clearing of the effusion may take six weeks or longer. Within two to three months the tympanic membrane should be entirely normal. If complete resolution has occurred and the episode represents the only known attack, the patient may be discharged. However, periodic follow-up is indicated for patients who have had recurrent episodes.

Persistent Middle Ear Effusion

If the middle ear fluid is persistent after the initial 10 to 14 days of antimicrobial therapy, one or more of the following treatment options have been advocated to hasten the resolution of the effusion during the next, *subacute,* phase:
1. Another 10 to 14 day course of the antimicrobial agent prescribed originally, since the ideal duration of therapy has yet to be established;
2. A course of an antimicrobial agent different from the initial one, based on the hope that if a resistant organism is present, the new antimicrobial agent may be effective;
3. A topical or systemic nasal decongestant or antihistamine, or a combination of these drugs;
4. Eustachian tube–middle ear inflation employing the method of Valsalva or Politzer.

Unfortunately, none of these commonly employed methods appear to be helpful; they have not been shown to be effective in randomized, controlled trials of children with subacute otitis media with effusion, and the combination of systemic decongestant and antihistamine has been shown to be ineffective for this stage of otitis media (Cantekin et al., 1983). At present, the best treatment for children who have asymptomatic otitis media with effusion still present after two weeks is watchful waiting with re-examination of the ears six weeks later (i.e., two months after the initial visit). At this time, most patients should have a middle ear that is effusion-free (see Table 4–3, Chapter Four, Epidemiology). However, treatment with another antimicrobial that is effective against possible resistant bacteria is a reasonable alternative. If the child still has otitis media with effusion after two or three months, the effusion is chronic and should be treated as described later under the heading "Otitis Media with Effusion" (page 127).

Recurrent Acute Otitis Media

It is not uncommon for an infant to have recurrent bouts of acute otitis media. Some children develop an acute episode with almost every respiratory tract infection, have more or less dramatic symptoms, respond well to therapy, and improve with advancing age. Others may have persistent middle ear effusion and suffer recurrent episodes of acute otitis media superimposed on the chronic disorder. The child with recurrent acute otitis media that completely clears between episodes may be managed as previously outlined. However, if the bouts are frequent and close together, prevention of further attacks is desirable, and the patient requires further evaluation. Several avenues of investigation are open: a search for respiratory allergy may prove fruitful; roentgenograms of the paranasal sinuses may reveal sinusitis; immunological studies may be of value if other organs are involved (the lung, for example). In addition, more thorough physical examination may reveal abnormalities, such as submucous cleft palate or a tumor of the nasopharynx, that require definitive management. If none of these conditions is present, then one or more of the popular methods of prevention may be attempted; however, the efficacy of these various modalities has yet to be proved in acceptable clinical trials. For infants and children who have frequent episodes (such as three or more episodes within the preceding six months) of acute otitis media without middle ear effusion in between the bouts, the most common non-surgical and surgical methods currently employed for prevention are (1) chemoprophylaxis with one or more of the following—antibiotics, topical or systemic nasal decongestants, or antihistamines; (2) myringotomy with or without insertion of tympanostomy tubes; (3) adenoidectomy with or without tonsillectomy. Pneumococcal vaccine is of limited efficacy in infants and should be considered only for children two years of age and older; *H. influenzae* type B vaccine is also effective for children two years of age and older, but the incidence of this organism as the cause of otitis media is only about one percent, and the vaccine is not effective for infants.

Chemoprophylaxis implies use of drugs in anticipation of infection, whereas treatment implies use of drugs after infection has taken place or signs of infectious disease are evident. Although indiscriminate use of antimicrobial agents for prophylaxis is to be avoided, many forms of chemoprophylaxis have been extensively tested and are of proven value. Recent studies suggest that chemoprophylaxis may be effetive in children with recurrent episodes of acute otitis media. Prophylaxis is discussed in the section on the use of antimicrobial agents in this chapter (page 163).

At present, there is no evidence that a topical or systemic nasal decongestant or antihistamine, either alone or in combination, administered daily or at the onset of an upper respiratory tract infection, prevents recurrent acute otitis media. Therefore, the use of such medications for prophylaxis is not recommended until their efficacy is proved.

Myringotomy as initial treatment for acute otitis media should only be considered in selected patients. Myringotomy with insertion of tympanostomy tubes is commonly performed to prevent recurrent episodes of acute otitis media. The procedure is usually performed after the signs and symptoms of the acute otitis media have resolved, but it may be performed during an acute episode if persistent otalgia or fever, or both, are present in a child who has had frequently recurrent episodes. A prospective randomized study by Gebhart (1981) was conducted in 95 children who had multiple episodes of acute otitis media. Comparison of infection rates was made between patients treated with conventional antibiotic therapy for each episode and patients who had tympanostomy tubes placed. Placement of tympanostomy tubes significantly decreased the number of episodes of acute purulent otitis media during a six-month observation period. However, children with and without middle ear effusions were admitted into the study.

Adenoidectomy with or without tonsillectomy is frequently advocated for the prevention of recurrent acute otitis media, but randomized, controlled studies reported in the past have not proved the efficacy of these procedures for this condition (Bluestone, 1979). However, some children may be benefited by adenoidectomy (and possibly tonsillectomy), whereas others fail to show a reduction in the number of subsequent episodes following these procedures, and still others improve with advancing age without being subjected to these procedures. At present, adenoidectomy, or tonsillectomy, or both procedures, must remain of uncertain benefit for children who have recurrent acute otitis media, and recommendations for these procedures should be individualized. For example, children who frequently have recurrent pharyngotonsillitis or moderate to severe airway obstruction secondary to tonsils-adenoids, would be more likely candidates than those who lack these conditions.

In summary, the parents of a child who has frequently recurrent episodes of acute otitis media in whom the effusion appears to clear between bouts should be offered the following management options: (1) antimicrobial treatment of each episode, (2) antimicrobial prophylaxis, (3) myringotomy and tympanostomy tube insertion, or (4) administration of pneumococcal vaccine if the patient is two years of age or older. The treatment option selected should involve the parents and possibly the child (if old enough) in the decision-making process. A few parents choose to watch and wait, usually if the episodes have been mild or relatively infrequent. At present, the decision should be between administering an antibiotic in a prophylactic dose or performing myringotomy and insertion of a tympanostomy tube. Since neither of these two procedures has been shown to be superior to the other, or even to watchful waiting, the decision should be based upon the parent's and (child's) willingness to have the child take daily medication as a preventative measure or to have surgery performed on the child's ear, which usually involves the administration of general anesthetic. The possibility of an adverse reaction occurring with either method should be discussed fully with the family. Usually a decision in favor of one of the treatment options is arrived at by this method, since some parents are unwilling to give a daily antibiotic or are concerned about the possible side effects of long-term antibiotic treatment, whereas other parents are concerned about the possible complications and sequelae of tympanostomy tube insertion or complications of a general anesthetic, or both. If the parents are undecided, then a trial of antimicrobial prophylaxis, such as amoxicillin or sulfisoxazole* given in one dose before bedtime, can be offered with the option to perform a myringotomy and tympanostomy tube insertion if the chemoprophylaxis fails to prevent recurrent otitis media or if the signs or symptoms of eustachian tube dysfunction persist. Antimicrobial prophylaxis, if effective, is recommended during winter and spring, the seasons of highest risk, and then

a period without prophylaxis can be tried to determine if indeed the child has improved.

For the rarely encountered child in whom tympanostomy tubes fail to prevent frequently recurrent acute otitis media (i.e., those who have otorrhea through the tube), the combination of both antimicrobial prophylaxis and tympanostomy tubes is usually effective in preventing the recurrent episodes.

The above management options should be offered only to those children in whom chronic middle ear effusion is not present between episodes (Fig. 8–2). If recurrent bouts of acute otitis media are superimposed on the chronic condition, the child should be treated as described below for management of chronic otitis media with effusion.

Otitis Media with Effusion

Infants and children who have otitis media with effusion ("secretory" otitis media) most likely have a condition that is an extension of an upper respiratory tract infection and that resolves spontaneously in most cases without active treatment. Treatment may be indicated in some children, since there are possible complications and sequelae associated with this condition. Since little information is currently available regarding the incidence of these complications and sequelae, and since the natural history of these effusions has not been studied formally, some thoughtful clinicians would take a watch-and-wait position and not actively treat such a child. However, hearing loss of some degree usually accompanies a middle ear effusion. Although the significance of this hearing loss is still uncertain, such a loss may impair cognitive and language function and result in disturbances in psychosocial adjustment. With these uncertainties in mind, the clinician should decide whether or not to treat or to watch, and, if treatment is decided upon, to choose one or more treatment options that appear to be most appropriate in eliminating the middle ear effusion in the individual child. Many factors should be considered in this decision-making process. A child with a unilateral, asymptomatic otitis media with effusion of recent onset, in whom there is only a mild hearing loss and in whom there are no serious secondary changes in the tympanic membrane, may be a candidate for watchful waiting. Conversely, a child with bilateral chronic middle ear effusions who has an associated marked hearing loss would be a more likely candidate for active treatment.

---

*Trimethoprim-sulfamethoxazole is not indicated for prophylaxis of otitis media (Physicians' Desk Reference).

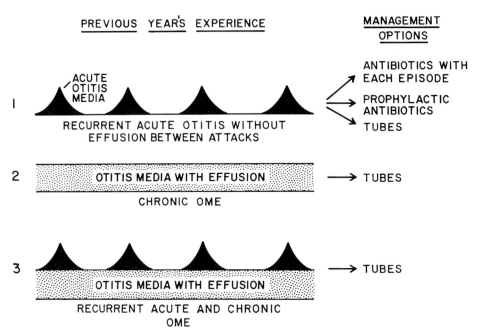

Figure 8–2. Three examples of children with recurrent acute or chronic otitis media, or both, related to available management options. (1) Patients with recurrent acute otitis media without middle ear effusion between attacks can be treated either with a prophylactic antimicrobial agent, tympanostomy tubes, or continuation of treatment of each episode. (2) Children with three or more months of chronic middle ear effusion should be considered to be candidates for tympanostomy tubes. (3) When recurrent acute otitis media is superimposed upon chronic otitis media with effusion, then tympanostomy tubes should be advised (see text).

Important factors that should be considered in addition to hearing loss when the decision is made to treat or not to treat (and which treatment) would be one or more of the following: (1) occurrence in young infants, since they are unable to communicate about their symptoms and may have suppurative disease; (2) an associated acute purulent upper respiratory tract infection; (3) concurrent permanent conductive or sensorineural hearing loss; (4) vertigo; (5) alterations of the tympanic membrane, such as severe atelectasis, especially a deep retraction pocket in the posterosuperior quadrant or the pars flaccida, or both; (6) middle ear changes, such as adhesive otitis or ossicular involvement; (7) effusion that persists for three months or longer; or (8) episodes that are frequently recurrent, resulting in an accumulation of an excessive duration of middle ear effusion during a given period of time, such as six out of 12 months.

Before a nonsurgical or surgical method of management of chronic effusion is begun, a thorough search for an underlying origin (i.e., paranasal sinusitis, upper respiratory allergy, submucous cleft palate, or nasopharyngeal tumor) should be attempted.

Of the many methods of management that are available for otitis media with effusion, only a few have been shown to be effective in acceptable clinical trials. However, the clinician is forced to make a decision regarding all possible nonsurgical or surgical treatment options that are reasonable and most appropriate for the individual child. If treatment is chosen, the most rational approach initially should be a trial of one or more of the nonsurgical methods, and if the effusion is still persistent, then periodic observation or surgical intervention should be considered; the decision between these latter options should be based upon the signs and symptoms present and should consider the potential complications and sequelae of both.

Probably the most popular method of management, a trial with an orally administered combination of a decongestant and antihistamine, has recently been shown to be ineffective in infants and children with acute, subacute, and chronic otitis media with effusion (Cantekin et al., 1983). The use of these agents for this disease in children is not recommended, but they may be effective in adolescents and adults or patients of all ages in whom there is evidence of upper respiratory allergy, since the study did not test the efficacy of this drug combination in these populations.

The efficacy of topical intranasal and systemic corticosteroid therapy has been tested, but convincing clinical trials showing benefit have not been reported; Maknin and Jones (1985) showed a lack of efficacy following treatment with systemically administered dexamethasone. In addition, some thoughtful clinicians consider that the risks of corticosteroid therapy for otitis media with effusion in children outweigh its possible benefits. Even though clinical trials have not tested the efficacy of immunotherapy and control of allergy in children with evidence of upper respiratory allergy, this method of management seems reasonable in children who have frequently recurrent or chronic otitis media with effusion. Likewise, inflation of the eustachian tube–middle ear system by using the method of Politzer or employing the Valsalva maneuver has been advocated for over a century. Inflation that achieves a positive middle ear pressure should enhance drainage of a thin (serous) middle ear effusion down the eustachian tube and into the nasopharynx. Unfortunately, no randomized controlled trials have been reported to establish the efficacy of such procedures and, therefore, it is seldom recommended, especially in children with chronic otitis media with effusion.

Of all the medical treatments that have been advocated, a trial of an antimicrobial agent appears to be most appropriate in those children who have not received therapy recently. Since bacteria similar to those found in acute otitis media have been isolated from a significant proportion of middle ear aspirates in children with chronic otitis media with effusion (Healy and Teele, 1977; Liu et al., 1976; Riding et al., 1978; Senturia et al., 1958; Stanievich et al., 1981), the antibiotic chosen and duration of treatment should be the same as recommended for children who have acute otitis media. In a study recently reported by Mandel et al. (1987), amoxicillin (40 mg/kg/day in three divided doses) given for 14 days was twice as effective as placebo. Therefore, amoxicillin would be a reasonable agent, but if the effusion is chronic and unresponsive to amoxicillin therapy, a trial with an antimicrobial agent effective against ampicillin-resistant bacteria might be of benefit prior to consideration for surgery.

Appropriate agents would be amoxicillin-clavulanate, erythromycin and sulfisoxazole, trimethoprim-sulfamethoxazole, or cefaclor; however clinical trials have not been reported that have shown these antimicrobials to be superior to amoxicillin for otitis media with effusion.

If nonsurgical methods of management fail, then surgical intervention should be considered. Myringotomy with aspiration of the middle ear effusions would appear to be appropriate in those children in whom the procedure can be performed without the aid of a general anesthetic, since a second myringotomy with or without the insertion of a tympanostomy tube would be indicated if the effusion is present soon after the myringotomy incision heals (i.e., if the disease is persistent). It is desirable to avoid the risk of administering a second general anesthetic: if myringotomy is elected and general anesthesia is required, a tympanostomy tube should be inserted at the time of the initial myringotomy to preclude, if possible, the necessity of performing a second procedure under general anesthesia should a tube later be required (Mandel et al., 1984). This method of management appears at present to be the most reasonable. Following spontaneous extubation of the tympanostomy tube, reinsertion for recurrence of effusion would be indicated only after antimicrobial treatment has failed and the effusion has persisted for three months. Adenoidectomy with or without tonsillectomy either alone or in combination with myringotomy and with or without tympanostomy tube insertion may also be of benefit. Maw (1984), and more recently, Paradise and coworkers (1987) reported the efficacy of adenoidectomy in reducing the recurrence rate of otitis media with effusion. However, some children failed to improve following the procedure, while still others improved without undergoing an adenoidectomy.

In some children myringotomy and placement of tympanostomy tubes must be repeated until the child grows older. For children who have had chronic otitis media with effusion that appears to be resistant to the methods of management described previously, mastoidectomy has been advocated (Proud and Duff, 1976), but this procedure is rarely indicated and should be reserved for those children in whom mastoid osteitis or a cholesteatoma is suspected, since almost all chronic effusions are at least temporarily eliminated after tympanostomy tube insertion.

Atelectasis of the Tympanic Membrane and High Negative Middle Ear Pressure

Atelectasis of the tympanic membrane can be either acute or chronic, localized or generalized, mild or severe, and may or may not be associated with abnormal negative pressure. Retraction of the tympanic membrane may be secondary to the presence of high negative pressure. However, a flaccid, atelectatic tympanic membrane may not be associated with high negative intratympanic pressure: the abnormal negative pressure may have been the original cause of such a condition of the membrane but may no longer be present. Localized atelectasis or a retraction pocket may be seen in the area of a healed perforation or at the site where a tympanostomy tube had been inserted ("atrophic scar" or dimeric membrane). A retraction pocket in the posterosuperior portion of the pars tensa or a pars flaccida retraction pocket is more frequently associated with the development of more serious sequelae (ossicular discontinuity or cholesteatoma) than is a retraction pocket in other areas of the tympanic membrane. These variations should be kept in mind when deciding how to manage atelectasis.

If a chronic middle ear effusion is present concurrently with atelectasis, then the child should be treated as previously outlined for patients with otitis media with effusion. However, whether or not a middle ear effusion is present, if a chronic severe retraction pocket of the posterosuperior area of the pars tensa or of the pars flaccida, or both, is present, myringotomy and insertion of a tympanostomy tube should be performed to prevent possible irreversible changes in the middle ear. After insertion of a tympanostomy tube, the tympanic membrane in the area of the retraction pocket should return to a more neutral position within several weeks or months, but if the retraction area remains adherent to the ossicles or middle ear, or both (see Fig. 9–13, Chapter Nine, Complications and Sequelae: Intratemporal), then adhesive otitis media is present, and tympanoplasty should be considered to prevent further progression of the disease process (such as ossicular discontinuity or cholestea-

toma formation, or both). Even though this method of management has not been tested in appropriately controlled clinical trials and the natural history of retraction pockets in these areas has not been studied adequately, this method of management would appear to be reasonable at present (Bluestone et al., 1977b).

For less severe cases in which the atelectasis of the tympanic membrane is apparently not associated with a middle ear effusion and a retraction pocket is not present in the posterosuperior portion or pars flaccida, the management options become less obvious and more controversial. Generalized atelectasis, or even a localized area that is retracted for only a short time (acute retraction), is usually secondary to transient high negative middle ear pressure associated with an acute upper respiratory tract infection (and occasionally due to barotrauma). This condition is quite common in children and usually is self-limited. No specific treatment should be directed toward the middle ear unless the child complains of severe otalgia, hearing loss, tinnitus, or vertigo. The atelectasis (and high negative intratympanic pressure) and associated symptoms, if present, will usually subside when the acute upper respiratory tract infection disappears. Treatment at this time should be directed toward relief of the nasal symptoms. Topical or systemic nasal decongestants may provide relief of these symptoms and may also relieve congestion of the eustachian tube, although their effectiveness in this latter area has not yet been shown. If the symptoms become severe enough, myringotomy may be necessary to provide relief by returning middle ear pressure to ambient levels. Inflation of the eustachian tube–middle ear system by employing the methods of Valsalva or Politzer has been advocated, but studies in animals indicate that these methods will not return the middle ear pressure to normal for a sustained period when the eustachian tube is obstructed (Cantekin et al., 1980c). Controlled trials in children have not been reported to demonstrate the efficacy of these methods.

When the atelectasis is chronic and there is no evidence of a deep retraction pocket in the posterosuperior quadrant or pars flaccida, a thorough search should be made for an underlying origin, as described previously for recurrent acute otitis media with effusion. If none is found, then the management options include only watchful waiting and active treatment. The decision for or against treatment should rest on the presence or absence of other, associated symptoms, and whether or not there is abnormal negative pressure within the middle ear. The presence of persistent or transient otalgia, hearing loss, vertigo, or tinnitus that is troublesome to the patient warrants active treatment. For chronic atelectasis in this case, a trial with a topical or systemic nasal decongestant with or without an antihistamine may be helpful; however, this type of treatment is often disappointing. Inflation of the eustachian tube and middle ear may provide temporary relief but usually must be repeated for permanent control of the symptoms and to maintain the tympanic membrane in a more normal position. For most children, myringotomy with insertion of a tympanostomy tube will usually be necessary to provide long-term relief. The procedure will prevent the sustained or transient high negative pressure secondary to eustachian tube obstruction that is responsible for the active retraction of the tympanic membrane. If the severely atelectatic tympanic membrane does not return to a more normal position after the insertion of the tympanostomy tube, or if the tube cannot be inserted owing to lack of a suitable aerated space within the middle ear, tympanoplasty should be considered.

When a flaccid tympanic membrane is passively collapsed upon the ossicles and middle ear and high negative middle ear pressure is not present, the nonsurgical and surgical management options described above may not be effective in restoring the tympanic membrane to a more normal position. Fortunately, symptoms of high negative middle ear pressure and eustachian tube obstruction are frequently absent, so no treatment may be necessary. Even myringotomy and tympanostomy tube insertion may not be beneficial, since the tympanic membrane is no longer actively being retracted by high negative middle ear pressure. In addition, at this stage, adhesive otitis media may also be present, and portions of the tympanic membrane may be adherent to the middle ear. The posterior or epitympanic (attic) portions of the middle ear may become separated from the anterior portion by adhesions, and subsequently, ventilation from the eustachian tube or a tympanostomy tube does not aerate the affected area. In such cases there are two management options: tympanoplasty or periodic (once or twice a year) observation.

Eustachian Tube Dysfunction

Otitis media with effusion and atelectasis with or without effusion are usually the result of dysfunction of the eustachian tube. However, abnormal function of the eustachian tube may cause otological symptoms without an apparent effusion or severe atelectasis. The tympanic membrane may have a normal appearance, and mobility may be unimpaired when tested with a pneumatic otoscope or by tympanometry. Two types of eustachian tube dysfunction can be present: obstruction or abnormal patency. When the eustachian tube is obstructed but no effusion is present, the tube periodically opens to ventilate the middle ear cavity but at less frequent intervals than normal; in this case high negative intratympanic pressure may be present for relatively long but transient periods. This type of intermittent middle ear ventilation may cause periods of otalgia, a feeling of fullness or pressure, hearing loss, popping and snapping noises, tinnitus, and even vertigo. Management of this situation should be similar to that described for generalized atelectasis of the tympanic membrane. If the condition is present only during an acute upper respiratory tract infection, medical treatment should be directed toward relief of the nasal congestion. If the symptoms are of a chronic nature, a search for an underlying cause should be attempted, and if found, appropriate management should be instituted. If no underlying cause is uncovered, then a trial with a decongestant or antihistamines, or both, may be helpful or eustachian tube–middle ear inflation may be tried, but if the nonsurgical methods are not successful, then myringotomy and insertion of a tympanostomy tube may be necessary.

At the other end of the spectrum of eustachian tube dysfunction is abnormal patency. In its extreme form, the hyperpatent eustachian tube is open even at rest (i.e., patulous). Lesser degrees of abnormal patency result in a semipatulous eustachian tube that is closed at rest but has low tubal resistance to airflow in comparison with the normal tube. A patulous eustachian tube may be caused by abnormal tube geometry or a decrease in extramural pressure, such as occurs as a result of weight loss or, possibly, mural or intraluminal changes. These last conditions may be seen when the extracellular fluid is altered by medical treatment of another unrelated condition. Interruption of the innervation of the tensor veli palatini muscle has also been shown to be a cause of a hyperpatent eustachian tube (Perlman, 1939).

Clinically, a patulous eustachian tube may be present in adolescents and adults but is less common in children. The patient frequently complains of hearing his or her own breathing in the ear or of autophony. Otoscopic examination reveals a tympanic membrane that moves medially on inspiration and laterally on expiration; the movement can be exaggerated with forced respiration. The condition is relieved when the patient is recumbent, since extramural pressure in the eustachian tube is increased by paratubal venous engorgement in this position. The patient should therefore be examined in the sitting position. The diagnosis can also be made by measuring the impedance of the middle ear (Bluestone, 1980). A tympanogram is obtained while the patient is breathing normally, and a second one is obtained while the patient holds his or her breath. Fluctuation in the tympanometric line should coincide with breathing. The fluctuation can be exaggerated by asking the patient to occlude one nostril and close the mouth during forced inspiration and expiration, or by performing the Toynbee or Valsalva maneuver.

Management of a patulous eustachian tube depends on first determining the cause of the problem. If the symptoms are of relatively short duration, the condition may subside without any active treatment. In children and teenagers this condition is usually self-limited and probably related to changes in the structure and function of the eustachian tube and adjacent areas secondary to rapid growth and development. When a medication can be identified as the agent responsible, cessation of the medication usually alleviates the problem. However, in most instances the condition is idiopathic. When the symptoms are disturbing and the condition is chronic, active treatment is indicated. Myringotomy with insertion of a tympanostomy tube may be performed but usually does not alter the symptoms in most cases and occasionally results in increasing the patient's discomfort. Insufflation of powders into the eustachian tube and instillation of 2 percent iodine or 5 percent trichloroacetic acid solution have also been advocated (Mawson, 1974). Infusion of an absorbable gelatin sponge solution has also been suggested (Ogawa et al., 1976), as has injection of polytetrafluorethylene (Teflon) into the para-

tubal area (Pulec, 1967), but all of these methods have major disadvantages. They are, for the most part, irreversible and may not improve the condition or may provide only temporary relief. Total obstruction of the eustachian tube can also be a complication. Stroud, Spector, and Maisel (1974) have suggested the transposition of the tensor veli palatini through a palatal incision, but the procedure has not been shown to be safe and effective in a large number of patients by other investigators.

At present, the most logical choice for relief when the discomfort becomes severe is a procedure that would alleviate the symptoms simply, reversibly, and without untoward reactions. A technique described by Bluestone and Cantekin (1981) has been used successfully in adults but is rarely indicated or necessary in children, since the patulous tube condition is usually self-limited. The procedure involves placement of a plastic catheter into the middle ear end of the eustachian tube.

ANTIMICROBIAL AGENTS

Decisions about optimal chemotherapy for otitis media are based on information about (1) the pathogens isolated from middle ear fluids; (2) the *in vitro* activity of antimicrobial agents against these pathogens; (3) the clinical pharmacological action of antimicrobial agents of value, including concentrations of drug achieved in middle ear fluid; and (4) the results of clinical and microbiological studies. These factors in choice of antimicrobial agents for treatment of children with otitis media with effusion will be discussed in this section.

Microbiology of Otitis Media: Therapeutic Implications

The preferred antimicrobial agent for the patient with otitis media must be active against *S. pneumoniae, H. influenzae,* and *B. catarrhalis,* the three most important bacterial pathogens in all age groups. Group A streptococcus and *S. aureus* are less frequent causes of acute otitis media. Gram-negative enteric bacilli must be considered when otitis media occurs in the newborn infant, the immunocompromised host, and suppurative complications or postoperative wound infections of the head and neck area. Anaerobic bacteria appear to have a limited role in chronic and a minimal role in acute otitis media. The bacterial pathogens are discussed further in Chapter Five, Microbiology.

Streptococcus pneumoniae

S. pneumoniae is markedly susceptible to penicillins, cephalosporins, erythromycin, clindamycin, and the combination of trimethoprim-sulfamethoxazole. Chloramphenicol and sulfonamides have moderate activity. Aminoglycosides are relatively ineffective.

Since the introduction of the penicillins more than 40 years ago, almost all strains of S. pneumoniae have been uniformly and markedly sensitive to penicillin G and other penicillins. In recent years, however, moderate and high resistance to penicillin G and other antimicrobial agents has appeared and in some cases has been responsible for clinical and microbiological failure. There are three facets to the problem: strains that are moderately resistant to penicillin G but susceptible to other antimicrobial agents, strains that are highly resistant to penicillin G and highly resistant to other antimicrobial agents, and strains that are sensitive to penicillin G but resistant to some other antimicrobial agents. The clinical and epidemiological aspects of

antibiotic-resistant pneumococci were reviewed by Ward (1981).

During the past 15 years, an increasing number of strains of S. pneumoniae have had decreased susceptibility to penicillins. The susceptibility of most strains of S. pneumoniae is less than 0.05 µg/ml, whereas moderately resistant strains are two to 20 times less sensitive to penicillin G, requiring 0.1 to 1.0 µg/ml of penicillin G for inhibition (Table 8–4). Since usual dosage schedules of penicillin G or V achieve concentrations of 0.2 µg/ml to 4 µg/ml in middle ear fluid, infection due to some moderately resistant strains may result in microbiological and clinical failure (Howard et al., 1976; Kamme, 1970). Clinical and microbiological failure in cases of pneumococcal meningitis due to moderately resistant strains treated with penicillin G has been reported (Mace et al., 1977; Paredes et al., 1976). Although the number of moderately resistant strains is now low (approximately 1–3 percent of pneumococcal isolates tested in our laboratory [Klein, unpublished data] and reported from laboratories in the United States and Western Europe), if the incidence of moderately resistant strains increases, physicians will have to reevaluate initial therapy or dosage schedules for treatment of otitis media.

Multiply-resistant strains of pneumococci

Table 8–4. SENSITIVITY OF *Streptococcus pneumoniae* AND *Haemophilus influenzae* ISOLATED FROM MIDDLE EAR EFFUSIONS OF CHILDREN WITH ACUTE OTITIS MEDIA, 1976–1979*

	Minimal Inhibitory Concentration (MIC) (µg/ml), Median†			
	S. pneumoniae		*H. influenzae*	
Antimicrobial Agent	*Sensitive***	*Resistant****	*Sensitive‡*	*Resistant§*
Penicillin G	0.01	0.4	1.6	100
Penicillin V	0.01	0.4	12.5	100
Ampicillin	0.03	0.1	0.8	100
Nafcillin	0.01	0.8	25	50
Cephalexin	3.2	3.2	100	50
Cefaclor	0.4	1.6	12.5	25
Erythromycin	0.05	0.03	3.1	3.1
Clindamycin	0.05	0.05	3.1	6.3
Chloramphenicol	3.2	3.2	0.4	0.8
Tetracycline	0.2	25	0.4	0.4
Trimethoprim	1.6	3.2	0.8	1.6
Sulfamethoxazole	100	100	100	100
Timethoprim-sulfamethoxazole‖	0.3/6	0.3/6	0.2/3	0.2/3

*From Teele, D. W., Norton, C. C., Mayer, J., Klein, J. O.: Unpublished data.
**Twenty-two strains with MIC for penicillin G, <0.1 µg/ml.
***One strain with MIC for penicillin G, $\geq$0.1 µg/ml.
†Inocula replicator method: 10^0 dilution for *S. pneumoniae*; 10^{-2} dilution for *H. influenzae*.
‡Beta-lactamase–negative strains, including three type b and 20 nontypable.
§Beta-lactamase–positive strains, including three type b and four nontypable
‖Trimethoprim-sulfamethoxazole = 1 part trimethoprim/19 parts sulfamethoxazole.

were noted in early 1977 by Appelbaum and colleagues (1977). These strains were highly resistant to penicillin G, requiring more than 4 µg/ml for inhibition, and were resistant to other drugs that serve as alternatives to penicillin G in pneumococcal disease, including other penicillins and cephalosporins, tetracyclines, chloramphenicol, erythromycin, clindamycin, sulfonamides, and rifampin. Some children with sepsis and meningitis due to a highly resistant pneumococcus died when treated with penicillin G alone. Since 1977, these strains have continued to appear in South Africa, mainly in Durban and Johannesburg, but have been reported rarely outside that country. Cases appearing elsewhere have usually been in immunosuppressed patients (Cates et al., 1978). The reason for the relative restriction of these strains to South Africa is unknown.

Strains of *S. pneumoniae* sensitive to penicillins but resistant to other antimicrobial agents are not uncommon. Resistance has been noted in some strains to tetracycline, chloramphenicol, sulfonamides, erythromycin, and lincomycin. Susceptibility testing should be considered for strains of *S. pneumoniae* causing otitis media that do not respond to an appropriate course of a usually effective antimicrobial agent.

Haemophilus influenzae

Strains of *H. influenzae* responsible for otitis media may be subdivided on the basis of susceptibility to ampicillin. Ampicillin-sensitive strains are only slightly less susceptible to penicillin G than they are to ampicillin, but they are much less susceptible to penicillin V and the penicillinase-resistant penicillins. "Second-generation cephalosporins"—cefoxitin, cefamandole, cefuroxime, and cefaclor—and the "third-generation cephalosporins"—moxalactam, cefoperazone, cefotaxime, ceftizoxime, cefixime, and ceftriaxone—have significant activity against *H. influenzae* and are effective against ampicillin-sensitive and resistant strains. The "third-generation" cephalosporins are the most active antimicrobial agents *in vitro* against *H. influenzae* (Table 8–5). Chloramphenicol and tetracycline are effective against both ampicillin-sensitive and ampicillin-resistant strains, as are less active agents such as aminoglycosides, erythromycins, and clindamycin. Addition of a beta-lactamase inhibitor, clavulanic acid, to ampicillin provides activity against *H. influenzae* without regard to production of the enzyme.

In recent years, ampicillin-resistant strains of both nontypable and type b *H. influenzae* have been reported throughout the United States. The resistance appears to be a new phenomenon; few resistant strains were detected before 1972. Resistance to ampicillin is based on production of penicillinase, a beta-lactamase that hydrolyzes the penicillin nucleus. Thus, all penicillins that are susceptible to beta-lactamase, including penicillin G, penicillin V, ampicillin, amoxicillin, and carbenicillin, are likely to be ineffective against infections caused by these strains (Table 8–4). At present in the United States, approximately 10 to 30 percent of strains of nontypable (Schwartz, 1982) and 5 to 20 percent of type b *H. influenzae* (Ward et al., 1978) isolated from children with disease are beta-lactamase–producing strains. Ampicillin-resistant strains of *H. influenzae* that do not produce beta-lactamase have been detected but are relatively uncommon. Children with suppurative life-threatening complications of otitis media (including sepsis or meningitis) in which *H. influenzae* may be the etiological agent must receive a drug of uniform efficacy, such as chloramphenicol. Chloramphenicol-resistant strains of *H. influenzae* (most of which are susceptible to ampicillin) are uncommon, but meningitis due to such a strain has been reported (Kinmonth et al., 1978). Resistance is based on production of an acetyltransferase capable of inactivating chloramphenicol. Strains of *H. influenzae* resistant to both ampicillin and chloramphenicol are rare in the United States, but a recent report notes a high incidence in Barcelona (Campos et al., 1984).

Ampicillin or amoxicillin alone is still appropriate therapy for children with mild to moderately severe disease of the respiratory tract, including otitis media. But if the patient fails to respond favorably, the presence of a resistant strain must be considered and therapy changed to include a drug effective against beta-lactamase–producing *H. influenzae* (amoxicillin-clavulanate, a sulfonamide, trimethoprim-sulfamethoxazole, cefaclor, or cefixime).

Beta-lactamase–producing organisms (including *H. influenzae*, *S. aureus*, and *B. catarrhalis*) may inactivate drugs that would be effective for other susceptible organisms present at the same site. This effect is more likely to occur on a mucosal surface (the pharynx) than in a body fluid, but it is possible that such an effect would occur in a middle ear fluid containing mixed cultures, including an ampicillin-resistant, beta-lacta-

Table 8–5. **THE CEPHALOSPORINS—1989**

Generic Name	Trade Name	Route
First Generation		
Cephalothin	Keflin	IM, IV
Cefazolin	Ancef, Kefzol	IM, IV
Cephapirin	Cefadyl	IM, IV
Cephalexin	Keflex	PO
Cephradine	Velosef	PO, IM, IV
Cefadroxil	Ultracef, Duricef	PO
Second Generation		
Cefamandole	Mandol	IM, IV
Cefoxitin	Mefoxin	IM, IV
Cefaclor	Ceclor	PO
Cefuroxime	Zinacef	IM, IV
Cefuroxime axetil	Ceftin	PO
Ceforanide*	Precef	IM, IV
Cefonicid*	Monocid	IM, IV
Cefotetan*	Cefotan	IM, IV
Third Generation		
Moxalactam	Moxam	IM, IV
Cefixime	Suprax	PO
Cefoperazone*	Cefobid	IM, IV
Cefotaxime	Claforan	IM, IV
Ceftizoxime	Cefizox	IM, IV
Ceftriaxone	Rocephin	IM, IV
Ceftazidime	Fortaz, Tazidime	IM, IV

*Not approved for use in infants and children.

mase–producing strain *(H. influenzae)* and an ampicillin-sensitive strain *(S. pneumoniae),* resulting in inactivation of the ampicillin and uninhibited growth of *S. pneumoniae* and *H. influenzae.*

Branhamella catarrhalis

Most current strains of *B. catarrhalis* produce beta-lactamase and are not susceptible to penicillin G and ampicillin. These strains are resistant to ampicillin, amoxicillin, and other beta-lactamase–susceptible penicillins but are susceptible to the combination of amoxicillin-clavulanate, various cephalosporins, erythromycin, chloramphenicol, and trimethoprim-sulfamethoxazole; about half of the beta-lactamase–producing strains are relatively resistant to cefaclor. Methicillin and other penicillinase-resistant penicillins and clindamycin are ineffective. As is the case with *H. influenzae,* the isolation of beta-lactamase–producing strains of *B. catarrhalis* was reported at the beginning of this decade. In 1970, Kamme reported that all 108 strains of *B. catarrhalis* isolated in the Department of Clinical Bacteriology in Lund, Sweden, were highly susceptible to penicillin G and ampicillin. In 1980, Kamme reported that 15 percent of strains of *B. catarrhalis* isolated in the same laboratory produced beta-lactamase. His *in vitro* studies showed that trimethoprim-sulfamethoxazole and erythro-

mycin were the preferred drugs for beta-lactamase–producing strains.

More recently, Shurin and coworkers (1984) and Kovatch and associates (1984) from Cleveland and Pittsburgh, respectively, reported that over 20 percent of isolates for acute middle ear effusion had *B. catarrhalis,* and that three fourths of those isolates produced beta-lactamase. Bluestone (1985) reported that amoxicillin-clavulanate was effective against beta-lactamase–producing strains of *B. catarrhalis.*

Groups A and B Streptococci

There are no known strains of group A and B streptococci that are resistant to the penicillins. These streptococci are markedly sensitive to the penicillins, cephalosporins, erythromycin, chloramphenicol, and clindamycin. They are relatively resistant to aminoglycosides and to sulfonamides. Trimethoprim-sulfamethoxazole in combination is more active than either component alone, but clinical efficacy is uncertain against group A streptococci.

Staphylococcus aureus and epidermidis

Most strains of *S. aureus* that cause otitis media in hospitalized patients produce penicillinase and are resistant to penicillin G and ampicillin; the number of strains of resistant staphylococci in patients who have community-acquired disease is lower but significant. Thus, the penicillinase-resistant penicillins are the drugs of choice for initial management of the patient with suspected or documented staphylococcal otitis media. Most cephalosporins are also effective against penicillinase-producing strains. The efficacy of erythromycins, clindamycin, chloramphenicol, and the aminoglycosides is variable, and tests of susceptibility should be used to guide the choice for the patient who is suspected or known to have a staphylococcal infection and is allergic to penicillin.

Disease due to methicillin-resistant staphylococci was reported shortly after the introduction of the drug. The strains are usually resistant to all penicillinase-resistant penicillins and to most cephalosporins. Bacterial resistance must be considered as a possible cause of therapeutic failure whenever a patient with staphylococcal disease who is on an adequate dosage schedule of a penicillinase-resistant penicillin does not respond favorably. Vancomycin is usually effective for these strains.

Most strains of *S. epidermidis* produce beta-lactamase that inactivates penicillin G, penicillin V, and ampicillin. *S. epidermidis* is also more resistant than *S. aureus* to the penicillinase-resistant penicillins, cephalosporins, erythromycin, and clindamycin. Vancomycin is usually effective against methicillin-resistant *S. epidermidis*.

Gram-negative Enteric Bacilli

The choice of antibiotics for infections due to gram-negative bacteria depends on the particular pattern of susceptibility in the hospital or community. These patterns vary in different hospitals or communities and from time to time within the same institution. In most areas, the most effective agents for *Escherichia coli*, *Proteus* (indole-positive and -negative) species, *Klebsiella* and *Enterobacter* species, and *P. aeruginosa* are the aminoglycosides tobramycin, gentamicin, netilmicin, and amikacin. Some of the new cephalosporins (cefoxitin, moxalactam, cefoperazone, cefotaxime, cefixime, ceftriaxone, and ceftazidime) have significant activity. Many gram-negative enteric bacilli are resistant to strep-

tomycin, tetracycline, ampicillin, and the early cephalosporins such as cephalothin. Since the susceptibility of gram-negative enteric bacilli is variable and unpredictable, isolates should be tested to determine optimal choice of antimicrobial agents.

Anaerobic Bacteria

Most anaerobic bacteria responsible for infection and disease in the upper respiratory tract, including anaerobic cocci, gram-positive nonsporulating anaerobic bacilli, and anaerobic gram-negative bacilli, are susceptible to penicillin G. Some strains of the gram-negative bacilli, such as *Bacteroides melaninogenicus*, are resistant to penicillin G. *Bacteroides fragilis* is an uncommon pathogen in the respiratory tract; most strains are resistant to penicillin G and susceptible only to clindamycin, chloramphenicol, or carbenicillin. Finegold (1981) has reviewed therapeutic implications for anaerobic infections in otolaryngology.

Chlamydia trachomatis

C. trachomatis is susceptible to erythromycin, sulfonamides, tetracyclines, and chloramphenicol. Since this organism is likely to be associated with infection of the respiratory tract, including otitis media, in young infants, erythromycin or sulfisoxazole has been recommended for documented or suspected infection. Although controlled trials of efficacy of these drugs in young infants with respiratory infection have not been performed, results of uncontrolled studies suggest that either shortens the course of the illness. No data are available about efficacy of any antimicrobial drugs for otitis media due to *C. trachomatis*.

Mycoplasma pneumoniae

Otitis media may accompany respiratory infection due to *M. pneumoniae*. The organisms are susceptible to erythromycin and tetracyclines. Controlled trials indicate that the duration of signs of lower respiratory tract infection such as cough, rales, and fever is less in patients receiving one of these drugs, but there are no data about efficacy of the antibiotics for otitis media due to *M. pneumoniae*.

Clinical Pharmacology of Antimicrobial Agents of Value in Therapy of Otitis Media and Its Suppurative Complications

The clinical pharmacological effects of orally administered antimicrobial agents of value in otitis media are discussed below. Parenterally administered drugs of value for suppurative complications of otitis media are also discussed in this chapter.

The Penicillins (Table 8–6)

Penicillin G and Penicillin V. It is remarkable that in the more than 40 years that this drug has been in use, some organisms have remained exquisitely sensitive to penicillin G and no resistant strains have emerged. Thus, there are no penicillin G–resistant strains of groups A or B streptococci. In contrast, the vast majority of strains of *S. aureus* and *S. epidermidis* are now resistant to penicillin G.

Oral preparations of buffered penicillin G and phenoxymethyl penicillin (penicillin V) are absorbed well from the gastrointestinal tract; the peak level of serum activity of penicillin V is approximately 40 percent (4 to 8 μg/ml), and that of buffered penicillin G is approximately 20 percent (1 to 4 μg/ml) of the level achieved by the same dose of aqueous penicillin G administered intramuscularly. Therefore, oral penicillins may be satisfactory for treatment of mild to moderately severe infections due to sensitive organisms. Penicillin V and penicillin G are of approximately equivalent efficacy *in vitro* against gram-positive cocci, but penicillin V is much less effective than penicillin G against *H. influenzae*. The efficacy of penicillin G against *H. influenzae in vitro* is only two times less than that of ampicillin (see Table 8–4).

Parenteral preparations include the salts potassium or sodium aqueous, and procaine and benzathine penicillin G, which modify absorption and thereby produce different patterns of peak and duration of antibacterial

Table 8–6. THE PENICILLINS—1989

Generic Name	Trade Name	Route
Traditional		
Penicillin G	Many	PO
Aqueous	Many	IM, IV
Procaine	Many	IM
Benzathine	Bicillin, Permapen	IM
Penicillin V	Many	PO
Penicillinase-Resistant		
Methicillin	Staphcillin, Celbenin	IM, IV
Oxacillin	Prostaphlin, Bactocill	PO, IM, IV
Nafcillin	Unipen, Nafcil	PO, IM, IV
Cloxacillin	Tegopen, Cloxapen	PO
Dicloxacillin	Dynapen, Pathocil, Veracillin	PO
Broad-Spectrum		
Ampicillin	Many	PO, IM, IV
Amoxicillin	Many	PO
Amoxicillin-clavulanate	Augmentin	PO
Bacampicillin	Spectrobid	PO
Cyclacillin	Cyclapen	PO
Extended-Spectrum		
Carbenicillin	Geopen, Pyopen	IM, IV
	Geocillin	PO
Ticarcillin	Ticar	IM, IV
Ticarcillin-clavulanate*	Timentin	IM, IV
Azlocillin	Azlin	IM, IV
Mezlocillin	Mezlin	IM, IV
Piperacillin*	Pipracil	IM, IV
Carbapenem		
Imipenem*	Primaxin	IM, IV

*Not approved for use in infants and children.

activity in serum and tissues. Aqueous penicillin G produces high peak levels of antibacterial activity in serum within 30 minutes after intramuscular administration but is rapidly excreted; thus, the concentration in serum is low within two to four hours after administration. If aqueous penicillin G is given by the intravenous route, the peak is higher and earlier, and the duration of antibacterial activity in serum is shorter (approximately two hours). Aqueous penicillin G, given intramuscularly or intravenously, is used for severe disease, including suspected sepsis and meningitis due to organisms known to be, or suspected to be, highly susceptible. In such cases the drug should be given at frequent intervals, usually every four hours, until the infection has been brought under control.

Procaine penicillin G given intramuscularly produces lower levels of serum antibacterial activity (approximately 10 to 30 percent of the peak level achieved by the same dose of the aqueous form), but activity persists in serum for as long as 12 hours. Intramuscular administration of procaine penicillin G should be reserved for the patient with mild to moderate disease who cannot tolerate oral penicillins (patients who are vomiting or have diarrhea, or the comatose patient) or the patient who requires the reliability of parenteral administration, although the disease is not severe enough to warrant frequent intramuscular or intravenous doses of aqueous penicillin G.

Benzathine penicillin G given intramuscularly is a repository preparation providing low levels of serum activity (approximately 1 to 2 percent of the peak level achieved by the same dose of the aqueous form). After administration of this drug, low concentrations of penicillin activity are measurable in serum for 14 days or more and in urine for several months. Significant pain at the site of injection is the major deterrent to widespread usage of this unique antibiotic. Combination of the benzathine and procaine salts (900,000 and 300,000 units, respectively) is less painful and comparable in efficacy to benzathine alone (1,200,000 units) for treatment of streptococcal pharyngitis (Bass et al., 1976). Benzathine penicillin G is appropriate only for highly sensitive organisms present in tissues that are well vascularized, so that the drug can diffuse readily to the site of infection. Thus, benzathine penicillin G is suitable for treatment of children with otitis media due to *S. pneumoniae* but not *H. influenzae*,

and it should not be used for otitis media alone unless the pathogen is known and is susceptible. The current place of intramuscular benzathine penicillin G in treatment and prevention of infections in infants and children was reviewed at a 1985 symposium; the proceedings were published in *Pediatric Infectious Disease* (Klein, 1985).

Penicillinase-Resistant Penicillins. Methicillin was the first penicillinase-resistant penicillin to be introduced and is available in parenteral form only. Oxacillin and nafcillin are available in both parenteral and oral preparations and have greater *in vitro* activity against gram-positive cocci. Cloxacillin and dicloxacillin are available in oral forms only and are absorbed more efficiently from the gastrointestinal tract than are the other oral drugs. Differences among these five penicillins include degree of binding to proteins, degree of degradation by beta-lactamases, and *in vitro* level of susceptibility; however, all are effective for treatment of staphylococcal disease, and clinical studies have shown them to be comparable when used according to appropriate dosage schedules. In addtion, all but methicillin have proved to be effective against infections due to *S. pneumoniae* and beta-hemolytic streptococci. The penicillinase-resistant penicillins can be used for initial therapy when the otitis is suspected to be due to *S. aureus*.

Broad-Spectrum Penicillins

Ampicillin and Amoxicillin. Ampicillin and amoxicillin are effective *in vitro* against a wide spectrum of bacteria, including gram-positive cocci (*S. pneumoniae*, beta-hemolytic streptococci, nonpenicillinase-producing strains of *S. aureus*, and oropharyngeal strains of anaerobic bacteria), gram-negative cocci, gram-negative coccobacilli (nonpenicillinase-producing strains of *H. influenzae*), and some gram-negative enteric bacilli (*E. coli* and *Proteus mirabilis*). The broad spectrum of activity of ampicillin and amoxicillin provides the basis for their use as a single agent for treatment of otitis media.

Both drugs are available for oral administration; ampicillin alone is available in a parenteral form. Amoxicillin provides levels of activity in serum that are higher and more prolonged than those achieved with equivalent doses of ampicillin; thus, amoxicillin can be given in lower doses and three times a day rather than four times, as required for ampicillin. An additional advantage of amoxicillin is that absorption is not altered when the antibiotic is administered with food, whereas absorption of ampicillin is decreased significantly when it is given with food.

Cyclacillin and Bacampicillin. These two new preparations are chemically and pharmacologically similar to ampicillin. Cyclacillin is an oral penicillin with a spectrum of activity similar to that of ampicillin. *In vitro* activity of cyclacillin against gram-positive and gram-negative micro-organisms, however, is 25 to 50 percent below that of ampicillin. Cyclacillin is inactivated by the beta-lactamase of *H. influenzae* and *S. aureus.* Peak serum concentrations of cyclacillin are three to four times greater than equivalent doses of ampicillin. Patients who received cyclacillin had fewer side effects, including diarrhea and rash, than did patients who received ampicillin in a double-blind clinical trial involving 2581 patients (McLinn et al., 1982).

Bacampicillin is a semisynthetic ester of ampicillin. After absorption, bacampicillin is completely hydrolyzed to yield ampicillin. The antibacterial activity of bacampicillin is similar to that of ampicillin. The drug is rapidly and completely absorbed after oral administration and achieves peak serum levels that are more than twice as high as those of ampicillin and approximately 30 percent greater than those of amoxicillin. Ingestion with food does not decrease or delay absorption. The peak serum level is achieved earlier than is the case with ampicillin, and the duration of activity is more prolonged. As a result of the more prolonged activity, dosage schedules require only two doses per day. The clinical usage and adverse effects are similar to those of ampicillin. Early clinical experience with bacampicillin was summarized in a series of articles published in 1981 (Craig and Kirby, 1981).

Amoxicillin-Clavulanate. Amoxicillin in combination with clavulanate potassium (Augmentin) was introduced in 1984 for oral administration. Clavulanate potassium is the salt of clavulanic acid, a beta-lactam antibiotic with poor *in vitro* activity against pathogenic bacteria but potent activity as an inhibitor of beta-lactamase enzymes. The combination drug is equivalent to amoxicillin alone in activity against amoxicillin-susceptible organisms. The addition of clavulanic acid extends the *in vitro* activity of amoxicillin to include beta-lactamase–producing strains of *S. aureus* (but not methicillin-resistant strains), *H. influenzae, B. catarrhalis, Neisseria gonorrhoeae, E. coli, Proteus* species, and anaerobic bacteria,

including *B. fragilis.* The pharmacokinetics of the two drugs are similar; both are rapidly absorbed and are not affected when taken with meals. Initial studies indicate that diarrhea, abdominal pain, and nausea are more frequent with the combination than with amoxicillin alone.

The combination of amoxicillin and clavulanate potassium may be considered if a beta-lactamase–producing organism is known or suspected to be the cause of otitis media. The combination may be of importance if the proportion of beta-lactamase–producing strains of *H. influenzae* increases or if these strains or those of *B. catarrhalis* (the majority of which are beta-lactamase producers), or both, are identified more frequently as pathogens in otitis media, sinusitis, and other respiratory tract infections.

Carbenicillin and Ticarcillin. These two agents are effective against gram-positive cocci *H. influenzae;* anaerobic bacteria, including *Bacteroides* species; and gram-negative enteric bacilli, including *Enterobacter* species, indole-positive *Proteus* species, and *P. aeruginosa.* High concentrations of these drugs are required to inhibit the gram-negative organisms, but this advantage is overcome in part by the low toxicity of the drugs, even when they are given in large intravenous doses. Combination of these penicillins with an aminoglycoside such as gentamicin or tobramycin produces synergistic activity against many gram-negative enteric bacilli. These combinations have been used effectively in initial therapy of sepsis of unknown origin or sepsis suspected to be due to gram-negative enteric bacilli in patients with malignancy or immunosuppressive disease (Kirby, 1970). An oral form of carbenicillin produces very low concentrations of drug in serum and should be restricted to therapy of infections of the urinary tract and not used for otitis media or its complications.

Ticarcillin is similar to carbenicillin, but it is more active against some strains of *P. aeruginosa* and less active against gram-positive cocci. Because of the increased activity, smaller dosages of ticarcillin than of carbenicillin may be used for treatment of disease due to gram-negative organisms (Fuchs et al., 1977). Ticarcillin in combination with potassium clavulanate was introduced in 1985. This combination drug extends the antibacterial activity of ticarcillin to include beta-lactamase–producing strains of *S. aureus, Klebsiella pneumoniae,* and *B. fragilis.* At present, the combination drug is not approved for children under 12 years of age.

Although ticarcillin and carbenicillin have no dose-related toxicity, both drugs are disodium salts; the large amounts in which they are given include significant quantities of sodium: 1 gm of carbenicillin contains 4.7 mEq, or 108 mg, of sodium per gram of drug; 1 gm of ticarcillin contains 5.2 mEq, or 120 mg, of sodium per gram of drug. The amount of sodium administered may be of concern in the treatment of certain patients with renal or cardiac disease.

For otitis media, the primary roles of carbenicillin, ticarcillin, or ticarcillin-clavulanate are in cases of chronic suppurative otitis media with perforation and discharge due to *P. aeruginosa* or *Proteus* species that are unresponsive to other forms of medical treatment, such as ototopical drops.

Piperacillin, Mezlocillin, and Azlocillin. These parenteral penicillins have a spectrum of activity similar to that of carbenicillin and ticarcillin but show greater activity *in vitro* against some gram-negative bacilli and anaerobic bacteria. Piperacillin and azlocillin are more active than carbenicillin, ticarcillin, or mezlocillin against *P. aeruginosa*. Piperacillin and mezlocillin are more active *in vitro* than carbenicillin or ticarcillin against susceptible strains of *E. coli* and *Klebsiella, Enterobacter,* and *Serratia* species. Each of these penicillins is inactivated by beta-lactamases. Combination with an aminoglycoside results in synergy against some gram-negative enteric bacilli.

Use of one of these penicillins (usually in combination with an aminoglycoside) in adults has included intra-abdominal, gynecological, and urinary tract infections and sepsis in patients with altered host defenses. The clinical experience with these drugs in infants and children is limited. The available data from children and adults indicate that each penicillin is effective against susceptible organisms, but the evidence is inadequate to demonstrate a significant advantage of any single drug (carbenicillin, ticarcillin, piperacillin, mezlocillin, or azlocillin). The last three drugs have half the sodium content per gram of carbenicillin or ticarcillin, a factor of some importance in patients who require large amounts of the penicillin and have cardiac or renal disease.

Bluestone and colleagues (Kenna et al., 1986) used azlocillin and other antipseudomonal agents for treatment of chronic suppurative otitis media due to *P. aeruginosa*. A

significant proportion of children were cured and did not require surgery. The results of this study suggest that use of a broad-spectrum penicillin may be effective alone for children with chronic suppurative middle ear infections (see Chapter Nine, Complications and Sequelae: Intratemporal).

Imipenem. Imipenem was introduced in 1985 as the first carbapenem antibiotic. Carbapenems have the same ring structure of the penicillins with the substitution of carbon for sulphur and presence of unsaturation in the five-member ring. The parent compound is thienamycin. Imipenem, the active thienamycin, is combined with cilastatin, which inhibits inactivation of imipenem. Imipenem has the broadest antimicrobial spectrum available among beta-lactam antibiotics, including gram-positive cocci, gram-negative cocci, gram-negative bacilli, and anaerobic bacteria. The uses include single-drug therapy for the immunocompromised patient with suspected sepsis, as an alternative to combination therapy for serious intra-abdominal infections, and for serious, hospital-acquired infections. The drug is not approved for use in children less than 12 years old. The role of the drug in infections of the head and neck is unclear.

Toxicity and Sensitization. The penicillins are unique among antimicrobial agents in having low dose-related toxicity. Seizures may occur under circumstances that result in high concentrations of penicillin in nervous tissues: rapid intravenous infusion of single large doses, large dosage schedules for prolonged periods in patients with impaired renal function, high concentrations given by an intrathecal route, or direct application of penicillin to brain tissue (as might occur inadvertently during a neurosurgical procedure). Nephritis has followed administration of some penicillins, most frequently after use of methicillin. The mechanism of the nephrotoxicity is uncertain, but recent data suggest that the renal injury is probably an immunological reaction and not a direct toxic effect (Barza, 1978). Thrombocytopenia with purpura due to drug-induced platelet aggregation has been noted after use of carbenicillin and penicillin G. These reports indicate a very low incidence of toxicity, so low as to preclude any change in the choice of therapy for the patient with an infection due to susceptible bacteria. However, when patients with impaired renal function are receiving prolonged parenteral courses of penicillin therapy (more than one week), the concentration of drug in serum should be determined to make certain that serum levels of the drug are not excessive.

If toxicity is not a significant concern with the penicillins, sensitization is a most important factor. Four types of reactions may occur after administration of a penicillin (or any drug or antigen):

1. Immediate or anaphylactic reactions occur within 30 minutes after administration and are life-threatening events. Clinical signs include hypotension or shock, urticaria, laryngeal edema, and bronchospasm. Acute anaphylaxis is rare after administration of penicillin (approximately one case per 20,000 courses of treatment in adults), but a significant number of fatalities occur each year because of the extensive use of these drugs. Children are believed to have fewer systemic reactions than adults, presumably because of less previous exposure to penicillin antigens. Oral preparations are less likely to result in an immediate reaction than are parenteral forms, perhaps because antigens are altered in the gastrointestinal tract or because of slower absorption.

2. Accelerated reactions occur from one to 72 hours after administration. The signs are similar to those of the immediate reaction but occur in a less severe form.

3. Late allergic reactions usually occur after three days. The major sign is skin rash. This is the most perplexing reaction to penicillin because it is nonspecific, and the rash may also be due to other drugs given at the same time or may be a sign of the infectious disease. Skin rash is associated with approximately 4 percent of courses of penicillins (up to 7 percent in the case of ampicillin).

4. Immune-complex reactions include serum sickness, hemolytic anemia, and drug fever. Penicillin-induced hemolytic anemia is associated with high and sustained levels of penicillin in blood. Circulating red blood cells are coated with a penicillin hapten, the patient makes antibody to the penicillin antigen, the antibody binds to the altered red cell surface, and the cell undergoes lysis or sequestration (Petz and Fudenberg, 1966).

Identification of the patient who will have a significant reaction if penicillin is administered is still difficult. Serological assays for detection of antibodies to penicillin have been considered; however, such assays lack specificity. Since the immediate reaction is largely mediated by IgE reagin or skin-sensitizing antibody, the patient who may subsequently respond with a life-threatening reaction could be identified by use of intradermal tests with appropriate antigens. Selection of the antigens to be used for skin testing, however, is an uncertain procedure because many different antigens play roles in the allergic reaction: at least 10 metabolic breakdown products of the penicillin nucleus have been identified, macromolecular impurities are present in solutions of the drug and high molecular weight penicillin polymers can be found in poorly buffered penicillin solutions standing for prolonged periods, side chains of the various penicillins may be responsible for reactions, and, finally, bacterial enzymes (amidases) used to prepare semisynthetic penicillins may cause an allergic reaction (Parker, 1972). Thus, investigators have had difficulty in choosing sensitive and specific antigens to use for skin-testing purposes.

The most promising studies of skin-test antigens have come from the laboratories of Levine (1966) at New York University and of Parker (1972) in St. Louis. Levine identified two materials for use in skin testing, penicilloyl polylysine, (Pre-pen, Kremers-Urban Co., Milwaukee, Wis.) and "a minor determinant mixture," a preparation of a dilute solution of aqueous crystalline penicillin G that includes metabolic breakdown products. In contrast, Parker used four skin-test antigens associated with penicillin and its products. A positive result is indicated by a wheal-and-flare reaction in 10 to 15 minutes and suggests a significant chance of reaction on subsequent administration of a penicillin; a negative result suggests that a significant allergic reaction will not take place. Although much effort has gone into clinical tests of these antigens, their prognostic value in children is still uncertain (Green et al., 1977; Levine et al., 1966).

At present, the physician must rely on the patient's history of an adverse reaction after administration of a penicillin to identify the patient who is likely to be allergic. If the reaction appears to be related to the administration of penicillin, the drug should be avoided for minor infections. If a life-threatening infection should occur and penicillin is clearly the drug of choice, as in the case of overwhelming disease due to *S. pneumoniae*, the physician may choose to administer the drug under carefully controlled conditions. A small dose may be injected initially in an extremity and may be followed by increasingly larger doses given every 30 minutes. Epinephrine, a tourniquet, and a tracheotomy set should be available in the event of a severe reaction during the testing period. All penicillins are cross-reactive in regard to sensitization, and allergy to any one implies sensitization to all.

Antimicrobial Agents Used as Alternatives to Penicillin

The Cephalosporins (see Table 8–5). The cephalosporins have a broad range of activity that includes gram-positive cocci, gram-negative enteric bacilli, and anaerobic bacteria. Most cephalosporins are relatively resistant to hydrolysis by beta-lactamases produced by *S. aureus*. At present, 19 cephalosporins are available in the United States, and many more are undergoing clinical trials. Some of the cephalosporins are of importance in therapy of otitis media and its complications. Many of the new products are introduced before clinical data on infants and children are available; physicians should read the package insert for current restrictions on usage in the pediatric age groups.

For simplicity, the cephalosporins have been categorized as first, second, and third generations (see Table 8–5), based on time of introduction and, to a lesser extent, similar *in vitro* activity. Most of the parenteral drugs can be administered by the intravenous or intramuscular routes, although for some, intramuscular injection is painful and intravenous administration is preferred. The oral products are absorbed well from the gastrointetinal tract, and the presence of food does not alter absorption.

The cephalosporins, like the penicillins, are safe for children and have almost no dose-related toxicity. Physicians should be alert for the uncommon reactions, including kidney problems, alcohol intolerance, serum sickness–like reactions, and bleeding. Nephrotoxicity has been reported in adults who received cephalothin in combination with gentamicin (Barza, 1978). A disulfuram-like response (Antabuse) occurred in patients taking alcoholic beverages following administration of cefamandole, moxalactam, and cefoperazone. Bleeding problems due to hypoprothrombinemia, thrombocytopenia, or platelet dysfunction have been associated with several cephalosporins but, in particular, moxalactam. If due to hypoprothrombinemia, bleeding was reversed by administration of vitamin K.

The cephalosporins may produce allergic reactions similar to those caused by the penicillins. There is cross-sensitization among the cephalosporins, and allergy to one implies (as is the case with the penicillins) allergy to all. Various degrees of immunological cross-reaction of penicillins and cephalosporins have been demonstrated *in vitro* and in animal models (Petz, 1978). Patients with a history of penicillin allergy have shown increased reactivity to cephalosporins. However, some patients who are allergic to penicillin have increased incidence of hypersensitivity to unrelated drugs, and it is still uncertain whether or not the penicillin-allergic patient reacts to a cephalosporin because of cross-allergenicity. Most patients who are believed to be allergic to penicillin may be given cephalosporins without an adverse reaction occurring. Although a cephalosporin may be used with caution as an alternative to penicillin in children who have an ambiguous history of skin rash, these cephalosporins should be avoided for the patient with a known immediate or accelerated reaction to a penicillin.

An unusual serum sickness–like reaction has been reported in children who received cefaclor (Murray et al., 1980). The children developed a generalized pruritic rash, similar to erythema multiforme; in some cases it was accompanied by purpura and arthritis with pain and swelling in knees and ankles. The signs appeared five to 19 days after the start of therapy with cefaclor and generally disappeared within four to five days after the drug was discontinued. The children had no prior history of allergy to a penicillin or a cephalosporin. Three hundred and eleven cases, including 289 children, were reported to the manufacturer by the winter of 1982. Approximately 3 million courses had been administered, suggesting a minimal (considering the likelihood of underreporting) incidence of one reaction per 10,000 courses. (Statistics provided by J. Getty, Marketing Plans Manager, Eli Lilly and Co., and published in Pediatric Infectious Disease Newsletter, edited by J.D. Nelson and G.H. McCracken, Jr., May/June, 1982, Vol. 8, No. 3.)

First-Generation Cephalosporins. The first-generation cephalosporins are effective against gram-positive cocci, including beta-lactamase–producing *S. aureus*, and have variable activity against gram-negative enteric bacilli. Six first-generation cephalosporins are currently available for use in infants and children: the parenteral drugs cephalothin, cefazolin, and cephapirin; the oral products cephalexin and cefadroxil; and cephradine, which is available in both oral and parenteral forms. Cephalothin and cephapirin are painful on intramuscular injection, and the intravenous route is preferred. Cefazolin produces higher concentrations in blood than the other parenteral first-generation drugs. The three oral preparations have comparable *in vitro* activity (Moellering and Swartz, 1976).

These drugs are alternatives to penicillin for disease caused by *S. aureus, S. pyogenes, S. pneumoniae,* and susceptible gram-negative enteric bacilli that are resistant to other drugs. Activity against *H. influenzae* is limited. First-generation cephalosporins are not the drug of choice for any pediatric infection but are of value for children with disease due to susceptible organisms who are known or suspected to be allergic to penicillin. Because of the uncertain aspects of cross-reactivity, cephalosporins should not be used if the patient has had an immediate or accelerated reaction to penicillin.

Second-Generation Cephalosporins. The second-generation cephalosporins consist of six parenteral drugs—cefamandole, cefoxitin, cefuroxime, ceforanide, cefonicid, cefotetan—and two oral preparations, cefaclor and cefuroxime. Ceforanide, cefotetan, and cefonicid are not approved for use in infants and children.

Cefoxitin has excellent activity against anaerobic organisms, particularly *B. fragilis,* and selective activity against gram-negative enteric bacilli. Cefoxitin has been effective for therapy of intra-abdominal, gynecological, and respiratory infections due to mixed bacterial pathogens, including anaerobic bacteria. Cefotetan was introduced in 1986 with an *in vitro* spectrum of activity and clinical usage similar to that of cefoxitin. Its safety and effectiveness have not been established in children.

Cefamandole is active against gram-positive cocci, including *S. aureus,* and was the first cephalosporin to be effective for infections due to *H. influenzae* (including beta-lactamase–producing strains). Reports of clinical and microbiological failure in a small number of cases of meningitis due to *H. influenzae* (presumably due to inadequate concentrations of drug in cerebrospinal fluid) indicate limited use of cephamandole for disease in which sepsis is not a concern.

Cefuroxime has an *in vitro* spectrum of activity similar to that of cefamandole but has been effective in meningitis due to *H. influenzae.* Cefuroxime is of value in the treatment of diseases in which gram-positive cocci, particularly *S. aureus* as well as *H. influenzae,* are the likely pathogens, as in septic arthritis, orbital cellulitis, and severe pneumonias. Cefuroxime offers the advantage of single-drug

therapy of these diseases, whereas previously, a combination of a penicillinase-resistant penicillin plus chloramphenicol was required. An oral form, cefuroxime axetil, has similar *in vitro* activity against pathogens of otitis media. At present the drug is not available in oral suspension, limiting its usage in infants.

Ceforanide possesses an antibacterial spectrum that is similar to that of cefamandole and cefuroxime; however, its *in vitro* activity is less. Experience in children is limited, and safety and effectiveness have not been established for children under one year of age. The main use in adults is perioperative prophylaxis.

Cefaclor is the only second-generation oral cephalosporin with activity that includes gram-positive cocci and *H. influenzae.* Clinical trials suggest efficacy in therapy of otitis media, sinusitis, and mild to moderate cases of pneumonia. Cefaclor is a suitable alternative to amoxicillin for treatment of the child with diseases due to susceptible bacteria and suspected allergy to penicillin or when a beta-lactamase–producing strain of *H. influenzae* is known or suspected to be a cause of disease.

Cefonocid has a spectrum of activity similar to that of cefamandole. The serum half-life is approximately five hours, and efficacy has been demonstrated for a single daily dose schedule. The drug is not approved for infants and children.

Third-Generation Cephalosporins. Cefoperazone, cefixime, cefotaxime, and moxalactam are very effective *in vitro* against gram-negative enteric bacilli and *H. influenzae* and have variable efficacy for gram-positive organisms. Cefoperazone has not been approved for use in children under 12 years of age. The *in vitro* activity of moxalactam and cefotaxime against *E. coli* and *S. pneumoniae* is greater than that from any other antibiotic now available. Moxalactam is not effective against group B streptococcus or *S. aureus,* and neither moxalactam nor cefotaxime is effective against *Enterococcus* species or *Listeria monocytogenes.* Moxalactam was equivalent to ampicillin or chloramphenicol for treatment of meningitis in children due to *H. influenzae* (Kaplan et al., 1984) and equivalent (when each was used in combination with ampicillin) to amikacin for treatment of meningitis in neonates that was caused by gram-negative enteric bacilli (McCracken et al., 1984). Moxalactam alone was successful in curing cases of chronic suppurative otitis media and malignant external otitis due to *P. aeruginosa* (Haverkos et al., 1982).

Ceftriaxone is effective against gram-positive cocci, including *S. aureus, S. pyogenes, S. pneumoniae,* and *H. influenzae,* and selected gram-negative enteric bacilli. The most unusual quality of ceftriaxone is the long duration of effective concentrations of drug in blood and tissues. The half-life in children is between 4.5 and 6.5 hours. Although meningitis due to *S. pneumoniae* and *H. influenzae* has been cured with regimens of ceftriaxone administered once per day, the recommended dosage schedule for treatment of serious disease is administration every 12 hours. For diseases requiring prolonged therapy, ceftriaxone may be of value for use outside the hospital. Once the acute signs of disease have diminished and the child remains in the hospital only for parenteral therapy, discharge and daily administration of ceftriaxone in the home or clinic may be considered (Higham et al., 1985).

Ceftizoxime has a spectrum of activity similar to that of cefotaxime and moxalactam. Clinical experience with the drug in children is limited.

Ceftazidime was introduced for clinical use in the United States in 1985. The drug is highly resistant to inactivation by a broad spectrum of beta-lactamases and has excellent activity *in vitro* against *P. aeruginosa,* including strains resistant to antipseudomonal penicillins. Its use in middle ear infections in children is likely to focus on chronic suppurative otitis media or other infections in which *P. aeruginosa* plays an important role.

Cefixime is an oral third-generation cephalosporin with broad gram-positive and gram-negative activity, including the bacterial pathogens responsible for otitis media. Its *in vitro* activity, clinical pharmacology, and use in patients with otitis media were reported in the proceedings of a conference held in March 1987 (Neu, 1987).

Use of the Cephalosporins in Infants and Children. Although many cephalosporins are available, there are relatively few infectious diseases in children for which one of these drugs offers a unique advantage over previously available antimicrobial agents. Some of the cephalosporins are appropriate alternatives when a previously available drug cannot be used (e.g., penicillin allergy), and some have potential advantages that have not been adequately studied in children. For treatment of otitis media and its complications, cephalosporins may be considered in the following circumstances: (1) Disease caused by *S. aureus, S. pyogenes,* and *S. pneumoniae* in children

with known or suspected allergy to penicillin—oral or parenteral first-generation cephalosporin. (2) Otitis media, sinusitis, and mild lower respiratory infections—cefaclor and cefixime. (3) Mixed infections, including anaerobic bacteria—cefoxitin. (4) Orbital cellulitis—cefuroxime or ceftriaxone. (5) Severe complications due to gram-negative enteric bacilli—cefotaxime or moxalactam. (6) Ambulatory therapy for patients requiring prolonged courses of therapy for disease—ceftriaxone. (7) Infections due to or suspected to be due to *P. aeruginosa*—ceftazidime.

Erythromycin. For otitis media, erythromycin is effective *in vitro* against the gram-positive cocci, *S. pneumoniae, S. pyogenes,* and penicillinase- and nonpenicillinase-producing strains of *S. aureus* but possesses only moderate activity against *H. influenzae.* Erythromycin is effective for infection due to chlamydia, a cause of otitis in young infants, and for infection due to *M. pneumoniae,* a possible cause of otitis in school-age children, adolescents, and young adults who have other respiratory manifestations of disease due to this organism.

Several preparations are available for oral administration. Because the erythromycin base is unstable in the acidic environment of the stomach, better-absorbed products were prepared by adding a protective enteric coating or by altering the chemical structure through formation of salts and esters. The derivatives of erythromycin are absorbed more efficiently from the gastrointestinal tract than is the base form; these derivations include the ethylsuccinate or propionate (esters), the stearate (a salt), and the estolate (salt of an ester). The estolate provides the highest concentration of antimicrobial activity in serum, but there is still controversy about which of the preparations provides the most biologically active drug at the site of infection. Since the base is the active component, all the erythromycin preparations must be hydrolyzed to the base after absorption.

Two erythromycin preparations are available for intravenous administration, the glucoheptonate (gluceptate) and the lactobionate forms. Intramuscular administration of these forms is painful and should be avoided. Phlebitis frequently occurs during intravenous administration and may limit the duration of use of these drugs.

The erythromycins administered by mouth are well tolerated, and all but the estolate are nontoxic. The estolate may give rise to a cholestatic jaundice that is believed to be due to a hypersensitivity reaction. Since this syndrome has been observed less frequently with other forms of erythromycin, the ester is thought to be responsible for the hepatotoxicity. The jaundice has been reported to occur almost exclusively in adults who receive the estolate for more than 14 days and to resolve usually when administration of the drug is stopped. Few cases of jaundice in children have been reported. At present, potential hepatotoxicity is not considered a contraindication to the use of the estolate in children. Nevertheless, physicians prescribing this preparation should limit duration of therapy to 10 days and should be alert for signs of liver toxicity (Braun, 1969).

Erythromycin may be considered for treatment of otitis media due to *S. pneumoniae, S. pyogenes,* and *S. aureus* (mild to moderate disease) in patients who are known or suspected to be allergic to penicillins. Serious disease due to *S. aureus* should be treated with a combination of erythromycin and another effective agent such as chloramphenicol because of the rapid development of resistance to erythromycin when prolonged use is required. Erythromycin has variable activity against *H. influenzae* and thus should not be relied on as the single antibiotic in treatment of otitis media (Table 8–4). *C. trachomatis* may be an important cause of otitis media in young infants (two weeks to six months of age); this disease appears to respond to therapy with either sulfonamides or erythromycin.

A fixed combination of erythromycin ethylsuccinate and sulfisoxazole is now available. Each 5 ml contains 200 mg of erythromycin activity and the equivalent of 600 mg of the sulfonamide. The combination provides activity against the pneumococcus and ampicillin-sensitive and -resistant strains of *H. influenzae.* The combination drug is of value for children who are allergic to penicillin or who fail initially when treated with ampicillin or amoxicillin and may have infection due to an ampicillin-resistant strain of *H. influenzae.*

Clindamycin and Lincomycin. These agents are effective *in vitro* against gram-positive cocci, including *S. pneumoniae.* Clindamycin is also active against a wide range of anaerobic bacteria, including penicillin-resistant *Bacteroides* species. Clindamycin provides higher levels of activity in serum than does lincomycin, and in contrast to lincomy-

cin, oral absorption is not decreased when the drug is taken with food.

Diarrhea and pseudomembranous enterocolitis may occur after use of clindamycin. Antibiotic-associated colitis has been reported in as many as 10 percent of patients after treatment with clindamycin. The epithelium of the colon undergoes necrosis, the mucous glands dilate and an inflammatory plaque forms and adheres loosely to the underlying epithelium. This disease has been associated with other antibiotics that alter intestinal flora, including ampicillin (Auritt et al., 1978), tetracycline, chloramphenicol, and lincomycin. Overgrowth of toxin-producing strains of *Clostridium difficile* is responsible for most cases of antibiotic-associated colitis. The antibiotic suppresses the normal flora in the colon, and the *C. difficile* organisms proliferate and produce an enterotoxin that is responsible for the disease. Most of these reactions have occurred in elderly patients, those with severe illness, or those receiving multiple antimicrobial agents (Gorbach and Bartlett, 1977). Clindamycin has been well tolerated by children. Diarrhea is a common side effect, but enterocolitis occurs rarely in this age group.

Clindamycin may be considered an alternative to penicillin for the patient who is believed to be allergic and has disease due to group A beta-hemolytic streptococci, *S. pneumoniae,* or *S. aureus.* Clindamycin should also be considered when infection is due to anaerobic bacteria, particularly *Bacteroides* species. Because of its limited activity against *H. influenzae,* clindamycin can be used as initial therapy for otitis only when combined with an agent, such as a sulfonamide, that is active against this organism.

The Sulfonamides and Trimethoprim-Sulfamethoxazole. The first sulfonamide (and the first drug of the modern antimicrobial era), Prontosil, was reported in 1935 by Domagk to be effective against infections due to beta-hemolytic streptococci. Sulfapyridine was introduced in 1938 and was the first antimicrobial agent effective against pneumococcal pneumonia. Soon after the introduction of these drugs, however, both streptococci and pneumococci developed resistance to the sulfonamides. Today, sulfonamides are used in the treatment of a wide variety of infections in children, including otitis media due to nontypable strains of *H. influenzae,* usually in combination with a penicillin or erythromycin to provide coverage for *S. pneumoniae*. Sulfisoxazole was used by Perrin and colleagues (1974) for prophylaxis in children with recurrent episodes of acute otitis media.

Trimethoprim-sulfamethoxazole is an antimicrobial combination with significant activity against a broad spectrum of gram-positive cocci and gram-negative enteric pathogens. Trimethoprim is more active than the sulfonamide, but the mixture is significantly more effective than either drug alone (see Table 8–4). The drugs act in synergy by blocking the sequence of steps by which folic acid is metabolized: the sulfonamide competes with and displaces *para*-aminobenzoic acid in the synthesis of dihydrofolate; trimethoprim binds dihydrofolate reductase, inhibiting conversion of dihydrofolate to tetrahydrofolate. The effect of sulfonamide in bacteria is circumvented in the mammal, which obtains folates from food sources. The reaction inhibited by trimethoprim is similar in bacteria and mammals but differs quantitatively in the extent of binding of the drug to the enzyme. Mammalian dihydrofolate reductase is 60,000 times less sensitive to trimethoprim than is the enzyme from *E. coli*.

Sulfamethoxazole was chosen as the sulfonamide to use in combination with trimethoprim because the drugs have similar patterns of absorption and excretion. Both are well absorbed from the gastrointestinal tract, and food does not affect absorption. A parenteral preparation is available. Rapid absorption and peak serum activity occur between one and four hours after oral administration; serum activity persists for more than 12 hours, but there is no significant accumulation after repeated doses given at 12-hour intervals

Adverse reactions to the combination include rashes similar to those previously associated with sulfonamides (maculopapular or urticarial rashes, purpura, photosensitivity reactions, and erythema multiforme bullosum) and gastrointestinal symptoms, primarily nausea and vomiting. Hematological indices have been carefully evaluated because of the antifolate activity of trimethoprim. Leukopenia, thrombocytopenia, agranulocytosis, and aplastic anemia have been associated with administration of trimethoprim-sulfamethoxazole, but the incidence of these adverse reactions is low. Hemolysis may occur in patients with erythrocyte deficiency of glucose-6-phosphate dehydrogenase.

The combination of trimethoprim and sulfamethoxazole in children has been effective in the treatment of acute otitis media due to *S. pneumoniae* or *H. influenzae* (including beta-lactamase–producing strains). However, the drug is not effective when *S. pyogenes* or *S. aureus* is the causative organism of acute otitis media. It also is not recommended for pharyngitis due to *S. pyogenes*. The combination has been used with success for children who are allergic to penicillins or who fail after an initial course of ampicillin due to beta-lactamase–producing strains of *H. influenzae* (Schwartz and Schwartz, 1980; Teele et al., 1981).

Vancomycin. Vancomycin is a parenterally administered antimicrobial agent with a spectrum of activity limited to gram-positive organisms. It is usually administered by the intravenous route because intramuscular injection causes pain and tissue necrosis. Ototoxicity and nephrotoxicity resulted from high concentrations in serum of early preparations, but improvements in the manufacturing process have resulted in a product that is believed to have lower toxicity. The principal uses in children are treatment of serious staphylococcal disease caused by strains resistant to the penicillinase-resistant penicillins and of sepsis caused by enterococci in the patient who has a significant history of allergy to penicillin. Vancomycin is one of the few drugs (rifampin, fusidic acid, and bacitracin are others) effective *in vitro* against the highly resistant strains of *S. pneumoniae* isolated recently in South Africa; it may become an important therapeutic agent if this strain becomes more widespread (Jacobs et al., 1978).

The Tetracyclines. Tetracyclines are effective against a broad range of microorganisms, including gram-positive cocci and some gram-negative enteric bacilli. Tetracycline should not be considered to be a substitute for penicillin for patients with otitis media due to or suspected to be due to gram-positive cocci, because a significant proportion of group A streptococci and some strains of *S. pneumoniae* are resistant.

Seven tetracycline compounds are available for oral administration in the United States: tetracycline, chlortetracycline, oxytetracycline, declomycin (demethylchlortetracycline), methacycline, doxycycline, and minocycline. Tetracycline, chlortetracycline, doxycycline, and minocycline are also available for intravenous administration. With few exceptions, there are only minor differences in the *in vitro* activity of the different preparations. However, minocycline may be effective against some strains of *S. aureus*, and doxycycline may inhibit strains of *B. fragilis* resistant to the other tetracyclines (Neu, 1978).

Tetracyclines are deposited in teeth during the early stages of calcification and cause dental staining. A relationship between the total dose and the degree of visible staining has been established. Tetracyclines cross the placenta, and discoloration of teeth has been seen in babies of mothers who received tetracycline or its analogues after the sixth month of pregnancy. The permanent teeth are stained if the drug is administered after six months and before six years of age. Other adverse effects include phototoxicity (particularly with declomycin), nephrotoxicity (with tetracycline hydrochloride, oxytetracycline, and declomycin), and vestibular toxicity (with minocycline).

There are few indications for administering a tetracycline to a young child; other effective drugs are available for almost all infections for which tetracycline might be considered. There is little reason to consider a tetracycline in the treatment of otitis media in children.

Drugs Effective Against Gram-Negative Enteric Bacilli

The Aminoglycosides. Aminoglycosides are drugs of value because they provide broad coverage against gram-negative enteric bacilli and some gram-positive organisms (such as *S. aureus*), are rapidly bactericidal, and are readily absorbed after administration. The major concerns in their use are nephrotoxicity, ototoxicity, and poor diffusion across biological membranes, including passage into cerebrospinal fluid. The aminoglycosides of current importance include streptomycin, kanamycin, gentamicin, tobramycin, netilmicin, and amikacin.

The *in vitro* activity of these antibiotics against gram-negative enteric bacilli varies and must be defined for each institution on the basis of current sensitivity tests. Streptomycin is not included in routine disk sensitivity tests nowadays because results for many years indicated that it is ineffective against a significant proportion of gram-negative enteric bacilli. The other aminoglycosides are active against most isolates of *E. coli* and *Enterobacter, Klebsiella,* and *Proteus* species. At present, gentamicin, tobramycin, netilmicin, and amikacin are the most active of the aminoglycosides against these organisms and against *P. aeruginosa.* The spectra of activity of gentamicin, netilmicin, and tobramycin are

similar, and strains resistant to one are usually resistant to the other. The major advantage of tobramycin is its activity against some strains of *P. aeruginosa* that are resistant to gentamicin. The spectrum of activity of amikacin is similar to that of gentamicin, netilmicin, and tobramycin, but there is little cross-resistance, and some gram-negative organisms resistant to these aminoglycosides are sensitive to amikacin.

The aminoglycosides have significant *in vitro* activity against *S. aureus* but are less effective for groups A and B beta-hemolytic streptococci and *S. pneumoniae*. A combination of a penicillin and an aminoglycoside results in more rapid killing and lower concentration of drug required to inhibit selected strains of gram-negative enteric bacilli and enterococci.

After parenteral administration, the aminoglycosides distribute rapidly in extracellular body water, with slow accumulation in tissues. Peak levels occur in serum between one and two hours after administration, and significant activity persists for six to eight hours. Penetration across biological membranes is variable, and diffusion into cerebrospinal fluid is limited (the concentration in cerebrospinal fluid is approximately 10 percent of the peak serum concentration).

All aminoglycosides may produce renal injury and ototoxicity. In general, gentamicin and tobramycin are more likely to affect vestibular function, and amikacin and kanamycin are more likely to damage the cochlear apparatus, but both functions may be affected by each drug. The cochlear effect may present as a high-frequency hearing loss or tinnitus; vestibular disturbances include vertigo, nystagmus, and ataxia. Some of the effects may be reversible, but permanent damage is frequent. Nephrotoxicity may present as albuminuria, the presence of white and red blood cells and casts in the urine sediment, or elevation of blood urea nitrogen or serum creatinine. Toxicity appears to be dose-related, although eighth nerve damage has followed the use of relatively small doses in patients with renal failure. Toxicity has not been a significant problem in children with normal kidney function who were treated with aminoglycosides according to currently recommended dosage schedules. Toxicity has usually been associated with administration of high doses for a long time, previous therapy with other aminoglycosides, administration of drugs to patients with impaired kidney function, or concurrent administration of other agents that are potentially nephrotoxic (e.g., the diuretics furosemide and ethacrynic acid).

Animal studies suggest that netilmicin has less ototoxicity and less nephrotoxicity than gentamicin. Comparable safety data in children are limited. The clinical role of netilmicin is probably similar to that of gentamicin, but assets over previously available aminoglycosides are yet to be demonstrated.

Concentrations of aminoglycosides in serum are variable and unpredictable. Patients who receive a prolonged course of aminoglycosides or who have impaired renal function require careful monitoring to determine safety as well as efficacy of the aminoglycoside. Blood should be obtained to determine drug concentration at the expected peak (one to two hours after parenteral administration) or trough (prior to the next dose, that is, eight or 12 hours after last administration). Specimens of blood should be obtained early in the course of therapy (within the first three days) to be certain that effective levels in serum are achieved and at subsequent intervals (every three to four days) to determine that the concentration of aminoglycoside in serum is below the level of toxicity (Evans et al., 1978). The desired peaks for the aminoglycosides are: gentamicin and tobramycin, 5 to 10 μg/ml; kanamycin and amikacin, 15 to 25 μg/ml. The trough should not exceed 2 μg/ml for gentamicin and tobramycin and 10 μg/ml for kanamycin and amikacin. The toxic ranges are considered to be 14 μg/ml for gentamicin and tobramycin and 40 μg/ml for kanamycin and amikacin. Dosage schedules should be modified if concentrations in serum are either too low, and therefore inadequate for optimal therapy, or too high and potentially toxic.

The major use of aminoglycosides for otitis media in children is for serious disease that is due to, or suspected to be due to, gram-negative enteric bacilli; these include infections of the neonate and suppurative complications of acute otitis media in the child with malignancy or immunological defect. Aminoglycosides may be of value alone or in combination with a broad-spectrum penicillin for chronic suppurative otitis media due to *P. aeruginosa*. The aminoglycosides may be administered by the intramuscular or intravenous (by slow drip over one to two hours) route. Oral preparations are not absorbed.

Published proceedings of symposia should be consulted for more specific information about the pharmacological actions and clinical uses of gentamicin (Finland and Hewitt, 1971), tobramycin (Finland and Neu, 1976), and amikacin (Finland et al., 1976).

Chloramphenicol. Chloramphenicol is active against many gram-positive and gram-negative bacteria and chlamydiae. Oral preparations are well absorbed. The intravenous route is preferred for parenteral administration, since lower levels of serum activity follow intramuscular use. The drug diffuses well across biological membranes even in the absence of inflammatory reaction. Approximately 70 percent of the concentration of chloramphenicol in serum is present in cerebrospinal fluid of patients with meningitis.

The major limiting factor in the use of chloramphenicol is its toxic effect on bone marrow. A dose-related anemia occurs in most patients receiving high-dosage schedules for more than a few days. The anemia is concurrent with therapy, ceases when the drug is discontinued, and is characterized by decreased reticulocyte count, increased concentration of serum iron, and cytoplasmic vacuolization of early erythroid and myeloid precursors in bone marrow (Scott et al., 1965).

Aplastic anemia is a rare (approximately one case per 20,000 to 40,000 courses of treatment) idiosyncratic reaction that is usually fatal. Most cases of aplastic anemia follow use of the oral preparation of chloramphenicol; few reports have been published of aplastic anemia that followed parenteral administration alone (Domart et al., 1961; Grilliat et al., 1966; Restrepo and Zambrano, 1968; Wallerstein et al., 1969). In some of these cases other drugs or the patient's disease could have been responsible for the aplastic anemia. Since very few patients receive chloramphenicol by the parenteral route only, as compared with the extensive world-wide oral usage of chloramphenicol (particularly in the many countries of Central and South America and Africa, where the oral drug is available without a prescription), and since the incidence of aplastic anemia is so low, we cannot be certain that aplastic anemia occurring almost exclusively after oral usage, rather than after parenteral administration, is a true event or one of statistical chance. Since cases of aplastic anemia following parenteral administration are extraordinarily rare, clinicians should not avoid use of intravenous chloramphenicol when it is indicated.

Because of the significant proportion of ampicillin-resistant strains of *H. influenzae,* chloramphenicol should be used in the initial treatment of severe and life-threatening complications of otitis media that are due to, or suspected to be due to, *H. influenzae* type b (such as meningitis). The initial regimen should be re-evaluated when results of cultures and susceptibility tests are available. Chloramphenicol may be an effective drug in the treatment of some cases of otitis media due to gram-negative enteric bacilli.

Wide variability occurs in concentrations of chloramphenicol in serum of infants and children. Peak serum concentrations should be 15 to 25 μg/ml to be safe and effective (Friedman et al., 1979).

The Polymyxins. Polymyxin and colistin are highly effective *in vitro* against a broad spectrum of gram-negative enteric bacilli, including *P. aeruginosa.* These drugs do not diffuse well across biological membranes, however, and are usually effective only when they are applied topically.

Antiviral Agents

Although three agents that have activity against respiratory viruses are available or under active investigation, no data are available about their efficacy in prevention or treatment of acute otitis media. Undoubtedly, this will change during the next few years.

Amantadine (Symmetrel), 1-adamantanamine hydrochloride, is active against influenza A and has been used extensively for prevention of illness. It has only modest therapeutic effect. The drug has little or no activity against influenza B, and higher concentrations that can be safely achieved in humans are required to inhibit rubella, parainfluenza, and respiratory syncytial viruses. Although the precise mode of action is unknown, antiviral activity appears to be due to interference with virus uncoating, rather than direct inactivation of infectious virus.

Ribavirin is a synthetic nucleoside that inhibits a wide variety of DNA and RNA viruses. Infants with bronchiolitis or pneumonia due to respiratory syncytial virus substantially improved with aerosolized ribavirin (Hall et al., 1983). The drug was introduced in the United States in 1986 (Virazole). Ribavirin is rapidly transported into cells, where it is converted by cellular enzymes to monophosphate, diphosphate, and triphosphate derivates that then inhibit viral or virally induced enzymes involved in viral nucleic acid synthesis.

Interferons are proteins that are released by cells in response to infection or other stimuli and induce a temporary antiviral state in uninfected cells. Until recently, only limited supplies of interferon were available; the drug was prepared by exposure of peripheral blood lymphocytes to a paramyxovirus. The interferon genes have been cloned into bacterial and yeast plasmids, and large quantities of interferon will be available now for investigational purposes. Alpha-2-interferon has been administered as an intranasal spray against infection due to rhinoviruses and coronaviruses, causes of the common cold. Recently published studies identify the efficacy of alpha-interferon administered as a nasal spray for short-term prophylaxis against the common cold in the household. Almost all the effect was against rhinovirus infections, with no preventive benefit for colds due to other agents (Douglas et al., 1986; Hayden et al., 1986).

Diffusion of Antimicrobial Agents into Middle Ear Fluids
(Tables 8–7 through 8–9)

Although studies of concentrations of various drugs in serum and middle ear fluid cited in Tables 8–7 through 8–9 differ in dosage schedules, time of collection, and methods of assay, the results indicate that most antimicrobial agents of value for treatment of acute otitis media achieve significant concentrations in middle ear fluid. Since the middle ear is embryologically, morphologically, and physiologically part of the respiratory tract, penetration of systemically administered antibiotics into middle ear mucosa and middle ear fluid provides a model for dynamics of diffusion of antibiotics in other areas of the respiratory tract.

The interested reader will find data about diffusion of the listed antimicrobial agent into middle ear fluid of patients with acute or chronic middle ear infection in these references:

penicillin G   Lahikainen, 1970; Silverstein et al., 1966

penicillin V   Howard et al., 1976; Kamme et al., 1969; Lundgren et al., 1979; Nelson et al., 1981

ampicillin	Coffey, 1968; Klimek et al., 1977 Lahikainen et al., 1977
amoxicillin	Klimek et al., 1977; Nelson et al., 1981
erythromycin estolate, ethyl succinate	Bass et al., 1971; Ginsburg et al., 1981 Nelson et al., 1981 Sundberg et al., 1979;
trimethoprim- sulfamethoxazole	Klimek et al., 1980; Kohonen et al., 1983 Nelson et al., 1981
cefaclor	Ginsburg et al., 1981; Lildholdt et al., 1981 Nelson et al., 1981
bacampicillin	Virtanen and Lahikainen, 1979
cefotaxime	Danon, 1980
oxytetracycline	Silverstein et al., 1966
metronidazole	Jokipii et al., 1978

These studies of penetration of systemically administered antibiotics have significant flaws in design:

1. Most include specimens obtained after a single dose, whereas Sundberg and coworkers (1979) showed that concentrations of erythromycin increased in middle ear fluids when specimens were obtained after multiple doses.

2. Standard curves of antibiotics are prepared in buffered solutions, which may not represent an adequate control for middle ear fluid.

3. Results of assays of materials obtained at various intervals after administration of drug give different concentrations in middle ear fluids and different ratios of middle ear fluid with simultaneously obtained serum. Peak values occur at different times for different drugs. Therefore, values taken at one sample time may not provide adequate indication of penetration into middle ear fluid.

4. Homogenization of mucoid or purulent middle ear fluid is difficult.

5. Specimens containing blood are not always excluded.

6. The condition of the mucosa is not accurately portrayed. Differences in penetration may vary, depending on the degree of inflammation of the mucosa, and this may not be identified or known by the investigator.

In spite of these significant limitations, data from assays of concentrations of drug in middle ear fluid provide useful information, which along with *in vitro* susceptibility data guide the choice of antimicrobial agents for otitis media.

Significant concentrations of each of the drugs tested appeared promptly in middle ear fluid. The concentrations of drug in the middle ear fluid were, in general, parallel though lower than concentrations of drug in serum. The peak activity in middle ear fluid was delayed when compared with peak activity achieved in serum, but duration of activity was similar in both serum and middle ear fluid. Concentrations of penicillin V and ampicillin in middle ear fluid of patients with

Table 8–7. CONCENTRATIONS OF ANTIMICROBIAL AGENTS IN SERUM (S) AND MIDDLE EAR FLUIDS (MEF/S) OF CHILDREN WITH ACUTE OTITIS MEDIA

Agent	Dosage (mg/kg)	Concentration (μg/ml)*			Reference
		S	MEF	MEF/S	
Penicillin V	13 PO	8.1	1.8	0.22	Kamme, Lundgren and
	26 PO	15.5	6.3	0.41	Rundcrantz, 1969
Ampicillin	10 PO	4.3	1.2	0.28	Lahikainen, Vuori, and
					Virtanen, 1977
Amoxicillin	10 PO	4.8	2.2	0.46	Howard et al., 1976
Bacampicillin	800 IM†	7.7	2.4	0.31	Virtanen and Lahikainen, 1979
Cefaclor	10 PO	7.0	1.3	0.19	Ginsburg, McCracken, and
					Nelson, 1981
Cefotaxime	25 IM/IV	5.8	2.1	0.36	Danon, 1980
Erythromycin					Ginsburg, McCracken, and
Estolate	15 PO	3.6	1.7	0.49	Nelson, 1981
Ethylsuccinate	15 PO	1.2	0.5	0.42	
Sulfonamide (trisulfapyrimidine)	30 PO	13.4	8.3	0.62	Howard et al., 1976

*Concentration achieved 0.5 to 2.5 hours after administration.

†Single dose administered to adults.

Table 8–8. **CONCENTRATIONS OF ANTIBIOTICS IN SERUM (S) AND MIDDLE EAR FLUIDS (MEF/S) OF CHILDREN WITH CHRONIC SEROUS OTITIS MEDIA***

Antibiotic (dose)†	Sample	Concentration (μg/ml)					
		Sample Time (minutes)					
		0–30	30–60	60–90	90–120	120–180	180–240
Amoxicillin	S	6.8	6.5	13.6	9.4	5.8	3.1
(15 mg/kg)	MEF	0.17	2.2	2.0	2.3	5.6	2.7
	MEF/S	0.03	0.34	0.15	0.24	0.97	0.87
Cefaclor	S	12.8	16.8	11.2	6.9	—	—
(15 mg/kg)	MEF	3.8	2.8	2.3	1.3	—	—
	MEF/S	0.30	0.17	0.21	0.19	—	—

*From Krause, P. J., Owens, N. G., Nightingale C. H., Klimek, J. J., Lehmann, W. B., Quintiliani, R.: Penetration of amoxicillin, cefaclor, erythromycin-sulfisoxazole, and trimethoprim-sulfamethoxazole into the middle ear fluid of patients with serous otitis media. J. Infect. Dis. 145:815–821, 1982.

†Specimens obtained after single dose.

chronic otitis media were lower than concentrations of fluid of patients with acute disease, but concentrations of amoxicillin, erythromycins, and cefaclor were similar in acute anc chronic effusions.

In children with chronic otitis media, concentrations of drug in purulent fluids had higher concentrations of drug than did mucoid or serous fluids, and concentrations were similar to those found in purulent fluids of children with acute otitis media (Nelson et al., 1981).

Penicillin V, ampicillin, bacampicillin, and cefaclor achieved concentrations in middle ear fluid that were approximately one fifth to one third of the levels present in serum. Approximately 50 percent of serum concentrations were achieved in middle ear fluid after administration of amoxicillin, erythromycins, and sulfonamides. Thus, usual dosage schedules of ampicillin, amoxicillin, bacampicillin, cefaclor, and trimethoprim-sulfamethoxazole produced concentrations of antimicrobial activity in middle ear fluid that were sufficient to inhibit *S. pneumoniae* and most strains of *H. influenzae* (excluding beta-lactamase–producing strains in the case of ampicillin, amoxicillin, and bacampicillin). The concentrations achieved in middle ear fluid after administration of penicillin V and erythromycins were sufficient to inhibit *S. pneumoniae* but were not adequate to inhibit most strains of *H. influenzae*.

Selected Aspects of Administration of Antimicrobial Agents

Dosage Schedules for Infants and Children

Dosage schedules of antimicrobial agents useful in otitis media are listed for infants (beyond the newborn period) and children in Table 8–3. Oral regimens are used for otitis media due to susceptible organisms in the absence of suppurative complications. Parenteral administration should be considered for severe infections due to less susceptible organisms and when sepsis or suppurative complications are present or imminent (Table 8–10).

Table 8–9. **CONCENTRATIONS OF ORALLY ADMINISTERED ANTIMICROBIAL AGENTS IN SERUM (S) AND MIDDLE EAR FLUIDS (MEF/S) OF CHILDREN WITH CHRONIC OTITIS MEDIA WITH EFFUSION**

Agent	Dosage	Concentration (μg/ml)*			Reference
		S	MEF	MEF/S	
Penicillin V	10 mg/kg	—	0.2	—	Nelson et al., 1981
Ampicillin	1 gm	22.4	1.5	0.07	Klimek et al., 1977
Amoxicillin	1 gm	15.3	6.2	0.41	Klimek et al., 1977
Trimethoprim	4 mg/kg	1.9	1.4	0.76	
Sulfamethoxazole	20 mg/kg	40.4	8.2	0.20	
Cefaclor	15 mg/kg	8.0	0.5	0.06	Lildholdt et al., 1981
Erythromycin	10 mg/kg				Nelson et al., 1981
Estolate		—	2.0	—	
Ethyl Succinate		—	0.3	—	

*Concentration achieved 0.5 to 2.5 hours after administration.

†Administered as the combination but assayed separately.

Table 8–10. **DAILY DOSAGE SCHEDULES FOR PARENTERAL ANTIMICROBIAL AGENTS OF VALUE IN INFANTS (OTHER THAN NEONATES) AND CHILDREN WITH SEPSIS OR SUPPURATIVE COMPLICATIONS OF OTITIS MEDIA**

Drug	Route	Dosage/kg/24 Hours*
Penicillin G	IV, IM	100,000–400,000 U in 4–6 doses
Methicillin	IV, IM	200 mg in 4–6 doses
Oxacillin	IV, IM	200 mg in 4–6 doses
Nafcillin	IV, IM	200 mg in 4–6 doses
Ampicillin	IV, IM	200–300 mg in 4–6 doses
Carbenicillin	IV, IM	400–600 mg in 4–6 doses
Ticarcillin	IV, IM	200–300 mg in 4–6 doses
Mezlocillin	IV	200–300 mg in 4–6 doses
Azlocillin	IV	200–300 mg in 4–6 doses
Cephalothin	IV, IM	100–150 mg in 4–6 doses
Cefazolin	IV, IM	50–150 mg in 4 doses†
Cefoxitin	IV, IM	80–160 mg in 3 doses
Ceftizoxime	IV, IM	150–200 mg in 3–4 doses
Cefuroxime	IV, IM	175–240 mg in 4–6 doses
Moxalactam	IV	150–200 mg in 3–4 doses
Cefotaxime	IV, IM	150–200 mg in 4 doses
Ceftriaxone	IV, IM	50–75 mg in 2 doses
Ceftazidime	IV	125–150 mg in 3 doses
Erythromycin	IV	50 mg in 4 doses†
Clindamycin	IM, IV	40 mg in 3–4 doses
Vancomycin	IV	40–60 mg in 4 doses
Chloramphenicol	IV	50–100 mg in 4 doses
Kanamycin	IV, IM	15 mg in 2–3 doses†
Gentamicin	IV, IM	5–7.5 mg in 3 doses†
Tobramycin	IV, IM	5 mg in 3 doses†
Amikacin	IV, IM	15 mg in 2 doses†
Sulfisoxazole	IV	120 mg in 4 doses
Trimethoprim-sulfamethoxazole	IV	8 mg TMP/40 mg SMZ in 2 doses

*Use high dosage schedule if meningitis is diagnosed or suspected.
†Administer in continuous drip or by slow infusion in 30 to 60 minutes or more.

Dosage Schedules for Newborn Infants (Table 8–11)

The clinical pharmacological action of antimicrobial agents administered to the newborn infant is unique and cannot be extrapolated from the results of studies done in older children or adults. Physiological and metabolical processes that affect the distribution, metabolism, and excretion of drugs undergo rapid changes during the first few weeks of life. The increased efficiency of kidney function after the first seven days of life requires a decrease in the interval between doses of penicillins and aminoglycosides to maintain high concentrations of drug in blood and tissues. Thus, different dosage schedules are provided for the first week of life and for subsequent weeks of the neonatal period. A recent monograph by McCracken and Nelson (1983) provides detailed information about the clinical pharmacological activity of antimicrobial agents in the newborn infant.

Food Interference with Absorption

The absorption of some oral antimicrobial agents is significantly decreased when the drug is taken with food or near mealtime. These drugs include unbuffered penicillin G, penicillinase-resistant penicillins (nafcillin, oxacillin, cloxacillin, and dicloxacillin), ampicillin, and lincomycin. Milk, milk products, and other foods or medications containing calcium or magnesium salts interfere with absorption of the tetracyclines. Absorption of penicillin V, buffered penicillin G, amoxicillin, cefixime, cephalexin, cefaclor, chloramphenicol, erythromycin, and clindamycin is only slightly affected by food. Antibiotics whose absorption is affected by concurrent administration of food should be taken one or more hours before or two or more hours after meals. A four-times-per-day dosage schedule should call for the drug to be given on arising, one hour before lunch, one hour before supper, and at bedtime.

Intravenous and Intramuscular Administration

After intravenous administration of most antimicrobial agents, there is a period when the concentration of drug in serum is higher than that following intramuscular administration. However, no therapeutic advantage of intravenous administration of antibiotics as opposed to intramuscular administration has been demonstrated. Intravenous administration should be used if the patient is in shock or suffers from a bleeding diathesis. If prolonged parenteral therapy is anticipated, the pain on injection and the small muscle mass of the young child preclude the intramuscular route and make intravenous therapy preferable.

Antibacterial concentrations in blood are similar after oral and intravenous administration of chloramphenicol and trimethoprim-sulfamethoxazole. Parenteral administration may be preferred because of hypothesized lesser bone marrow toxicity of chloramphenicol and ease of administration for the patient unable to take oral trimethoprim-sulfamethoxazole.

Chloramphenicol, the tetracyclines, and erythromycin should be administered parenterally by the intravenous, rather than the intramuscular, route. Chloramphenicol has variable absorption from intramuscular sites. The intramuscular injection of parenteral tetracyclines and erythromycin causes local irritation and pain.

The physician must be alert for thrombophlebitis that may result from prolonged intravenous administration and sterile abscesses that may follow intramuscular administration. The technique and complications of intramuscular injections were reviewed by Bergeson and colleagues (1982). In general, the site of injection in young infants is the upper lateral thigh, in children over two years of age it is the gluteal area, and for older children, the deltoid muscle. After selection of the proper site and insertion of the needle into the muscle, negative pressure is applied by pulling back on the plunger to be certain that the needle is not in a blood vessel.

Table 8–11. **DAILY DOSAGE SCHEDULE FOR PARENTERAL ANTIBACTERIAL AGENTS FOR NEWBORN INFANTS WITH SEPSIS OR SUPPURATIVE COMPLICATIONS OF OTITIS MEDIA**

Drug	Route	Dosage/kg/24 Hours* Seven Days of Age	Seven to 28 Days of Age
Penicillin G, crystalline	IV, IM	50,000–75,000 U in 2–3 doses	75,000–100,000 U in 3–4 doses
Penicillinase-Resistant Penicillins			
Methicillin	IV, IM	50–75 mg in 2 doses	75–100 mg in 3 doses
Oxacillin	IV, IM	50–75 mg in 2 doses	75–100 mg in 3 doses
Nafcillin	IM	50–75 mg in 2 doses	75–100 mg in 3 doses
Broad-Spectrum Penicillins			
Ampicillin	IV, IM	50–75 mg in 2 doses	75–100 mg in 3–4 doses
Carbenicillin	IV, IM	200–300 mg in 2–3 doses	300–400 mg in 3–4 doses
Ticarcillin	IV, IM	150–225 mg in 2–3 doses	225–300 mg in 3–4 doses
Cephalosporin			
Moxalactam	IV	100 mg in 2 doses	150 mg in 3 doses
Cefotaxime	IV, IM	100 mg in 2 doses	150 mg in 3 doses
Ceftazidime	IV, IM	60 mg in 2 doses	90 mg in 3 doses
Aminoglycosides†			
Kanamycin	IV,‡ IM	15 mg in 2 doses	15 mg in 3 doses
Gentamicin	IV,‡ IM	5 mg in 2 doses	7.5 mg in 3 doses
Tobramycin	IV,‡ IM	4 mg in 2 doses	6 mg in 3 doses
Amikacin	IV,‡ IM	15 mg in 2 doses	15 mg in 3 doses
Chloramphenicol†	IV	Premature—25 mg in 1 dose	Premature—25 mg in 2 doses
		Term—25 mg in 1 dose	Term—50 mg in 2 doses
Vancomycin	IV§	20 mg in 2 doses	30 mg in 3 doses

*The higher dose is recommended in the treatment of meningitis.
†Serum concentrations should be assayed to determine the optimal dose.
‡Intravenous administration given in a 20- to 30-min interval.
§Intravenous administration given in a 30- to 60-min interval.

Use of Drugs for Children in School or Group Day-Care Centers

Infants and children may return to the school or day-care center during a course of antimicrobial therapy. Because of the problems with administration of drugs outside the home, physicians should use medications that are given infrequently and need only simple directions. Drugs that are administered once or twice a day are preferred. Use of chewable tablets, when available, may be of value in reducing the need for the school or day-care provider to measure specific amounts of liquid suspension. Single-dosage regimens, such as intramuscular benzathine penicillin G for group A streptococcal infections, may be advantageous. Guidelines for administration of medications in school have been published recently by the Committee on School Health of the American Academy of Pediatrics and may also serve as a model for the physician who is prescribing drugs to be administered in day care (Zanga et al., 1984). Administration of medications in day care is addressed in a recent monograph, *Infectious Diseases in Child Day Care* (Smith and Aaronson, 1986).

Patient Compliance

The most frequent drug-related factor in failure of antibiotic therapy is inadequate compliance. Physicians overestimate the degree of compliance of their patients. Unacceptable taste or odor of drugs may result in poor compliance. Penicillin V, amoxicillin, and ampicillin are somewhat bitter, but acceptance is usually not a problem. Erythromycin preparations, alone or in fixed combination with sulfonamide, cefixime, and cefaclor are well accepted. Trimethoprim-sulfamethoxazole and the oral penicillinase-resistant penicillins have a bitter aftertaste, and compliance problems should be anticipated in instructions to parents (Nelson and McCracken, 1980; Schwartz and Schwartz, 1980). Diarrhea leads to discontinuance of courses more frequently with ampicillin than with amoxicillin or trimethoprim-sulfamethoxazole (Feder, 1982) and is a particular problem with amoxicillin-clavulanate.

Mattar, Markello, and Yaffe (1975) evaluated treatment given at home for children with otitis media. Full compliance with prescribed medications occurred in only five of 100 patients. Factors limiting compliance included incorrect dosage schedules (36 per-

cent), early termination (37 percent), inadequate dispensing of medication at drugstores (15 percent), spilled medicine (7 percent), and a series of other errors by physician, pharmacist, and parent (Table 8–12). Compliance improved to more than half when hospital pharmacy personnel gave patients and parents verbal and written instructions for administration of medications that were dispensed with a calibrated measuring device and a calendar to record doses taken.

Other drug-related factors include inappropriate dosage schedule and inadequate duration of therapy. Some antimicrobial agents deteriorate on prolonged storage. Adherence to expiration dates recommended by the manufacturer safeguards against inadequate potency of the drug.

Pharmacological Interactions

Concurrent administration of an antimicrobial agent and a second drug may result in altered pharmacokinetics of either drug.

The tubular secretion of penicillins and most cephalosporins is blocked by probenecid. This effect can be exploited by coadministration of probenecid (in a dose of 10 mg/kg four times a day in children to a maximum dose of 500 mg/kg four times a day) to

Table 8–12. **FACTORS IN FAILURE OF PATIENTS TO COMPLY WITH PRESCRIBED MEDICATION***

Physician Errors
Action of drugs and possible side effects not explained to parent
Dosage schedule ambiguous or incorrect
Instructions absent or incomplete
Multiple drugs prescribed, resulting in confusion
Cost of expensive trade brand used exceeds Medicaid reimbursement rate

Pharmacist Errors
Misleading or incorrect labels
Underfilling of prescriptions

Community Factors
Drugstores not open at time of day when parents seek medication

Parent and Home Factors
Difficulty in giving medication—two people often necessary to administer drug
Use of household teaspoon unsatisfactory
Bottles broken or spilled
Schedule of administration unrealistic for parent—baby sitter inadequate to dispense medication

*After Mattar, M. E., Markello, J., and Yaffe, S. J.: Pharmaceutic factors affecting pediatric compliance. Pediatrics 55:101–108, 1975.

produce a higher peak and more sustained level of antimicrobial activity.

Administration of chloramphenicol succinate with the anticonvulsant drugs phenobarbital and phenytoin leads to significant changes in concentrations of the antibiotic in serum: lower serum concentrations of chloramphenicol resulted when phenobarbital was coadministered, whereas higher serum concentrations of chloramphenicol were detected when phenytoin was coadministered. Phenobarbital may have induced the activity of hepatic endoplasmic reticulum, thereby increasing the metabolism of chloramphenicol, resulting in decreased concentrations of active antibiotic in serum and tissues. Phenytoin may cause induction of hepatic microsomal enzymes and compete with chloramphenicol for binding sites, resulting in elevated serum concentration of one or both drugs, possibly to toxic levels. Patients who receive chloramphenicol and anticonvulsant therapy require monitoring of serum concentrations to be certain of the safety and efficacy of the antibiotic (Krasinski et al., 1982).

Erythromycin interferes with the hepatic metabolization of theophylline, resulting in increased serum concentrations of theophylline that may produce nausea, vomiting, and other signs of toxicity. Coadministration of the two drugs is frequent in children with asthma. An alternative antibiotic should be considered, and if a suitable alternative is not optimal therapy, the dosage schedule of theophylline should be reduced and serum levels monitored (Prince et al., 1981).

Ototopical Use of Antimicrobial Agents

Ototopical antimicrobial agents are used for otitis media when a perforation of the tympanic membrane (or tympanostomy tube)

and a discharge are present. Neomycin, polymyxin B, chloramphenicol, and gentamicin are the most commonly used drugs. All of the agents are potentially ototoxic and should be used only when absolutely necessary. Sensitization does not appear to be an important problem with topical antibiotics, although some patients with chronic dermatoses may react to certain agents, such as neomycin.

Results of Clinical Trials of Antimicrobial Agents for Otitis Media

Assessment of Efficacy of Antimicrobial Agents

The efficacy of antimicrobial agents for otitis media may be assessed in terms of clinical, microbiological and immunological results (Table 8–13). Clinically, we expect effective drugs to produce a significant decrease in signs and symptoms of disease in 48 to 72 hours, to limit the duration of time of middle ear effusion, and to prevent complications of disease that occur by extension to adjacent tissues. Studies by Mandel and colleagues (1982) and McLinn (1980) indicate that more children who received cefaclor were free of effusion at 14 days after onset of therapy than children who received amoxicillin. The basis for this effect is unknown, but the data suggest that time to resolution of middle ear effusion should be included in assessment of antimicrobial agents evaluated for use in otitis media.

The major microbiological criterion for efficacy of antimicrobial drugs is sterilization of the middle ear infection. Studies by Howie and Ploussard (1969) attest to the value of the information provided by this "in vivo susceptibility test." Recent studies indicate that bacterial antigens persist in middle ear fluid, although the antibiotic may have rid the ear of viable organisms. Pneumococcal polysaccharide has been identified in the vast majority of fluids in which the organism is isolated and in many specimens that have no bacterial growth. The role of these bacterial products in diseases and the effect of antibacterial drugs in processing and eliminating the antigens are unknown but may be important in dealing with the problem of effusion that persists after acute infection.

The immunological process of otitis media is incompletely understood, and little information is available about the effect of antimicrobial agents on the development of local

---

Table 8–13. EFFICACY OF ANTIMICROBIAL AGENTS FOR TREATMENT OF OTITIS MEDIA

Clinical Efficacy
Resolution of acute signs
Decrease in duration of middle ear effusion
Prevention of complications

Microbiological Efficacy
Sterilization of infection
Elimination of microbial antigens

Immunological Efficacy
Development of local and systemic immunity

and systemic immunity after acute or chronic otitis media. Do antibiotics limit the immune response to infection in the middle ear? Do antibiotics differ in their effect on local or systemic immunity of the middle ear? How will these features of the immune response affect the duration of fluid in the middle ear? How will these features affect type-specific protection against the same bacteria? Antimicrobial agents undoubtedly play a role in modulating the immune response of the mucosa of the middle ear, but little is known about that role.

History of Clinical Trials

The design of clinical trials for evaluation of efficacy of antimicrobial agents in children with acute otitis media has undergone significant changes in the past 30 years. Prior to 1960, most American studies were performed without tympanocentesis and, thus, without a specific microbiological diagnosis. Often large numbers of children were enrolled to evaluate two or more drugs, the definition of otitis media was broadly stated and included such signs as inflammation of the tympanic membrane (which most experts now do not accept as a suitable sole criterion for otitis media with effusion), the drugs were assigned by some random method, and results of therapy were presented in general terms such as "good response" or "therapeutic failure." The results were usually ambiguous and demonstrated only minimal differences between the drugs studied (Stickler and McBean, 1964). A review of such articles today would yield little information of value in assessment of use of various antimicrobial agents available for management of acute otitis media.

Tympanocentesis to define the etiological agent in the middle ear fluid of children with otitis media with effusion had been common to clinical trials by Scandinavian investigators, but it became customary in American studies only in the 1960s. About this time, more investigators, both in the private practice of pediatrics and in academic centers, became interested in various aspects of infection of the middle ear, including evaluation of antimicrobial agents. The study designs were more precise—many studies were double-blind, sterilization was defined in some studies by reaspiration of persisting middle ear fluid, compliance was evaluated by assessment of use of the drug (weighing of returned bottles of medication or assay of urine for antimicrobial activity), the clinical course

was followed with precise endpoints, and side effects and toxicity of the antimicrobial agents were carefully assessed by clinical evaluation and laboratory tests.

Are Antimicrobial Agents Indicated for Acute Otitis Media?

Prior to the introduction of sulfonamides in 1936, management of acute otitis media included watchful waiting or, when the suppurative process produced severe clinical signs or complications, use of myringotomy to drain the middle ear abscess. Spread of infection to the mastoid, meninges, or other intracranial foci was a feared complication of otitis media.

After the advent of sulfonamides and later of penicillin and other antibiotics, the frequency of complications of otitis media showed a dramatic decline. In 1938, the frequency of mastoidectomy associated with acute otitis media was 20 percent; by 1948 it was 2.5 percent (Sorensen, 1977). In some studies it dropped to zero (Herberts et al., 1971). Mortality from acute otitis media was a concern prior to the advent of use of antimicrobial agents (Sorensen, 1977).

Most experts agree that acute otitis media should be treated with antimicrobial agents. This consensus is based on the facts that susceptible organisms, predominantly bacterial pathogens, are isolated from the majority of middle ear effusions of children who have acute otitis media and that there has been a significant decline in the incidence of suppurative intratemporal and intracranial complications of otitis media since the advent of use of antimicrobial agents. On the other hand, some physicians believe that antimicrobial therapy is used too frequently and should not be instituted for episodes of otitis media with minimal symptoms, that instead, it should be reserved for severe cases, for otitis media associated with suppurative complications, for effusions that become chronic, or for otitis media in certain high-risk children (Diamant and Diamant, 1974; van Buchem et al., 1981, 1985). Participants in a panel discussion at the Third International Symposium on Recent Advances in Acute Otitis Media with Effusion held in May of 1983 concluded that "there may be some merit in withholding antimicrobial therapy in selected patients who have acute otitis media, but the criteria for identifying patients for whom this type of management will be safe have not been defined." They recommended appropriate clinical trials to answer the question but, for the time being, concluded that an antimicrobial agent was indicated for treatment of acute otitis media (Bluestone et al., 1984).

Results of Therapeutic Trials Including Children Who Receive a Placebo

Many children with acute otitis media improve without use of antimicrobial agents. The use of a placebo group in a comparative trial with one or more antimicrobial agents has been studied by many investigators in the past 30 years. Some of these studies yield important information on the course of infection of the middle ear unmodified by an antimicrobial agent (at least, at onset).* Results from representative studies provide important insights into the value of antimicrobial agents and use of myringotomy alone or in combination with a drug. Only studies that used a method of aspiration of middle ear fluid to define the microbiological agents will be cited.

1. Rudberg (1954) evaluated 1365 patients with acute, uncomplicated otitis media treated as inpatients or outpatients at the Ear, Nose, and Throat Department of Sahlgrensk Sjukhuset, Gothenberg between January, 1951, and May, 1952. All patients were confined to bed and had their ears drained by syringe daily, as long as discharge was present. If spontaneous perforation did not occur, myringotomy was performed. Four regimens of antimicrobial agents were used: penicillin G tablets or a triple sulfonamide preparation alone or in combination, or an IM injection of a combintion of benzathine and procaine penicillin G. A fifth group received none of the drug regimens. The criteria for efficacy included the duration of discharge and incidence of complications. Between 236 and 333 cases were included in each group. The results were as follows:

Duration of ear discharge was significantly shortened in infections due to the pneumococcus and *H. influenzae* in patients who received penicillin or sulfonamide preparations, when compared with those who received placebo. Infections due to *S. aureus* and beta-hemolytic streptococcus were favorably altered by use of penicillin, but the

*These studies should not be considered to describe the natural course of otitis media, since all include a procedure that drains variable amounts of fluid: tympanocentesis (aspiration) or myringotomy (incision and drainage). In some cases, the procedure was repeated at frequent intervals.

results in the sulfonamide group were not significantly different from those for the placebo group. Complications, including exacerbation of clinical signs, mastoiditis, and failure of the infection to subside, occurred significantly more often in the placebo group than in the groups receiving penicillin, but the complications in patients receiving a sulfonamide were not significantly different from those of the placebo group. Mastoiditis occurred in 44 of 254 (17 percent) of patients receiving placebo, in four of 267 patients treated with sulfonamides, and in none of 844 patients managed with one of the penicillin regimens. The highest incidence of complications occurred in patients with disease due to beta-hemolytic streptococcus and *H. influenzae*.

2. In 1953 Lahikainen reported a study of children who were managed by use of myringotomy alone or in combination with penicillin G. The duration of discharge was significantly decreased in the group who received the antibiotic. No complications occurred in the penicillin-treated group, but nine of 153 patients who had myringotomy alone developed complications, including seven cases of mastoiditis, one case of meningitis, and one case of sinus thrombosis and brain abscess.

3. Van Dishoeck, Derks, and Voorhorst (1959) reported that 50 percent of 400 children treated with eardrops alone recovered in seven to 17 days, but 13 children developed mastoiditis requiring operation.

4. Halstead and colleagues in 1968 identified clinical improvement in a majority of untreated patients with suppurative otitis (almost all had cultures that were positive for *S. pneumoniae* or *H. influenzae*), but one third of the children (13 of 19) continued to be ill.

5. Howie and Ploussard (1972) evaluated various antimicrobial agents and included a group without antimicrobial therapy. Clinical and microbiological resolution occurred without use of antibiotics in a small number of patients with otitis media due to *S. pneumoniae* (nine of 45, 20 percent) and in a larger number of those with disease due to *H. influenzae* (nine of 21, 43 percent).

6. Lorentzen and Haugsten (1977) evaluated 505 children, and from these, three treatment groups were defined: myringotomy, penicillin V, and penicillin V in combination with myringotomy. Significantly more failures occurred in the myringotomy group (15 percent) than in the penicillin group (4 percent) or the penicillin plus myringotomy

group (5 percent). Thus, penicillin V was more efficacious than myringotomy alone, but myringotomy did not add to the effectiveness of the drug.

7. Van Buchem, Dunk, and van't Hof (1981) reported that antimicrobial therapy had no effect on the outcome of children with acute otitis media. The investigators treated 171 children in a double-blind study of four regimens: amoxicillin alone, amoxicillin plus myringotomy, myringotomy alone, and neither drug nor surgery. Children aged two to 12 years were enrolled by 12 general practitioners in or near Tilburg, The Netherlands. The results suggested that the clinical course (pain, temperature, otoscopic appearances, and recurrence rate) was not different in any of the groups, although ears had discharge for a longer time and eardrums took longer to heal (neither difference significant) in the children treated without antibiotics. The authors concluded that "symptomatic therapy with nosedrops and analgesics seems a reasonable initial approach to acute otitis media in children" (van Buchem et al., 1981).

The study has been discussed extensively in Letters to the Editor following publication of the article in The Lancet in October, 1981, and it was criticized in a Commentary in the Journal of the American Medical Association (Saah et al., 1982). The critics of the study identify flaws in the study design and analysis of results and question the validity of the conclusions. In general, the criticisms focus on the age of the patients (excluding infants, who have the highest age-specific incidence of disease), the small number of patients in each treatment group, the methods of statistical analysis, the absence of microbiological data, the absence of definition of disease, the failure to assess observer reliability for the many participating physicians, and the failure to consider important variables of disease in randomization for therapy.

Van Buchem and colleagues performed a second trial in which 4860 children two years of age or older with acute otitis media were treated with nose drops and analgesics alone for the first three to four days. Children whose condition took "an unsatisfactory course" (high temperature, otalgia, or persistent discharge) were treated with antimicrobial drug alone or in combination with myringotomy (van Buchem et al., 1985). More than 90 percent of the children recovered within a few days using this regimen, but two developed mastoiditis. Group A

Table 8–14. REASONS FOR RESOLUTION OF EFFUSION IN ACUTE OTITIS MEDIA WITHOUT USE OF ANTIMICROBIAL AGENTS

Effusion is due to nonbacterial organism
Effusion is due to a noninfectious cause
Effusion persists from a prior episode of otitis media
Effusion is cleared by:
  drainage through eustachian tube
  drainage through spontaneous perforation of tympanic membrane
  absorption by middle ear mucosa

streptococci was cultured from ear fluids of 39 percent of the children with the "unsatisfactory course" who underwent myringotomy; S. pneumoniae was cultured from 17 percent, but H. influenzae was cultured from only one child (1.4 percent).

These studies suggest that many cases of infection of the middle ear resolve spontaneously or with the assistance of surgical drainage. The reasons for resolution are listed in Table 8–14. Many cases improve because the contents of the middle ear infection are discharged through the eustachian tube or after spontaneous perforation of the tympanic membrane. In addition, many children have acute otitis media due to viruses or other microorganisms that are not susceptible to currently used antimicrobial drugs. The major advantages of antimicrobial agents as compared with placebo (the latter usually including some drainage procedure) are (1) the duration of drainage and other signs of clinical disease are decreased, and (2) the incidence of complications, though low, is significantly decreased, almost to zero.

Results of Recent Clinical Trials

A summary of results of selected clinical trials of various antimicrobial agents in children with acute otitis media is given in Table 8–15. The reports were published between 1969 and 1985, and the list includes only studies that identified the bacterial cause by aspiration of middle ear fluid. The clinical results were consistent with the results that would be expected based on in vitro studies of the activity of antimicrobial agents (see Table 8–4) and data about concentrations of drug achieved in middle ear fluid (see Tables 8–7 through 8–9).

Because of the marked susceptibility of the pneumococcus for all drugs tested (with the sole exception of sulfonamides), clinical results of drugs for otitis media due to S. pneumoniae were uniformly satisfactory. The efficacy of the drugs for infections due to H. influenzae was variable. Ampicillin, amoxicil-

Table 8–15. **SELECTED TRIALS OF ANTIMICROBIAL AGENTS FOR ACUTE OTITIS MEDIA—CLINICAL RESPONSE TO THERAPY***

Investigator	Drugs	Clinical Efficacy	
		Streptococcus pneumoniae	*Haemophilus influenzae*
Nilson et al., 1969	Penicillin V	+	−
	Penicillin V Trisulfapyrimidines	+	+
	Ampicillin	+	+
Howie and Ploussard, 1972	Placebo	−	−
	Ampicillin	+	+
	Erythromycin esolate (E)	+	−
	Trisulfapyrimidines (S)	−	+
	E & S	+	+
Feigin et al., 1973	Ampicillin	+	+
	Clindamycin	+	−
Howie et al., 1974	Ampicillin	+	+
	Amoxicillin	+	+
Howard et al., 1976	Amoxicillin	+	+
	Penicillin	+	−
	Erythromycin esolate	+	−
	E & S	+	+
Stechenberg et al., 1976	Ampicillin	+	+
	Cephalexin	+	−
Shurin et al., 1980	Ampicillin	+	+
	Trimethoprim-sulfamethoxazole	+	+
Mandel et al., 1982	Amoxicillin	+	+
	Cefaclor	+	+
Berman and Laver, 1983	Cefaclor	+	+
	Amoxicillin	+	+
Blumer et al., 1984	Trimethoprim-sulfamethoxazole	+	+
	Cefaclor	+	+
Marchant et al., 1984	Trimethoprim-sulfamethoxazole	+	+
	Cefaclor	+	−
Odio et al., 1985	Amoxicillin-clavulanate	+	+
	Cefaclor	+	+
Rodriguez et al., 1985	Erythromycin-sulfamethoxazole	+	+
	Amoxicillin	+	+

*For purposes of this table, clinical results are defined as satisfactory (+) or unsatisfactory (−).

lin, cyclacillin, cefaclor, sulfonamides, and trimethoprim-sulfamethoxazole were effective. Penicillin V, erythromycins, and clindamycin were ineffective. Cephalexin was ineffective in a dosage of 50 mg/kg/day (Stechenberg et al., 1976) for infections due to *H. influenzae*, but McLinn (1980) noted that improved results occurred when 100 mg/kg/day was used. Cases of acute otitis media due to beta-lactamase–producing *H. influenzae* either were not present (such strains were first identified in 1974), were not identified, or were of limited number.

A small number of cases of otitis media due to *S. aureus* were treated successfully with clindamycin (Feigin et al., 1973). As had been noted in earlier studies, sulfonamides (in this case trisulfapyrimidines) failed to alter the course of acute otitis media due to group A streptococcus (Howie and Ploussard, 1972).

Relapse and Recurrence

The reasons for antimicrobial failure were addressed in two studies. Children whose clinical signs did not resolve after initial therapy of a 10-day course of ampicillin, amoxicillin, or erythromycin-sulfonamide mixture were evaluated (Schwartz et al., 1981). Middle ear fluid was aspirated and cultured for bacteria: ampicillin-resistant *H. influenzae* was found in about one third (31 percent), ampicillin-susceptible strains of *S. pneumoniae* or *H. influenzae* were identified in about one half (51 percent), and no bacterial growth was found in the other fluids. Boston children who failed to respond to therapy were studied in a similar fashion with the following results: 19 percent had organisms resistant to initial therapy, and 57 percent had no bacteria isolated from the middle ear fluids (Teele et al., 1981). Some children who fail clinically do so because of a bacterial pathogen resistant to initial therapy, but many children have bacteria that are susceptible to the drug, and some have negative bacterial cultures and presumably have a nonbacterial microorganism as the cause of otitis media or some other reason for the persistent fever. The child who fails to respond to therapy in 48 to 72 hours, or later relapses, should receive a new antimicrobial regimen that provides effective activity against organisms that might be resistant to the initial therapy (i.e., beta-lactamase–producing organisms that would inactivate ampicillin).

The bacteriological features of middle ear infection in children who have recurrent episodes of acute otitis media are, in general, similar to those found in first episodes: the predominant pathogens are *S. pneumoniae* (though of different serotypes) and nontypable strains of *H. influenzae*. Thus, the child with recurrent episodes of otitis media may be treated initially with the same antimicrobial regimens as the child with a first episode of middle ear infection.

Sterilization of Middle Ear Fluids by Antimicrobial Agents

Drs. Virgil Howie and John Ploussard, pediatricians in practice in Huntsville, Alabama, have contributed significant information about the epidemiology, diagnosis, and management of otitis media. The *in vivo* sensitivity test is one of their most valuable studies (1969). The middle ear fluid of children with acute otitis media was aspirated and cultured prior to the start of therapy with various antimicrobial agents. All drugs were prescribed in usual dosage schedules, and patients were advised to return in two to five days. If fluid was still present at the second visit, a culture of the fluid was obtained by needle aspiration. The results of these cultures are listed in Table 8–16. Their studies are consistent with expected results based on *in vitro* data (see Table 8–4) and achievable concentrations of drug in middle ear fluid (see Tables 8–9 and 8–10). Penicillins G and V, intramuscular benzathine penicillin G, and erythromycin were successful in eradicating *S. pneumoniae* from middle ear fluid. Sulfonamides and tetracyclines did not eradicate *S. pneumoniae*. *H. influenzae* was eradicated by ampicillin but not by penicillin V, intramuscular benzathine penicillin G, and erythromycin. The high minimum inhibitory concentration of penicillin V for *H. influenzae*

Table 8–16. **RESULTS OF ANTIMICROBIAL THERAPY IN OTITIS MEDIA—THE *IN VIVO* SENSITIVITY TEST**

Drug	Number of Patients from Whom Organism Was Recovered during Therapy*/ Number of Patients with Bacterial Otitis Media		
	Streptococcus pneumoniae	*Haemophilus influenzae*	*Branhamella catarrhalis*
Data from Howie and Ploussard, 1969			
Phenoxymethyl penicillin	0/2	7/7	N/A
Phenoxymethyl penicillin with sulfonamides	0/17	2/6	N/A
Ampicillin	1/20	0/17	N/A
Benzathine, procaine, aqueous penicillin	1/9	7/7	N/A
Erythromycin ethylsuccinate	1/15	17/20	N/A
Erythromycin ethylsuccinate plus triple sulfonamide suspension	3/8	2/7	N/A
Triple sulfonamide suspension	8/18	3/8	N/A
Data from McLinn, 1980†; McLinn and Serlin, 1983‡; Marchant et al., 1984§			
Amoxicillin†	4/37	3/14	0/6
Amoxicillin‡	0/35	0/23	0/4
Cyclacillin†	0/40	0/18	1/5
Trimethoprim-sulfamethoxazole§	0/19	1/14	0/9
Cefaclor,§ three times daily	1/37	3/20	0/2
Cefaclor,§ twice daily	4/20	8/18	0/8

*Two to 10 days after beginning therapy.
†Reaspiration of middle ear fluid two days after therapy.
‡Reaspiration of middle ear fluid two to three days after therapy.
§Reaspiration of middle ear fluid three to six days after therapy.

and the relatively low concentrations of benzathine penicillin G achieved in serum (and by extrapolation in middle ear fluid) are the probable reasons for failure of these two penicillins to sterilize *H. influenzae* from the middle ear fluid. An oral form of penicillin G was not studied.

Three recent studies using the methods of the *in vivo* sensitivity test add information about additional antimicrobial agents (McLinn, 1980; McLinn and Serlin, 1983; Marchant et al., 1984). Amoxicillin, cyclacillin, trimethoprim-sulfamethoxazole, and cefaclor (administered in the recommended dosage schedule of three times a day) were effective in sterilizing middle ear fluids two to six days after identification of otitis media due to *S. pneumoniae*, *H. influenzae*, and *B. catarrhalis*. Cefaclor administered twice a day was less effective than the other regimens for otitis media due to *S. pneumoniae* and *H. influenzae*.

Effect of Antimicrobial Agents on Duration of Effusion

The primary role of antimicrobial agents is to eradicate the local infection and to prevent spread to continuous and distant tissues. Recent studies demonstrating the persistence of middle ear effusions after acute infection suggest a need to consider duration of fluid in the middle ear among the criteria for efficacy of an antimicrobial agent. Few investigations have been designed to answer this question. Mandel and colleagues (1982) compared the results obtained by cefaclor and amoxicillin in children with acute otitis media. Fourteen days after onset of therapy, more children who received cefaclor had aeration of the middle ear (59 percent of 106 = 55.7 percent) than did children who received amoxicillin (40 percent of 97 = 41.2 percent; p=0.05). On day 42, the proportion of children with normal aerated ears was the same, 68.9 percent for cefaclor and 67.5 percent for amoxicillin. McLinn demonstrated similar findings in a study of ampicillin and cefaclor. It is possible that the differences on day 14 were related to differing effects of the antimicrobial drugs on the inflammatory response in the middle ear, whereas, by day 42, host factors were dominant and little difference would be expected, irrespective of the antibiotic used.

Effect of Antimicrobial Agents on Chronic Otitis Media with Effusion

Bacterial pathogens are identified in about one third of children with chronic otitis media with effusion (see Chapter Six, Microbiology). The role of the bacteria in persistence of fluid in the middle ear is uncertain. One hypothesis is that the bacteria or their products are a factor in the continued production of fluid. Would a course of an appropriate antimicrobial agent assist in ridding the ear of fluid? Healy administered trimethoprim-sulfamethoxazole (8 mg trimethoprim and 40 mg sulfamethoxazole kg/day in two doses) or control for four weeks to 200 children two to five years of age with middle ear effusion present for longer than 12 weeks. The proportion of children who were free of effusion at the four-week observation was significantly higher for the antibiotic group (58 percent), as compared with the observation group (6 percent) (Healy, 1984).

A similar benefit of cefaclor for treatment of otitis media with effusion was identified by Ernston and Anari (1985). Children with chronic otitis media with effusion were randomized to receive cefaclor (20 mg/kg/twice daily) or no antimicrobial therapy during the 10 days preceding the day appointed for surgery. On the day scheduled for surgery, 24 of 46 treated children had resolved the middle ear effusion, compared with five of 45 untreated children (p < 0.001). Eighteen of the 24 primarily healed children remained unoperated upon at a follow-up period with median of 20 months.

In a study of 488 children with middle-ear effusion, Mandel and coworkers (1987) reported that those treated with amoxicillin for two weeks had higher rates of resolution at two and four weeks after initiation of treatment than did placebo-treated controls. These data are sufficiently compelling to warrant consideration of a 10- to 14-day course of an appropriate antimicrobial agent, such as amoxicillin, prior to consideration of placement of ventilating tubes or adenoidectomy, or both.

Strategy for Management of Acute Otitis Media

Choice of Antimicrobial Agents

At present, antimicrobial agents should be administered to children who have acute otitis media (see Fig. 8–1). Since the same bacteria found in acute middle ear effusions have been isolated from ears of children who lack the classic signs and symptoms of acute otitis media and also from ears of children with chronic effusions, all children who have otitis media, regardless of the stage, should be considered candidates for a course of an antimicrobial agent if one has not been given during the recent past. However, in asymptomatic children who have otitis media with effusion of recent onset, spontaneous resolution can occur 90 percent of the time (Casselbrant et al., 1985).

Amoxicillin or ampicillin is the currently preferred drug for initial treatment of acute otitis media, since they are active both *in vitro* and *in vivo* against *S. pneumoniae* and *H. influenzae*. The current incidence of strains of ampicillin-resistant *H. influenzae* is low (only 3 to 8 percent of all cases of acute otitis media), and occurrence of ampicillin-resistant *B. catarrhalis* is variable from community to community; these resistance patterns do not require a change in recommendations for initial therapy (see Fig. 5–1). Other regimens that are satisfactory include trimethoprim-sulfamethoxazole, cefaclor, cefixime, amoxicillin-clavulanate, and combinations of a sulfonamide with benzathine penicillin G (administered by the intramuscular route as a single injection), oral penicillin G or V, clindamycin, or erythromycin. For the child who is allergic to penicillins, trimethoprim-sulfamethoxazole, cefaclor, or erythromycin or clindamycin combined with a sulfonamide provide equivalent antimicrobial coverage.

Intramuscular benzathine penicillin G is an alternative choice if the child is vomiting, if there is difficulty in oral administration, or if there is doubt concerning patient compliance with the prescribed regimen. This agent is effective against *S. pneumoniae* and *S. pyogenes* but must be combined with a sulfonamide for coverage of *H. influenzae*.

For neonates, immunosuppressed children, or those in whom an unusual organism has been isolated from the middle ear culture, the appropriate antimicrobial agent should be selected according to the results of sensitivity testing.

Dosage Schedules

Dosage schedules have been determined on the basis of studies of clinical pharmacology and results of clinical trials (see Table 8–7). Oral ampicillin, 50 to 100 mg/kg/24 hr, in four divided doses for 10 days, is recommended. Amoxicillin, 40 mg/kg/24 hr, is equally effective, can be given in three divided doses, and has fewer side effects, such as diarrhea. Ten days of treatment is recommended. If the child is allergic to the penicillins, then a combination of oral eryth-

romycin, 40 mg/kg/24 hr, and sulfisoxazole, 120 mg/kg/24 hr, trimethoprim-sulfamethoxazole, 8/40 mg/kg/24 hr, are suitable alternatives. The availability of a fixed combination of these two antimicrobial agents (Pediazole) makes the combination an attractive choice, since patient compliance is improved when only one medication need be given instead of two. If beta-lactamase–producing *H. influenzae* or *B. catarrhalis* is suspected or documented by tympanocentesis, then appropriate choices would be amoxicillin-clavulanate (dosage based on amoxicillin content), erythromycin and sulfisoxazole, trimethoprim-sulfamethoxazole (8/40 mg/kg/24 hr), cefaclor, 40 mg/kg/24 hr, in three divided doses, or cefixime, 8/mg/kg/day.

Failure to Respond to Initial Therapy

With appropriate antimicrobial therapy, most children with acute bacterial otitis media are significantly improved within 48 to 72 hours. The physician should be in contact with the patient to ascertain that improvement has occurred. If the patient does not respond to initial therapy with ampicillin or amoxicillin, infection with a resistant strain of *H. influenzae* should be considered. Toxicity with persistent or recurrent fever or otalgia, or both, should prompt the clinician to recommend tympanocentesis or myringotomy, or both, to identify the causative organism; a specific antimicrobial agent may then be chosen on the basis of the results of the culture of the middle ear effusion and sensitivity testing. However, if signs persist but the child has no toxic symptoms and aspiration to culture the middle ear effusion is not performed, the initial antimicrobial agent should be changed to a regimen to which most uncommon organisms, such as a beta-lactamase–producing *H. influenzae* or *S. aureus*, would be sensitive. If ampicillin or amoxicillin was initially given, then the combinations of erythromycin-sulfisoxazole, amoxicillin-clavulanate, cefixime, or cefaclor should be administered. Trimethoprim-sulfamethoxazole (8/40 mg/kg/24 hr in three divided doses) appears to be effective when ampicillin-resistant *H. influenzae* is present or suspected to be present. However, trimethoprim-sulfamethoxazole is usually not effective when *S. pyogenes* or *S. aureus* is the causative organism.

Duration of Therapy

Physicians must rely on empirically derived schedules of therapy to plan drug regimens that lead to rapid and complete resolution of disease but are of minimal risk in terms of clinical or microbiological failure or drug toxicity. For treatment of otitis media, opinions vary and the data are not easy to interpret. The dosage schedules presented in Table 8–7 appear appropriate for a 10-day course on the basis of currently available data.

Other dosage schedules (longer or shorter) than the traditional 10- to 14-day course may be as good, if not better. Recent studies compared the results of three- and 10-day courses of amoxicillin (Chaput de Saintonge et al., 1982), treatment with penicillin V for two and seven days (Meistrup-Larsen et al., 1983), and penicillin V administered for five or 10 days (Ingvarsson and Lundgren, 1982). In each study, the shorter course was similar in clinical results to the longer course. Methodological problems, including absence of microbiological diagnosis, limit the validity of the results. Nevertheless, there is reason to believe that for most children shorter courses may be as appropriate as 10 to 14 days, but the efficacy of longer courses, as yet not tested, may be superior to that of shorter courses.

Chemoprophylaxis for Recurrent Acute Otitis Media

Chemoprophylaxis implies use of drugs in anticipation of infection, whereas treatment implies use of drugs after infection has taken place or signs of infectious disease are evident. Although indiscriminate use of antimicrobial agents for prophylaxis is to be avoided, many forms of chemoprophylaxis have been extensively tested and are of proven value. Recent studies suggest that chemoprophylaxis may be effective in children with recurrent episodes of acute otitis media.

Criteria for Use of Chemoprophylaxis

Since prolonged courses of any drug may have harmful effects, the physician must be assured that the benefits of freedom from infection outweigh the risk of a prolonged course of a modified dosage schedule of drug. For any form of chemoprophylaxis, the following criteria should be considered:

1. The patient is at risk if infection occurs.
2. The microorganisms are known and are consistent causes of disease.

3. The microorganisms are unlikely to develop resistance to the drug used for a prolonged course.
4. The drug is well tolerated and can be administered in a convenient dosage and form.
5. The drug has limited side effects or toxicity.

We believe otitis media is a disease of sufficient importance to warrant chemoprophylaxis. The bacteriological aspects of otitis media are well documented, and *S. pneumoniae*, *B. catarrhalis*, and nontypable strains of *H. influenzae* are the major bacterial pathogens in all studies. Resistance has not occurred during prolonged use of sulfonamides or ampicillin. The experience with penicillins and sulfonamides for prevention of streptococcal infections in patients with rheumatic heart disease may provide some support for the concept that resistance of the upper respiratory flora is unlikely to occur. The sulfonamides and penicillins are available in a variety of convenient forms that are well tolerated in infants and older children. Drug toxicity is not a problem, although allergic reactions are to be expected in a small number of children. Parents must be made alert for signs indicative of known side effects or toxicity.

Children are at risk for recurrent episodes of acute otitis media during a relatively short period of life: most episodes occur between six and 24 months of age. If the child who is susceptible to recurrent otitis media could be protected from infection during this period, the morbidity of middle ear disease might be avoided. Thus, the concept of prophylaxis is a worthy one and deserves careful study by investigators, and it may be helpful when used appropriately by physicians who care for children.

Published Reports

Eight controlled trials suggest the value of chemoprophylaxis in children with recurrent episodes of acute otitis media.

Maynard, Fleshman, and Tschopp (1972) studied Alaskan Eskimo children. Ampicillin or a placebo was administered for one year to children under seven years of age living in Alaskan Eskimo villages. The children received a daily dose of oral ampicillin—125 mg for those up to two and one half years of age and 250 mg for older children. Otitis media was defined as a new episode of otorrhea by history or observation of a research

Table 8–17. **EFFECTS OF CHEMOPROPHYLAXIS ON RECURRENCE OF OTITIS MEDIA***

Drug	Number of Children (n = 54)	Number of Episodes	
		None	One or More
First Trial (12/72 to 2/73)			
Sulfisoxazole	28	25	3
Placebo	26	14	12
Second Trial (3/73 to 5/73)			
Sulfisoxazole	26	25	1
Placebo	28	19	9

*From Perrin, J. M., Charney, E., MacWhinney, J. B., Jr., McInerny, T. K., Miller, R. L., and Nazarian, L. F.: Sulfisoxazole as chemoprophylaxis for recurrent otitis media: A double-blind crossover study in pediatric practice. N. Engl. J. Med. 291:664–667, 1974.

nurse who made monthly visits to the villages. The incidence of otorrhea was reduced by approximately 50 percent in the 173 children receiving ampicillin, compared with the incidence in 191 children who received a placebo.

Perrin and coworkers (1974) administered sulfisoxazole or a placebo to 54 children in Rochester, New York, who were 11 months to eight years of age and had histories of recurrent episodes of acute otitis media (three or more episodes in the previous 18 months, or a total of more than five episodes). Children received a placebo or 500 mg of sulfisoxazole twice a day for three months. They were then switched to the alternate regimen for another three-month period. No specific criteria for otitis media were used by the participating pediatricians (a four-physician group practice in suburban Rochester). A significant decrease in new episodes of acute otitis media occurred in the group of children receiving the antimicrobial agent. The older children, six to eight years of age, showed minimal or insignificant decrease in incidence of otitis media when on the prophylactic regimen. The results of the study are given in Table 8–17.

Biedel (1978) evaluated the effectiveness of sulfonamides (sulfisoxazole or trisulfapyrimidine in a dosage of 100 to 130 mg/kg/24 hr, or sulfamethoxazole in a dosage of 55 mg/kg/24 hr) used at the onset of signs of infection of the upper respiratory tract. Children were enrolled in the program after recovery from a recent acute episode of otitis media. They were placed alternately into treatment (sulfonamide) or control (decongestant) groups when parents called the physician and reported any sign of a new upper respiratory tract infection. Treatment was prescribed for a minimum of six days, and any new episodes of otitis media that occurred during the eight weeks following recovery from the original episode were recorded. Otitis media was found to recur with a new upper respiratory infection more frequently in children receiving decongestants than in children receiving sulfonamide.

Five other studies of prophylaxis for recurrent acute otitis media published between 1981 and 1985 by Schwartz and colleagues—Liston, Foshee, and Pierson (1983); Schuller (1983), Versans and colleagues (1985), and Persico and associates (1985)—corroborated the results in the initial studies. Of the eight studies, six used a sulfonamide (sulfisoxazole in five and sulfamethoxazole in one) and two used a penicillin (ampicillin or penicillin V in one each). Reduction in number of episodes of acute infection in children in the prophylactic group, when compared with results for the controls, varied from 47 percent (Maynard et al., 1972) to 90 percent (Schuller, 1983). These additional features were noted in one or more of the studies:

1. Age was an important factor—infants under two years of age were most likely to be benefited by chemoprophylaxis.

2. Compliance was critical to success of the program.

3. A carry-over effect was noted in some of the studies (Liston et al., 1983; Schwartz 1982). Children had less disease in the months after conclusion of the prophylactic regimen.

4. No increase in drug resistance of organisms in the upper respiratory tract occurred. The data about bacterial resistance are limited, and we must continue to monitor these results in studies in progress.

5. No significant incidence of side effects occurred when sulfonamides or ampicillin was used.

6. Duration of middle ear effusion was not significantly different in treated and control children.

Plan for Prophylaxis

Although the available studies do not provide conclusive evidence of the validity of chemoprophylaxis, the data are persuasive that children who are prone to recurrent episodes of acute infection of the middle ear are benefited. While we await definitive studies of usage of chemoprophylaxis, we believe it is reasonable to consider the following program:

Who?

Children who have had three documented episodes of acute otitis media in six months or four episodes in 12 months should be considered for the program.

Which Drugs?

Sulfisoxazole and ampicillin (amoxicillin is preferable) were the agents used in published studies and provide the advantages of demonstrated efficacy, safety, and low cost.

What Dosage?

Half the therapeutic dose should be administered once a day (usually at bedtime offers maximal compliance, but any single time during the day would be satisfactory). Dosage is amoxicillin 20 mg/kg or sulfisoxazole 50 mg/kg.

How Long?

During the winter and spring period, when respiratory tract infections are most frequent, treatment should be given for a period up to six months.

What Type of Follow-up?

Children should be examined at one-month intervals when free of acute signs to determine if middle ear effusion is present. Management of prolonged middle ear effusion should be considered separately from prevention of recurrences of acute infection (see Fig. 8–2).

How Should Acute Infections Be Treated?

Acute infections should be treated with an alternative regimen. Amoxicillin-clavulanate would be a suitable alternative irrespective of the drug used for prophylaxis. If a sulfonamide was used for prophylaxis, ampicillin or cefaclor would also be appropriate choices for treatment. If ampicillin or amoxicillin was used for prophylaxis, erythromycin-sulfisoxazole, trimethoprim-sulfamethoxazole, or cefaclor would be adequate to treat the acute infection.

OTHER MEDICAL THERAPIES

Decongestants and Antihistamines

Nasal and oral decongestants, administered either alone or in combination with an antihistamine, are currently among the most popular medications for the treatment of otitis media with effusion. The common concept is that these drugs reduce congestion of the mucosa of the eustachian tube; however, the efficacy of this mode of therapy for otitis media with effusion has not been demonstrated.

A number of investigators have evaluated decongestants with or without antihistamines, but the quality of design of the programs has varied and therefore the results are difficult to interpret.

1. Collipp (1961) evaluated the use of phenylephrine hydrochloride nose drops in treating acute purulent otitis media with effusion in 180 children aged two to 14 years. Half of the children were treated with nasal spray by their parents four times per day; the other half received no decongestant. All subjects were given an initial injection of procaine penicillin G and a 10-day course of sulfisoxazole, chlorpheniramine maleate, and phenylephrine hydrochloride. No statistical differences were noted in the otological status of the children who received the nasal spray and those who did not.

2. Rubenstein and coworkers (1965) treated 462 episodes of otitis media with effusion using several antimicrobial agents and the decongestant pseudoephedrine. Although some improvement was noted to be the result of treatment with the antimicrobial agents, the addition of pseudoephedrine to the medication regimen did not appear to improve treatment results significantly.

3. Miller (1970) evaluated the effect of a decongestant mixture containing carbinoxamine maleate and pseudoephedrine hydrochloride on 13 children with tympanostomy tubes that had been inserted to treat recurrent otitis media with effusion. The study used drug or placebo in a limited double-blind crossover design. The success of the placebo or drug was determined by the results of eustachian tube function tests that measured the ability to equilibrate applied

negative middle ear pressures. An almost equal number of patients demonstrated "suggestive" positive response or no response to the drug, whereas none of the children showed any response to the placebo.

4. Stickler and colleagues (1967), in a follow-up to Rubenstein's study (1965), evaluated the effects of penicillin and antihistamine (chlorpheniramine maleate), of penicillin alone, and of penicillin with sulfonamides on otitis media with effusion. Although sulfonamides did not improve the effects of the penicillin, the addition of the antihistaminic agent to penicillin did produce better results.

5. Olson and coworkers (1978) evaluated the efficacy of pseudoephedrine hydrochloride by studying the response to treatment of 96 children who had had acute otitis media with effusion that had not responded to treatment for two weeks. Following a double-blind protocol that compared the effects of the drug with those of the placebo, the children were treated for up to four or more weeks and were re-examined by pneumatic otoscopy and tympanometry. No significant differences between the treatment groups were found. Although the findings were not statistically significant, these researchers did note that males and children with an allergic history did worse on the decongestant.

6. Holmquist (1977) reported the effect of a combination of ephedrine and antihistamine compared with that of a placebo in a double-blind study on eustachian tube function in 58 patients (62 ears). The eustachian tube function was evaluated by means of air-pressure equalization and tympanometry. In the 28 ears of patients who received the drug, a "positive effect" was noted in 16 (57 percent), whereas of the 34 ears of subjects who received the placebo, a "positive effect" was reported in only 6 (18 percent); the difference was statistically significant at the 95 percent confidence level.

7. Fraser, Mehta, and Fraser (1977) compared ephedrine nose drops; a combination of brompheniramine maleate, phenylephrine hydrochloride, and phenylpropanolamine hydrochloride; autoinflation; and no treatment in children with otitis media with effusion and found no difference in tympanic membrane compliance, middle ear pressure, or audiometric findings among the treatment groups. In addition to problems associated with documentation of otitis media with effusion, the investigators had eight treatment regimens with only 10 or 11 subjects in each group, which leads one to question the design and statistical analysis of the study.

8. In a double-blind study, Roth and coworkers (1977) showed that pseudoephedrine hydrochloride decreased nasal resistance in adults who had an upper respiratory infection.

Past studies, employing a modified inflation-deflation manometric technique to assess eustachian tube function in children who had had recurrent or chronic otitis media with effusion, showed that the obstruction of the eustachian tube was functional rather than mechanical (Bluestone et al., 1974; Cantekin et al., 1976). However, further studies during periods of upper respiratory infection showed that eustachian tube function was decreased from the baseline measurements at these times (Bluestone et al., 1977a). This decrease was attributed to intrinsic mechanical obstruction superimposed on the functional obstruction.

9. In an attempt to determine the effect of an oral decongestant with or without an antihistamine on the ventilatory function of the eustachian tube, two separate studies were conducted in 50 children who had had chronic or recurrent otitis media with effusion and in whom tympanostomy tubes had been inserted previously (Cantekin et al., 1980a). The first was a double-blind study that compared the effect of an oral decongestant, pseudoephedrine hydrochloride, with that of a placebo in 22 children who developed an upper respiratory infection during an observation period. Certain measures of eustachian tube function were significantly elevated above baseline values during the upper respiratory infection, which was attributed to intrinsic mechanical obstruction of the eustachian tube. It was found that oral decongestants tended to alter these parameters of eustachian tube function in the direction of the baseline (before upper respiratory infection) values. Even though the effect was statistically significant, the favorable changes in measurements of tubal function were only partial and were more prominent on the second day of the trial, after the subjects had received four doses of the decongestant. However, the administration of a nasal spray of 1 percent ephedrine had no effect on eustachian tube function in these children.

The second study was a double-blind crossover design. In this study of 28 children who did not have an upper respiratory infection, the effect of a decongestant-antihistamine combination (pseudoephedrine hydrochloride and chlorpheniramine maleate) was compared with that of a placebo. When the subjects were given the decongestant-antihistamine medication, there were favorable changes in certain eustachian tube function measures that were not observed when the children received the placebo. Again, the response differences between the two groups were statistically significant. Even though these two studies indicated that an oral decongestant appeared to affect favorably the eustachian tube function of children who had an upper respiratory infection and that the combination of an oral decongestant and antihistamine had a similar effect on tubal function in children without an upper respiratory infection, an evaluation of the efficacy of these commonly employed medications must await the results of controlled clinical trials in children with otitis media with effusion.

10. Lildholdt and coworkers (1982) evaluated the effect of a topical nasal decongestant spray on eustachian tube function in 40 children with tympanostomy tubes. Five parameters of tubal function were assessed, employing a modified-inflation test and forced-response test before and after spraying the nose with either oxymetazoline hydrochloride or placebo, according to a double-blind study design. The results showed no significant differences between the two treatment groups of the study children who had severe functional tubal dysfunction, as documented by the constrictions of eustachian tube lumen during swallowing.

11. Cantekin, Mandel, Bluestone, and coworkers (1983), in a double-blind, placebo-controlled, randomized clinical trial of an oral decongestant and antihistamine combination in 553 infants and children with otitis media with effusion, showed *no* efficacy of these drugs. In addition, side effects such as irritability and sleepiness were more common in children in the drug group than in subjects who received placebo.

12. Mandel et al. (1987) reported that amoxicillin was effective when compared with placebo, in the treatment of otitis media with effusion. However, the addition of a combination of an oral decongestant and antihistamine to amoxicillin provided no additional benefit over amoxicillin alone; more side effects were noted in children who received the decongestant and antihistamine combination.

The conclusion from these studies is that topical or systemic decongestants and antihistamines for otitis media with effusion are not warranted but may be effective for less severe conditions such as eustachian tube obstruction (Cantekin et al., 1980a). In children receiving these agents, however, side effects are common, and some, such as visual hallucinations, are quite disturbing.

Corticosteroids

The administration of adrenocorticosteroids in the form of either a topical nasal spray or a systemic preparation has been advocated for treatment of otitis media with effusion for the past two decades. Heisse (1963) reported excellent results with depomethylprednisone in 30 allergic patients who had otitis media with effusion. Oppenheimer (1968, 1975) recommended a short-term trial of corticosteroids in children. Shea (1971) also reported success in treating allergic children who had middle ear effusions with a four-day course of prednisone. Persico, Podoshin, and Fradis (1978) treated one group of 160 children with prednisone and ampicillin and another group of 116 children with ampicillin only. They reported a 53 percent resolution of the effusion in the group that received the steroid and ampicillin treatment, as compared with 13 percent in the group that was treated only with the antibiotic. However, none of these studies was a randomized, controlled trial.

Schwartz, Puglese, and Schwartz (1980) reported 70 percent success in treating 41 children with a seven-day course of prednisone in a double-blind, placebo-controlled, crossover study. The steroid appeared to be equally effective in those children who did and in those who did not have a history of allergy. However, Macknin and Jones (1985) conducted a controlled trial in children with either otitis media with effusion or persistent middle ear effusion after acute otitis media who were randomly assigned to enter a course of dexamethasone or placebo. The study was stopped before the trial was completed, since the investigators found no benefit in giving the drug.

Studies have been reported that have evaluated the effects of administering a topical corticosteroid nasal spray. However, Schwartz, Puglese, and Schwartz (1980) noted that when beclomethasone dipropionate spray was given to 10 children with otitis media with effusion, it was only effective in three. Lildholdt (1982), in a double-blind study employing beclomethasone nasal spray in children with otitis media with effusion, failed to show efficacy.

If, indeed, adrenocorticosteroid therapy is effective in the treatment of otitis media with effusion, the mode of action remains only speculative at this time but may be related to the anti-inflammatory action of the drug. Persico, Podoshin, and Fradis (1978) postulated that the drug altered surface tension forces within the lumen of the eustachian tube. Schwartz, Puglese, and Schwartz (1980) suggested that steroids may shrink the lymphoid tissue around the eustachian tube, acting on mucoproteins to decrease the viscosity of the middle ear effusion by reducing tubal edema or reversing metaplasia of the middle ear mucosa.

From these few studies it appears that a short course of systemic adrenocorticosteroid therapy is of uncertain efficacy in alleviating the problems of otitis media with effusion in children. At this time, the potential adverse side effects associated with the administration of a systemic adrenocorticosteroid for otitis media does not appear to justify its use in infants and children.

Immunotherapy and Allergy Control

Since the precise role of allergy in the development of otitis media with effusion has not been documented, and since at times it is difficult to establish or confirm the diagnosis of allergy with certainty, it is not possible at this time to quantify the relative efficacy of allergic management of otitis media with effusion in children. This topic is discussed further in the section on allergy and eustachian tube obstruction (page 24). In spite of this dilemma, owing to a lack of information, there are clinicians who advocate allergy management for infants and children who have recurrent or chronic otitis media with effusion. Other physicians doubt that allergy plays any part in the origin of otitis media with effusion and rarely, if ever, consider directing their treatment of a patient with this problem to a possible underlying allergy. For example, Bluestone and Shurin (1974) and Paradise (1980), in extensive reviews of otitis media in infants and children, did not include control of allergy as a management option. On the other hand,

there are those who include allergy in the differential diagnosis if there are one or more of the following: (1) past or present atopy in the child, (2) family history of allergy, or (3) signs of upper respiratory allergy present at the time of the clinical examination. These investigators have employed various regimens in their management of allergies, but all have reported obtaining good results from such treatment (Draper, 1967, 1974; Fernandez and McGovern, 1965; Kjellman et al., 1976; Phillips et al., 1974; Rapp and Fahey, 1973; Whitcomb, 1965).

Clemis (1976) considers inhalant allergy easiest to identify and treat and therefore advocates searching for inhalant sensitivities before looking for allergies to foods and chemicals. In his experience, house dust is the most frequent inhalant allergen identified. When house dust is identified as the problem, he advises "dust-proofing" the child's environment (especially the child's bedroom) and using electrostatic air filters. If environmental control measures are not successful in reducing symptoms, then hyposensitization to house dust may be considered. Mold spores are the second most common aeroallergen responsible for nonpollen allergy, for which he advocates environmental control, and if unsuccessful, hyposensitization. The treatment of choice when an adverse food reactivity is suspected is total dietary elimination of that food. In Clemis's experience, pollinosis plays a much less dominant role than that of dusts, molds, and foods in causing otitis media, but when pollinosis is present, he recommends hyposensitization. Pets may also be a source of allergy, but in this case, hyposensitization is not as successful as exclusion of the offending pet from the house. In Clemis's (1976) view, antihistamines are not of benefit in treating otitis media caused by allergy, and he advises against the use of cortisone, in either the systemic or topical intranasal forms, for therapy. Waickman (1979) agrees with Clemis that house dust is the most common allergic offender in patients who have otitis media with effusion that persists for two weeks or longer and has been unresponsive to adequate therapy for infection. Other inhalant antigens are considered to be less common offenders than dust, but for all inhalants the Rinkel (1962, 1963) method of immunotherapy is advocated.

In a double-blind, crossover study by Friedman and coworkers (1983) that involved adult volunteers without otitis media, eustachian tubes became obstructed when the subjects were challenged intranasally with the antigen to which they were sensitive but not when they were challenged with a placebo (i.e., an antigen to which they were not sensitive).

Unfortunately, none of these studies was based on randomized, controlled trials in children with otitis media. Nevertheless, there does appear to be some evidence that chronic and recurrent otitis media with effusion may be associated with upper respiratory tract allergy. Therefore, until our knowledge of the origin, method of diagnosis, and management of allergy in relation to otitis media with effusion increases, when a child has recurrent or chronic middle ear disease and evidence of upper respiratory tract allergy, management of the allergy should be considered as a treatment option. A history of itching of the eyes, nose, or throat; of paroxysms of sneezing; and of chronic or frequently recurrent watery rhinorrhea in the presence or absence of the classical signs of nasal allergy should prompt the clinician to evaluate further the possibility that the child has an upper respiratory tract allergy. However, since no convincing clinical trials of the treatment options have been reported, no single method of treatment can be recommended. It does not seem favorable at present to treat for allergy those children who have recurrent or chronic or both types of middle ear effusion and who lack the signs and symptoms of upper respiratory tract allergy. This could change, however, in the event that convincing data were presented to establish that the middle ear is a shock organ.

SURGICAL AND MECHANICAL THERAPIES

Myringotomy and Tympanocentesis

Myringotomy, or the incision of the tympanic membrane for acute otitis media, was first described by Sir Ashley Cooper in 1802 (Alberti, 1974). This procedure became increasingly popular until the 1940s, when antimicrobial agents came into wide use. Nowadays, myringotomy is reserved only for selected cases and performed primarily by otolaryngologists and a handful of primary care physicians; the indications are usually limited to those children who have severe otalgia or suppurative complications, or both. However, facing an apparent recent increase

in the prevalence and incidence of acute and chronic otitis media with effusion, there has been considerably more effort to study the efficacy of myringotomy in the management of this disease. The potential benefit from more liberal use of the procedure in cases of acute otitis media might be relief of otalgia and a decrease in persistence and recurrence rates. When chronic otitis media with effusion is present, myringotomy may be as effective in eliminating the middle ear effusion as when the procedure is followed with the insertion of a tympanostomy tube, with its attendant complications and sequelae (assuming a surgical procedure is indicated at all).

The results of studies conducted in the past to determine the efficacy of myringotomy for acute otitis media are shown in Table 8–18. In the study by Roddey and coworkers (1966), all 181 children received an antimicrobial agent, and in approximately half of the subjects, myringotomy was performed as well. The only significant difference between the two groups—judged by otoscopy at two, 10, 30 and 60 days and by audiometry at three to six months—was more rapid pain relief among a small group who had severe otalgia initially. Fewer children who had the myringotomy and antimicrobial therapy had middle ear effusion at the end of six weeks than did those who received antimicrobials alone, but the difference was not statistically significant. However, if a larger number of children had been involved in the study, the difference might have achieved statistical significance. Herberts and colleagues (1971) found no difference in the percentages of children with persistent effusion 10 days after either myringotomy and antimicrobial therapy or antimicrobial therapy alone. Lorentzen and Haughsten (1977) found the "myringotomy only" group to have the same recovery rate (88 percent) as both the group treated with penicillin V alone and the group treated with penicillin V and myringotomy. Puhakka and coworkers (1979) repeated the same study with 158 children and found that four weeks after the onset of acute otitis media, 71 percent of the children who did not undergo myringotomy but were treated with penicillin V were cured, whereas 90 percent of the group that had myringotomy and penicillin V treatment had the same outcome, indicating that "myringotomy clearly accelerates the recovery rate from acute otitis media." Qvarnberg and Palva (1980) reported results of their study of 248 children in which they compared the efficacy

Table 8–18. **PERCENTAGE OF PATIENTS WITH PERSISTENT MIDDLE EAR EFFUSION FOLLOWING INITIAL MYRINGOTOMY AND ANTIMICROBIAL THERAPY, COMPARED WITH THOSE RECEIVING ANTIMICROBIAL THERAPY ALONE FOR ACUTE OTITIS MEDIA**

| Investigator | Procedure* | Number of Subjects | Percentage With Persistent Effusion After: | | | Statistical Significance Achieved |
			10 to 14 Days	4 Weeks	6 Weeks	
Roddey et al., 1966	AB	121	35	7	2	No
	AB&M	94	24	9	1	
Herberts et al., 1971	AB	81	10	—	—	No
	AB&M	91	18	—	—	
Lorentzen and Haugsten, 1977	AB	190	16	6		No
	AB&M	164	20 (Est)	6		
Puhakka et al. 1979	AB	90	78	29	—	Yes
	AB&M	68	29	10	—	
Qvarnberg and Palva, 1980	AB	151	50	—	—	Yes
	AB&M	97	28	—	—	
Schwartz and Schwartz, 1980	AB	361	47	—	—	No
	AB&M	415	51	—	—	

*Key: AB = antibiotic; AB&M = antibiotic and myringotomy.

of penicillin V and myringotomy, penicillin V alone, and amoxicillin, and concluded that if the first attack of acute otitis media is treated with myringotomy and antibiotics (penicillin V or amoxicillin), cure is the rule, but that if antibiotics alone (either one) are used, 10 percent of the patients will run a prolonged course. Schwartz, Rodriguez, and Schwartz (1981) treated 776 children with a variety of antimicrobial agents, half of whom also had myringotomy (without aspiration), and found no difference in the relief of pain or in the percentage with persistent effusion 10 days after myringotomy therapy.

Unfortunately, all of these studies had design and methodological flaws that make interpreting their results and answering the question of the value of myringotomy for acute otitis media difficult. For example, in the study conducted by Puhakka and coworkers (1979), myringotomy was performed along with aspiration of the middle ear effusion, but it was a nonrandomized trial. However, children who received a myringotomy had a significantly shorter course of their disease than those who did not have a myringotomy. On the other hand, Schwartz, Rodriguez, and Schwartz (1981) failed to find a difference between those children who did and those who did not receive a myringotomy. There was no attempt to aspirate the middle ear effusion, and the children were not randomly assigned into the two treatment groups.

Indications

In spite of the lack of convincing evidence to support the routine use of myringotomy for *all* children with acute otitis media, there are certain indications for which there is consensus at present:

Suppurative Complications. Whenever a child has acute mastoiditis, labyrinthitis, facial paralysis, or one or more of the intracranial suppurative complications such as meningitis, myringotomy and aspiration should be performed as an emergency procedure. Tympanocentesis should precede myringotomy to identify the causative organism. In addition, in such cases the insertion of a tympanostomy tube should be attempted to provide prolonged drainage.

Severe Otalgia Requiring Immediate Relief. Even though some studies have failed to show that myringotomy alleviated earache (Schwartz et al., 1981), Roddey, Earle, and Haggerty (1966) did show that acute pain was relieved in those children who received myringotomy. Culture of the effusion is reasonable, since the middle ear is being opened, but it is not absolutely necessary if there is no reason to suspect the presence of an unusual organism.

Tympanocentesis and Myringotomy. Although not as compelling as the above indications, whenever diagnostic tympanocentesis is indicated, myringotomy for drainage may follow the needle aspiration, especially when a copious amount of middle ear effusion is identified by the tympanocentesis. Myringotomy may then reasonably follow tympanocentesis when acute otitis media is present and (1) when the child is critically ill; (2) when there is persistent or recurrent otalgia or fever, or both, in spite of adequate and appropriate antimicrobial therapy; (3) when acute otitis media occurs during the course of antimicrobial therapy given for another infection, and when the agent should be effective against the most common organisms causing otitis (for example, amoxicillin or ampicillin); (4) when otitis media occurs in the neonatal period; and (5) when it occurs in the immunologically compromised host.

(The specific indications and techniques for tympanocentesis are completely discussed in Chapter Seven, Clinical Diagnosis of Otitis Media.)

The benefit of performing myringotomy on all infants and children with acute otitis media is uncertain at present but it is a reasonable procedure, especially if otalgia is present. If a middle ear effusion persists after 10 to 14 days of antimicrobial therapy, myringotomy may also be appropriate if the child is still symptomatic, but if the child is relatively asymptomatic, the indications for the procedure would be less valid, since most effusions at this stage would be expected to clear spontaneously during the next several weeks. If the middle ear effusion persists for longer than three months, surgical drainage would appear to be a reasonable choice. If the procedure can be performed without the need of a general anesthetic, myringotomy alone would seem appropriate, with the physician reserving the insertion of a tympanostomy tube in case the effusion recurs soon after the myringotomy incision heals. However, if a general anesthetic is required to perform the surgical drainage of chronic otitis media with effusion, myringotomy and tympanostomy tube insertion would seem a valid option at present. This recommendation is appropriate, since Mandel and coworkers (1984) showed that myringotomy with insertion of a tympanostomy tube was more effective than myringotomy alone in a control group. The study was conducted in over 100 children who had chronic otitis media with effusion, which was unresponsive to amoxicillin treatment.

Tympanocentesis is a needle aspiration of the middle ear contents for diagnostic purposes, but myringotomy is a procedure in which an incision of the tympanic membrane by a myringotomy knife is made to provide adequate drainage (see Fig. 8–3). To accomplish this goal, the incision should be large enough to provide not only adequate and prolonged drainage into the external auditory canal but also aeration of the middle ear to enhance drainage down the eustachian tube. When acute otitis media is present in the infant or young child, adequate restraint

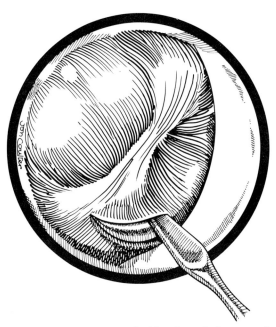

Figure 8–3. Myringotomy incision through the tympanic membrane for drainage of the middle ear.

employing a sheet or board especially designed for restraining children may be all that is needed; sedation is not necessary. However, for older children, sedation or even general anesthesia may be required. Iontophoresis does not effectively provide anesthesia of the tympanic membrane when acute otitis media is present. However, when myringotomy is to be performed for a middle ear effusion when acute disease is not present, iontophoresis may be a satisfactory method. The use of a topical solution of phenol gently applied to the exact spot on the tympanic membrane to be opened may be all that is necessary in older children and teenagers. The myringotomy incision should be a wide circumferential incision encompassing both inferior quadrants of the tympanic membrane in order to provide adequate drainage, and an attempt should be made to aspirate as much of the middle ear effusion as possible. Frequently, insertion of the suction tip through the incision on the tympanic membrane will enhance removal of the effusion and provide a larger opening which, it is hoped, will remain open longer than just an incision alone.

The procedure can be performed through an otoscope with a surgical head attached, or, for better magnification and binocular vision, the otomicroscope is desirable. For the routine case, the otoscope is quite adequate and makes the procedure readily available to the clinician in settings other than an operating room or otological outpatient area, where an otomicroscope would be available. By becoming proficient with the otoscope in performing myringotomy, the physician can perform the procedure in emergency rooms, inpatient pediatric floors, the child's home, or any other setting in which a child is examined and is in need of myringotomy.

In almost all conditions in which myringotomy is performed, diagnostic tympanocentesis may precede it. In such instances, the procedure should be performed as described in Chapter Seven (page 103).

The complications of performing a myringotomy properly are few. The persistent otorrhea that follows the procedure and is the most common finding after myringotomy can hardly be considered a complication, since it is the desired outcome; however, the discharge may become profuse and cause an eczematoid external otitis. If this occurs, meticulous cleaning of the external auditory canal with a cotton-tipped applicator; instillation of otic drops containing hydrocortisone, neomycin, and polymyxin; and insertion of a small piece of cotton (which should be changed frequently) in the outer canal will usually eliminate the problem. Dislocation of the incudostapedial joint, severing the facial nerve, and puncturing an exposed jugular bulb are dreaded complications but are so rare in experienced hands that they should not deter the trained practitioner from employing the procedure when indicated. The most common sequelae of the procedure are persistent perforation, atrophic scar, or tympanocentesis at the site of the incision. Even though the incidence of these conditions has not been systematically studied in a prospective manner, the risk of any or all occurring should not outweigh the benefits of myringotomy when indicated. The incidence of these sequelae occurring would rise in children who require repeated myringotomy, and in these patients, a tympanostomy tube should be considered, even though this is not without complications and sequelae.

Inflation of the Eustachian Tube

Procedures that force air through the eustachian tube and into the middle ear and mastoid cavities have been employed for over one hundred years in an effort to normalize negative intratympanic pressure and elimi-

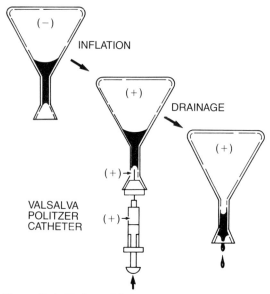

Figure 8–4. Flask model showing the rationale of how inflation of the middle ear promotes drainage down the eustachian tube. The eustachian tube–middle ear–mastoid air cell system can be likened to an inverted flask with a long, narrow neck (see text).

nate middle ear effusion. The methods of Valsalva and Politzer are the most commonly used in children (Politzer, 1909; Valsalva, 1949). Catheterization of the eustachian tube has also been utilized but is of limited usefulness in children, since the procedure can be frightening and is technically difficult to perform in young patients. All three of these methods are also crude tests of eustachian tube patency and have been described in detail in Chapter Three: Physiology, Pathophysiology, and Pathogenesis.

From a physiological standpoint, inflation of the eustachian tube, middle ear, and mastoid has merit. Figure 8–4 shows the flask model of the nasopharynx–eustachian tube–middle ear system: liquid is shown in the body and narrow neck of an inverted flask. Relative negative pressure inside the body of the flask prevents the flow of the liquid out of the flask. This is analogous to an effusion in a middle ear that has abnormally high negative pressure. If air is insufflated up into the liquid, through the neck and into the body of the flask, the negative pressure is converted to ambient or positive pressure and the liquid will flow out of the flask. However, if the liquid is of high viscosity, the likelihood of air being forced through the liquid into the body of the flask is remote, especially if the thick liquid completely fills the chamber. Therefore, in the human sys-

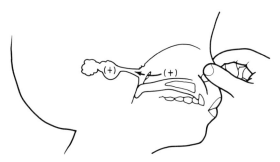

Figure 8–5. Self-inflation of the eustachian tube–middle ear, employing the method of Valsalva.

tem a thin, or serous, effusion would be more likely to flow out of the middle ear and down the eustachian tube than would a thick, mucoid effusion that fills the middle ear and mastoid cavities. The method probably is not effective in maintaining normal middle ear pressure in children who have atelectasis caused by eustachian tube obstruction (i.e., high negative pressure), since experiments in animals have shown inflation of the middle ear not to be effective (Cantekin et al., 1980c).

Theoretically, then, inflation of the eustachian tube and middle ear should be an effective treatment option for children with certain types of otitis media with effusion or atelectasis, or both; however, in reality, there are several problems with this method of management. The self-inflation method of Valsalva is somewhat difficult for children to learn, since it is a technique involving forced nasal expiration with the nose and lips closed. Cantekin, Bluestone, and Parkin (1976) tested 66 children between the ages of two and six years who had had chronic or recurrent otitis media with effusion and who had functioning tympanostomy tubes in place. They asked each subject to try to blow his or her nose with the glottis closed (Fig. 8–5). None of these children could passively open their eustachian tubes and force air into the middle ear by the Valsalva method, even though they developed a maximum nasopharyngeal pressure of 538.8 ± 237.0 mm H_2O. It was concluded that the Valsalva method of opening the eustachian tube in this age group was not successful owing to possible tubal compliance problems. Unfortunately, children in this age group have a high incidence of otitis media; for infants, who have the highest incidence of otitis media, the procedure cannot be used at all.

Politzer's method of opening the eustachian tube involves inserting the tip of a rubber air bulb into one nostril while the other nostril is compressed by finger pressure (Fig. 8–6) and then asking the child to swallow while the rubber bulb is compressed. Some children complain of a sudden "pop" in the air as the positive pressure is forced up the eustachian tube and have discomfort with the procedure. However, this method is also extremely difficult to perform in infants.

The major difficulty with both methods is determining whether the middle ear is actually inflated by the procedure. If a child hears a "pop" or has a pressure sensation in the ear, there is only presumptive evidence of passage of air into the middle ear. Auscultation of the ear (listening for the sound of air entering the middle ear during the procedure) is helpful in determining whether or not the procedure is successful, but a sound may be heard even when air does not enter the middle ear. Objective otoscopic evidence that the middle ear is actually inflated would be constituted by the presence of bubbles or a fluid level behind the tympanic membrane when these findings were not present prior to inflation. Another excellent method for determining objectively if the inflation is successful is to obtain a tympanogram before and after the procedure: the compliance peak should shift toward or be in the positive pressure zone after inflation (Fig. 8–7). If none of the results of these presumptive or objective methods of determining the success of inflation is definitive, then the clinician cannot be certain that the procedure has been therapeutic. Failure to

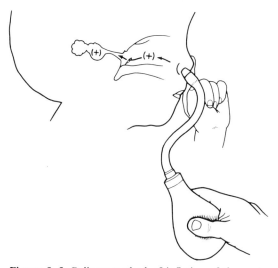

Figure 8–6. Politzer method of inflation of the eustachian tube–middle ear.

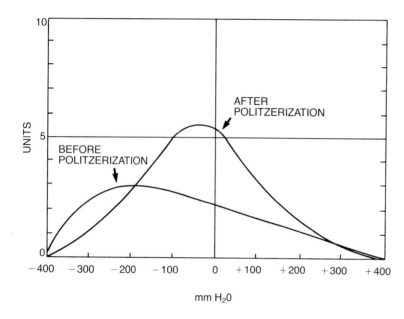

Figure 8–7. Tympanogram demonstrating objective evidence that inflation of the middle ear is successful. Before inflation, the compliance peak is in the negative zone (an effusion pattern), whereas after inflation, the peak is shifted toward the positive pressure zone.

achieve a successful result may be related to (1) inability of the patient to learn the method; (2) insufficient nasopharyngeal overpressure to open the eustachian tube passively; (3) eustachian tube abnormality; or (4) a middle ear filled with a very thick, mucoid effusion.

Unfortunately, the beneficial effect of the Valsalva and Politzer methods of inflation for treatment of otitis media with effusion or atelectasis has not been subjected to any acceptable randomized, controlled trials. Most of the evidence has been anecdotal. Gottschalk (1966, 1980) described remarkable success with a modification of the Politzer method in over 12,000 patients; the average course of treatment was a minimum of 12 inflations in the office on three separate days. Schwartz, Schwartz, and Redfield (1978) have shown that it is possible to inflate the middle ears of children at home by the Politzer method; they documented the results of the method by tympanometry but did not test its efficacy. The only controlled trial of this method was reported by Fraser, Mehta, and Fraser (1977), and they were not able to demonstrate that it was efficacious.

Until well-controlled clinical trials are reported, it would appear reasonable to use the Politzer method of inflating the middle ear for the following conditions. Barotrauma (following flying or swimming) should respond ideally to the Politzer procedure if atelectasis with high negative pressure or otitis media with effusion or both are present.

Inflation of the middle ear should be helpful under these circumstances, since this condition is usually not due to chronic eustachian tube dysfunction, and inflation may resolve the acute, subacute, or chronic disorder rapidly. When a middle ear effusion not due to barotrauma is found in a patient who only occasionally has a problem and in whom frequently recurrent or chronic disease is not suspected, then the procedure may also be successful, especially if a small amount of serous effusion is visible behind a translucent tympanic membrane. However, it is unlikely that a mucoid or purulent effusion could be evacuated by this technique, and if it could be, it would probably recur immediately after the procedure. Atelectasis of the tympanic membrane and middle ear, with or without high negative pressure, can also be treated by repeated autoinflation (Valsalva) or the Politzer method, but even if the middle ear is successfully inflated, the benefit is usually only of short duration and the procedure must be repeated frequently. Therefore, it is unlikely that inflation will be successful in alleviating for any length of time frequently recurrent or chronic eustachian tube dysfunction. There is also a remote possibility that bacteria can be forced into the middle ear from the nasopharynx during this procedure.

In conclusion, these procedures may be worthwhile for children with barotitis and for children who have an occasional episode of otitis media with effusion or atelectasis, but they are probably not helpful in children who have chronic or frequently recurrent middle ear effusion or atelectasis, or both.

Tympanostomy Tubes

Myringotomy with insertion of tympanostomy tubes is currently the most common surgical procedure performed in children that requires general anesthesia. The use of tympanostomy tubes was first suggested by Politzer over 100 years ago (1868), but they did not become readily available until they were reintroduced by Armstrong in 1954. Since then they have become increasingly popular. It has been estimated that in 1976 two million tubes were manufactured and, presumably, inserted through the tympanic membranes of probably more than one million patients (Paradise, 1977).

Several studies have addressed the question of the efficacy of myringotomy and the insertion of tympanostomy tubes for the treatment of otitis media with effusion.

1. Shah (1971) performed a myringotomy and aspiration in one ear and a myringotomy and aspiration with tympanostomy tube insertion on the opposite ear of children with bilateral mucoid otitis media with effusion. Adenoidectomies were performed on all of these children at the time that ear surgery was performed. Shah found that the hearing in the ears into which the tympanostomy tubes had been inserted was better than the hearing in the other ears six to 12 months after the procedures.

2. Kilby, Richards, and Hart (1972) also performed bilateral myringotomies (and inserted a tympanostomy tube into only one ear) in a series of children but did not perform an adenoidectomy at the same time. These investigators found no difference in the hearing in the two ears of these children two years after surgery, when all the tubes had been extruded.

3. Kokko (1974) compared findings in the ears of children who had undergone adenoidectomy, myringotomy, and tympanostomy tube insertion with the findings in the ears of those who had undergone adenoidectomy and myringotomy without insertion of tubes. He found, four and a half years after the procedures, no differences in the pathological conditions of the tympanic membranes or in the degree of hearing loss in the two groups.

4. Yagi (1977) compared 100 children who underwent an adenoidectomy, myringotomy, and tympanostomy tube insertion with 100 children who underwent only adenoidectomy. There were no significant differences between the two groups in (1) the number of children whose hearing problems were "cured" without further surgery, (2) the number of those requiring insertion of tubes due to recurrence of problems after initial treatment, (3) the number of patients having abnormal tympanic membranes, and (4) the number of patients with more than a 20-dB hearing loss 18 months after treatment.

5. Mawson and Fagan (1972) performed adenoidectomy, myringotomy, and tympanostomy tube insertion on a number of children and found that the degree of hearing loss and the number of tympanic membrane abnormalities (such as tympanosclerosis) noted increased the longer the children were followed. They reported that 76 percent of the children in their study required insertion of another tympanostomy tube within four years of initial treatment.

6. Tos and Poulsen (1976) performed adenoidectomy, myringotomy, and tympanostomy tube insertion on 108 children. During a five- to eight-year follow-up period, they reported that only 2.5 percent of the children into whose ears tympanostomy tubes had been placed had hearing losses, but that scarring was a frequently observed abnormality.

7. Marshak and Neriah (1981) did a retrospective study on 58 children, half of whom had undergone adenoidectomy and myringotomy for chronic otitis media with effusion and the other half of whom had only had tympanostomy tubes inserted. Only 20.7 percent of the adenoidectomized children had normal hearing and aerated middle ears during a two-year follow-up, whereas 59 percent of the children who had had tympanostomy tubes inserted had normal hearing and aerated middle ears at the same period.

8. Mandel, Bluestone, and coworkers (1984) conducted a study in 109 children who had chronic otitis media with effusion that had been unresponsive to antimicrobial therapy and randomly assigned subjects to receive either (1) myringotomy, (2) myringotomy and tube, or (3) no surgery (control). During the first year of the trial, subjects who had tympanostomy tubes inserted had less middle ear disease and better hearing than either children who had only myringotomy or those subjects in whom no

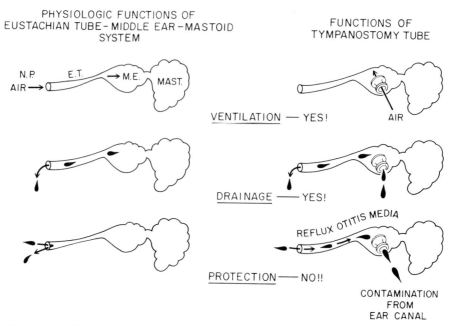

PHYSIOLOGIC FUNCTIONS OF
EUSTACHIAN TUBE-MIDDLE EAR-MASTOID
SYSTEM

FUNCTIONS OF
TYMPANOSTOMY TUBE

VENTILATION — YES!

DRAINAGE —— YES!

PROTECTION—NO!!

Figure 8–8. Physiological functions of the eustachian tube that are related to the middle ear. *NP*, nasopharynx; *TVP*, tensor veli palatini; *ET*, eustachian tube; *ME*, middle ear; *TM*, tympanic membrane; *EC*, external auditory canal; *MAST*, mastoid (see text).

surgery had been performed. In addition, half of the subjects in the myringotomy group had to have tympanostomy tubes inserted during the year, owing to an excessive number of myringotomies to control their disease. Likewise, half of the subjects in the control group required tympanostomy tube insertion during the course of the year because of development of "significant" hearing loss associated with their chronic middle ear effusion, even though none of the children had this degree of hearing loss when they entered the trial. This study is continuing at the Children's Hospital of Pittsburgh, since the long-term complications and sequelae of tympanostomy tube insertion must also be assessed.

Rationale for the Use of Tympanostomy Tubes

Even though the completed controlled clinical trials have not been reported, tympanostomy tube insertion would appear to be beneficial, since hearing is restored and permanent structural changes within the middle ear may be prevented. The rationale for the procedure may be found in certain physiological and pathophysiological aspects of the nasopharynx, eustachian tube, middle ear, and mastoid air cell system that are related to the pathogenesis of otitis media. The eustachian tube has three important physiological functions in relation to the middle ear (Fig. 8–8): (1) middle ear pressure regulation, (2) drainage of secretions down the eustachian tube, and (3) protection of the middle ear from the entrance of unwanted nasopharyngeal secretions (Bluestone and Beery, 1976).

A functioning tympanostomy tube would maintain ambient pressure within the middle ear and mastoid and provide adequate drainage both down the eustachian tube and through the tympanostomy tube. Therefore, two physiological functions of the eustachian tube are fulfilled by the tympanostomy tube. However, the protective function of the eustachian tube may be impaired by tympanostomy tube insertion, since all of the conventional tympanostomy tubes used leave an opening in the tympanic membrane, and the physiological middle ear air cushion is not present if the tympanic membrane is open. Therefore, reflux of nasopharyngeal secretions into the middle ear may be enhanced when a tympanostomy tube eliminates the middle ear air cushion, a situation that can result in "reflux otitis media" and otorrhea.

The ideal eustachian tube prosthesis would be a transtympanic tube that fulfilled all three of the important physiological functions of the eustachian tube: pressure regulation, drainage, *and* protection.

Recommended Indications for Insertion of Tympanostomy Tubes

Even though the efficacy of tympanostomy tubes has not been established, current indications for their use seem reasonable in selected cases until such controlled studies are reported.

Chronic Otitis Media with Effusion. Patients who have had otitis media with effusion that has been unresponsive to a course of antimicrobial therapy for at least three months are reasonable candidates for the insertion of tympanostomy tubes. The use of antimicrobial agents is based on results of several studies that have demonstrated the presence of bacteria in chronic middle ear effusions (Healy and Teele, 1977; Liu et al., 1975; Riding et al., 1978; Senturia et al., 1958). If antimicrobial therapy is unsuccessful, then removal of the middle ear effusion through a myringotomy incision is warranted. Persistence of otitis media with effusion immediately following myringotomy and aspiration of the effusion would be a compelling indication for the use of a tympanostomy tube. It would seem reasonable to attempt a myringotomy and aspiration of the middle ear effusion prior to insertion of a tympanostomy tube in both children and adults who do *not* require general anesthesia. However, if general anesthesia is necessary to perform a myringotomy, insertion of a tympanostomy tube at the same time would appear to be reasonable.

Removal of a middle ear effusion that is asymptomatic, especially when significant hearing loss is not present, is questionable. If air is visualized behind a translucent tympanic membrane (i.e., bubbles or a fluid level are visible), the condition would appear to be less severe. However, all such children have some degree of conductive hearing loss, and the short- or long-term effects of even modest degrees of hearing loss on the development of a child have not been measured adequately (Hanson and Ulvestad, 1979). In addition, it is not known what chronic irreversible changes such as adhesive otitis media, tympanosclerosis, ossicular discontinuity, or cholesteatoma might occur in the middle ear space if such an effusion is not treated. Therefore, the ultimate decision for use of tympanostomy tubes for chronic otitis media with effusion must be based on many factors, most of which remain arbitrary. At present, however, it seems to be reasonable to insert tympanostomy tubes to restore hearing and prevent possible complications and sequelae of recurrent and chronic otitis media with effusion.

Recurrent Acute Otitis Media. Many children, especially infants, have recurrent episodes of acute otitis media that respond to medical therapy or resolve spontaneously, and in these children the middle ear effusion does not become chronic. However, it would still be desirable to prevent these episodes when they occur frequently over a relative short period of time, since hearing is affected when the middle ear effusion is present and the child may be uncomfortable because of accompanying otalgia and fever. At present, there are three popular treatments for such episodes: (1) antimicrobial prophylaxis (Biedel, 1978; Ensign et al., 1960; Maynard et al., 1972; Perrin et al., 1974), (2) adenoidectomy with or without tonsillectomy (Bluestone et al., 1972, 1975), and (3) myringotomy with insertion of tympanostomy tubes (Gebhart, 1981).

In spite of the relative lack of proof of their efficacy, tympanostomy tubes may reasonably be assumed to prevent acute otitis media. Presumably, the tube could prevent aspiration of infected nasopharyngeal secretions into the middle ear, since ambient, rather than negative, middle ear pressure would be present. Absence of negative middle ear pressure could also prevent accumulation of a noninfected middle ear effusion. In addition, a nonintact tympanic membrane would allow for excellent drainage down the eustachian tube of any secretions entering the middle ear. However, in children with semipatulous eustachian tubes, reflux of nasopharyngeal secretions could be enhanced when the tympanic membrane is not intact, resulting in otorrhea secondary to reflux otitis media. Studies of appropriate design to test these hypotheses are lacking. Although data are not available, myringotomy with insertion of a tympanostomy tube appears to the authors to be helpful for children who suffer frequent, recurrent attacks of acute otitis media. Three or more episodes during the preceding six months, or at least four episodes during the preceding year (with the last episode occurring during the preceding six months), would be indications for performing this procedure. However, for such children a trial of antimicrobial prophylaxis would be an acceptable alternative management option, and myringotomy with insertion of tympanostomy tubes should be reserved for those children in whom chemo-

prophylaxis has failed. Antimicrobial prophylaxis should be considered only in those
children who have *no* evidence of a middle
ear effusion between the acute attacks. For
those children who have recurrent acute episodes superimposed on a chronic otitis media with effusion, tympanostomy tubes
should be inserted.

**Eustachian Tube Dysfunction and Atelec-
tasis of the Tympanic Membrane.** Tympanostomy tubes may restore normal middle
ear pressure in patients who have eustachian
tube dysfunction but who do *not* have a
middle ear effusion when one or more of the
following conditions is present: (1) otalgia,
(2) significant and symptomatic conductive
hearing loss, (3) vertigo, or (4) tinnitus. If
these signs and symptoms are believed to be
due to eustachian tube obstruction and not
related to a condition that can be improved
by medical treatment (e.g., sinusitis), then
tympanostomy tubes often provide relief.
This is not usually the case in patients with a
patulous or semipatulous eustachian tube.
When an abnormally patent eustachian tube
is suspected, a trial with just myringotomy
should first be attempted. If the patient is
symptom-free when the tympanic membrane
is not intact, a tympanostomy tube can then
be inserted. However, if the symptoms are
not eliminated or become worse, a tympanostomy tube should not be inserted. While
the tympanic membrane is open, a test of
eustachian tube function should be performed in an effort to determine the specific
type of dysfunction present. If the function
of the eustachian tube is normal, another
cause of the symptoms (e.g., inner ear disease) should be sought.

Atelectasis of the middle ear may be the
result either of passive collapse of the tympanic membrane, due to lack of stiffness of
the drum, or of active retraction of the tympanic membrane secondary to high negative
middle ear pressure. Atelectasis may either
be generalized or localized, or both, and may
be accompanied by a retraction pocket in the
pars flaccida or posterosuperior portion of
the tympanic membrane. These two portions
of the tympanic membrane are the most
compliant areas of the drum (Khanna and
Tonndorf, 1972). A severe retraction pocket
in the posterosuperior portion of the tympanic membrane may cause irreversible destruction of the incus, with resultant conductive hearing loss. Progression of such a
retraction pocket may also result in a choles-

teatoma. This sequence of events has been
shown to be associated with eustachian tube
dysfunction (Bluestone et al., 1977b) and may
be reversed by insertion of a tympanostomy
tube. However, if the retraction pocket is
associated with adhesive otitis media in which
the tympanic membrane is adherent to the
incudostapedial joint and the surrounding
area, restoration of normal intratympanic
pressure with a tympanostomy tube may not
be successful in returning the tympanic membrane to its neutral position. Following tympanostomy tube insertion, persistence of such
a retraction pocket in the attic or in the
posterosuperior quadrant, or in both, may
require a tympanoplastic procedure in an
effort to prevent progressive disease. However, when tympanoplasty is performed in
such ears and eustachian tube function is
abnormal, insertion of a tympanostomy tube
should be considered postoperatively to
maintain normal middle ear regulation of
pressure, which should prevent recurrence
of the retraction pocket and possibly the
development of a cholesteatoma (Bluestone
et al., 1978, 1979).

Surgical Technique and Type of Tube Employed

Insertion of a tympanostomy tube into the
posterosuperior quadrant of the tympanic
membrane is not advised, since this is the
most compliant part of the pars tensa and
may result in a permanent perforation or an
atrophic scar with subsequent retraction
pocket. A retraction pocket could lead to
necrosis of the incus or formation of a cholesteatoma, or both. Insertion of a tympanostomy tube under the annulus also may result
in a cholesteatoma. It seems more appropriate to insert the tube into the anterior portion
of the pars tensa. In fact, when there is severe
generalized atelectasis, the anterosuperior
portion may be the only area into which a
tympanostomy tube can be inserted (Fig.
8–9).

The type of tube employed varies with the
surgeon. The short, double-flanged tubes appear to provide adequate middle ear aeration
without a high incidence of obstruction of
the lumen by mucus or cerumen, but water
can more readily enter the ear through a
short tube. However, when the longer type
of tube is used, there is a greater chance of
obstruction of the lumen. The size of the

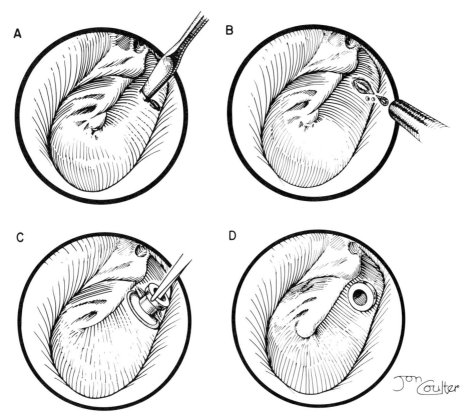

Figure 8–9. Method of insertion of a tympanostomy tube. *A*, Radial incision in the tympanic membrane. *B*, Middle ear effusion aspirated. *C*, Short, biflanged tympanostomy tube (Armstrong type) inserted using alligator forceps. *D*, Tube position in anterosuperior portion of tympanic membrane.

lumen of the tube is quite variable, but, again, if the lumen is too small, obstruction is a problem, and if the lumen is too large, removal or spontaneous extrusion of the tube could result in a persistent perforation. Tubes are made of various materials, but no data are available to show the superiority of one type of biocompatible material over another.

Much controversy exists concerning the indications for insertion of tympanostomy tubes that are more or less "permanent." Insertion of such tubes may be warranted in selected patients: those in whom tympanostomy tubes have frequently been tried and in whom eustachian tube dysfunction appears to be not only chronic but also not likely to improve in the near future. "Permanent" tubes may also be used in adults with long-standing chronic otitis media with effusion or severe atelectasis. However, these tubes should not be used in children, since the incidence of otitis media with effusion and atelectasis of the tympanic membrane progressively decreases with advancing age

during childhood. This is true even for children with cleft palates who have had repeated myringotomies. On the infrequent occasions when permanent tympanostomy tubes are used in children, the function of the eustachian tube should be tested periodically to determine when or if there is evidence of improvement so that the tube may be removed.

Even though many ways to assess eustachian tube function have been tried, there is currently no known method that surpasses observation of the middle ear when the tympanic membrane is intact. Therefore, the best way to determine if a patient needs another tympanostomy tube after the tube extrudes spontaneously is to examine the ears frequently.

When Should Tympanostomy Tubes Be Removed?

In general, once tubes have been inserted, they should be permitted to extrude spontaneously into the external auditory canal and not be removed surgically. The rationale for such management is based on experience rather than on any controlled clinical trials: in children with tympanostomy tubes in place, eustachian tube function has not been shown to change significantly, even after several years (Beery et al., 1979).

There are, however, some exceptions to this generalization. Serial eustachian tube function tests should be carried out, and if significant improvement does occur, then the tympanostomy tube may be removed.

Most tympanostomy tubes remain in the tympanic membrane for six to 12 months, although some have been known to have remained in place for years. In children in whom tympanostomy tubes have been inserted bilaterally and in whom one tube subsequently extrudes but the other remains in place for a prolonged period, the remaining tube can usually be removed if the opposite middle ear remains free of high negative middle ear pressure or middle ear effusion, or both, for at least one year after the spontaneous extrusion of the opposite tube. This method of management is based on the observation that eustachian tube function is usually about the same in both ears in children. If high negative middle ear pressure or otitis media with effusion, or both, occur during the observation period, the tube in the opposite ear should not be removed. Unfortunately, this method of management cannot be employed in adults, since eustachian tube function may not be symmetrical.

Complications and Sequelae

Complications of insertion of tympanostomy tubes include scarring of the tympanic membrane (tympanosclerosis) and localized or diffuse membrane atrophy, with or without retraction pockets, or atelectasis, or both (Kokko, 1974; Lildholdt, 1981; Mawson and Fagan, 1972; Muenker, 1980). Much less commonly, a perforation may remain at the insertion site following extrusion of the tube, or a cholesteatoma may develop. Other complications include secondary infection accompanied by otorrhea through the tube and dislocation of the tube into the middle ear cavity.

The most common complication of tympanostomy tube insertion is otorrhea through the lumen of the tube. This is usually the result of reflux of nasopharyngeal secretions into the middle ear. Otorrhea occurs in two thirds of infants with unrepaired cleft palates

who have had tympanostomy tubes inserted to treat chronic otitis media with effusion and who are followed during the first two years of life (Paradise and Bluestone, 1974). However, otorrhea may also occur in children without cleft palates in whom tubes have been inserted. When this occurs, a culture should be obtained from the middle ear by obtaining an aspirate through the tympanostomy tube. A preliminary culture of the ear canal and meticulous cleaning of the ear canal should precede the aspiration of the middle ear. Oral systemic antimicrobial therapy should be guided by the results of the middle ear culture and susceptibility studies; the same pathogens that cause acute otitis media in the community are usually isolated. Treatment in the absence of results from a culture would be the same as recommended when the tympanic membrane is intact, e.g., amoxicillin (see pp. 121–124). Topical antimicrobials and irrigation of the middle ear with a variety of agents has been advocated, but the ototoxic effect of these medications must be considered (see section on chronic suppurative otitis media, page 216).

When frequently recurrent episodes of acute otitis media occur despite the presence of a functioning tympanostomy tube, antimicrobial prophylaxis should be given to prevent the recurrent middle ear infection and otorrhea. The selection of antibiotic and dose would be the same as recommended for antimicrobial prophylaxis alone (see the section on prevention, page 163).

Protection of the Ear When Tubes Are in Place

Water from bathing or swimming should not be allowed to enter the middle ear through the tympanostomy tube, since contamination usually results in otitis media and discharge. During bathing or hair washing, a wad of either lamb's wool or cotton covered with petroleum jelly should be inserted into the external auditory meatus. Ear defenders (Mine Safety Appliance Co., Pittsburgh, Pa.) are usually effective in protecting the middle ear and may be used to permit the patient to swim; surface swimming is recommended only, as diving or swimming deeply under water may lead to contamination of the middle ear.

Conclusions

It is extremely important to continue to determine the efficacy of insertion of tympanostomy tubes in patients with recurrent acute or chronic otitis media with effusion, as well as with certain related conditions such as atelectasis of the tympanic membrane and middle ear. However, the apparent beneficial results obtained by this technique warrant its continued use. It does not seem that the use of tympanostomy tubes is a modern fad that will become obsolete in the near future. Recurrent acute otitis media and chronic otitis media with effusion are extremely prevalent in infants and young children but are conditions that are highly age-related. Since hearing loss secondary to otitis media during infancy and early childhood may impair language or cognitive development, and since insertion of tympanostomy tubes permits hearing preservation and probably prevents many of the complications and sequelae of otitis media while the tubes are in place, their use is advocated despite the fact that otitis media usually improves with increasing age.

Until randomized clinical trials are conducted and reported, tympanostomy tubes are indicated in the following types of cases: (1) chronic otitis media with effusion that has been present for at least three months and is unresponsive to or not improving progressively with nonsurgical methods of management (e.g., antimicrobial therapy), and whose duration is either documented or evident from the history; (2) at least three episodes of recurrent acute otitis media within the preceding six months, the frequency documented or evident from the history, especially when antimicrobial prophylaxis has failed or is not deemed feasible or desirable; (3) eustachian tube dysfunction resulting in one or more of the following: significant and symptomatic hearing loss, otalgia, vertigo, tinnitus, or severe atelectasis, especially in those ears in which a deep retraction pocket is present in the posterosuperior quadrant or pars flaccida, or both; (4) following tympanoplasty, when eustachian tube function is known to be poor; and (5) when a suppurative complication is present, such as facial paralysis, since tympanostomy tubes can provide drainage of the middle ear.

Tonsillectomy and Adenoidectomy

Adenoidectomy performed either separately or in combination with tonsillectomy is the most common major surgical procedure employed to prevent otitis media; myringotomy with tympanostomy tube insertion is the most common minor surgical procedure for otitis media with effusion (Paradise, 1977).

Tonsil and adenoid surgery are the most common major operations performed in the United States; approximately one fourth of all children are subjected to tonsillectomy and adenoidectomy during childhood. Such operations account for about one half of all major surgical operations performed on children, one fourth of all hospital admissions of children, and 10 percent of hospital bed-days utilized by children. In 1983, about 450,000 procedures on the tonsils and adenoids were performed in the United States, which, as shown in Figure 8–10, represents a significant reduction from the over one million such operations performed 10 years earlier.

However, this decrease in the total number of tonsil and adenoid operations may be related to a change in demography, since the total reduction during the same period in the number of children in the age group concerned was approximately 20 percent. Although the number of adenoidectomies without tonsillectomy remained relatively small in comparison with the number of tonsillectomies performed either separately or in combination with adenoidectomy, there was more than a twofold increase in the performance of adenoidectomy without tonsillectomy. Also, there appears to be a wide variation in the rate of performance of these operations by region of the country; the rates for adenoidectomy vary the most widely (National Center for Health Statistics, 1974). However, there are no data available related to the indications for which these operations were performed. Certainly, for many, otitis media was one of the indications, and in many instances the only indication, for adenoidectomy either with or without tonsillectomy.

Clinical Trials

Despite the high frequency of their performance, it has never been established through controlled scientific studies that the benefits of tonsil and adenoid surgery for otitis media exceed their cost in any age group of children. In the past, there have been only a few prospective clinical trials of tonsillectomy and adenoidectomy. The following is a summary of the results of these studies as they relate to the efficacy of the surgical procedures for prevention of otitis media. In 1930, Kaiser reported the results of following 4400 children, on one half of whom tonsillectomy and adenoidectomy were performed (the indications for surgery were not reported). Even though there was no

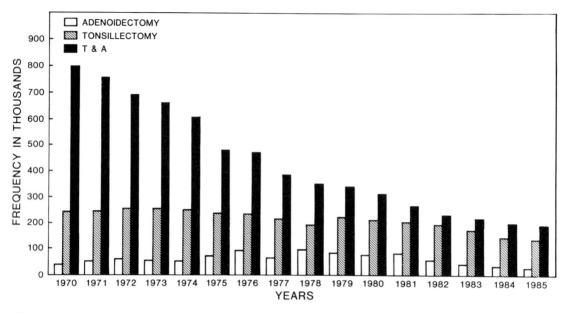

Figure 8–10. Frequency of tonsillectomies and adenoidectomies in all United States nonfederal, short-term hospitals (estimated in the Hospital Record Study, 1986).

difference in incidence of purulent otorrhea in the children who had been operated on and those who had not, the study cannot be considered to indicate conclusively the lack of efficacy of tonsillectomy and adenoidectomy in preventing otitis media since (1) the two groups may not have been similar at the outset, (2) they were not randomized, (3) the analysis was retrospective, and (4) only purulent otorrhea was considered as a measurement of the effectiveness of tonsillectomy and adenoidectomy.

The first truly prospective clinical trial of tonsillectomy and adenoidectomy was reported by McKee (1963a). The criterion for entry into the study was a history of at least three episodes of "throat infection" or of acute upper respiratory tract infection with cervical adenitis during the preceding year.

The mean incidence of otitis media among control subjects was twice as high as among children having the tonsillectomy and adenoidectomy during the first year of the trial, but during the second year there was no difference in incidence of otitis media in the group that had been operated on and the control group. However, this study was based on the occurrence of sore throats and not on the presence of middle ear disease in the year preceding the study. In fact, subjects were initially excluded from the study if they had "marked deafness, or recurrent or chronic otitis media." In addition, the follow-up evaluation was based solely on interview data,

with no objective examinations being made, and no attempt was made to detect asymptomatic otitis media with effusion or impairment of hearing.

In a second study, McKee (1963b) attempted to distinguish the effects of tonsillectomy from those of adenoidectomy. The criterion for entry into the study was the same as in the first study and, again, children with deafness and otitis media were excluded. Two hundred children were randomly assigned to undergo either tonsillectomy and adenoidectomy or adenoidectomy only. The mean incidence of otitis media in each of the two surgical groups was approximately the same.

Therefore, McKee concluded from the two studies that otitis media was infrequent after adenoidectomy or tonsillectomy and adenoidectomy and that the combined operation did not offer any particular advantages in the prevention of the disease. Even though the studies did not select children with a high morbidity of otitis media, McKee stated that it was reasonable to infer that adenoidectomy without tonsillectomy was indicated for the prevention of otitis media with effusion.

In 1967, Mawson, Adlington, and Evans reported their prospective study of tonsillectomy and adenoidectomy. The design of their experiment was similar to that of the first McKee study in that an unspecified number of children who were severely affected were excluded and operated upon. Minimal

Table 8–19. **RELATIVE FREQUENCY OF EARACHE AND OTITIS MEDIA IN 404 CHILDREN RECEIVING TONSILLECTOMY AND ADENOIDECTOMY, COMPARED WITH CONTROL GROUP***

Number of Episodes	Relative Frequency (%)					
	Year Prior to Trial		First Year of Trial		Second Year of Trial	
	Tonsillectomy and Adenoidectomy	Control	Tonsillectomy and Adenoidectomy	Control	Tonsillectomy and Adenoidectomy	Control
0	63	65	59	57	58.5	57.5
1	5	4.5	7.5	15	7	9.5
2 to 3	19	22.5	15.5	18	9	11
4 to 6	6	3	3.5	2	1	1.5
More than 7	5	4		2.5		1

*From Mawson, S. R., Adlington, R., and Evans, M.: A controlled study evaluation of adeno-tonsillectomy in children. J. Laryngol. Otol. 81:777–790, 1967.

criteria for entry were not described. Table 8–19 shows the relative incidence of earache and otitis media before and one and two years after randomization of 404 children into either the tonsillectomy and adenoidectomy or control group.

There was no apparent difference at any age between the two groups. However, as can be seen from Table 8–19, over one half of the children did not have otitis media prior to entry, and the occurrence of asymptomatic otitis media with effusion or the incidence of hearing loss was not reported.

In a study from New Zealand, using an experimental design similar to McKee's, Roydhouse reported his findings in 1970. In addition to the group of children who were referred for tonsillectomy and adenoidectomy and who were randomized into surgical and no-surgery groups, a third matched group of children who were presumably normal were followed during the trial. Table 8–20 shows the mean incidence of otitis media in the three groups: tonsillectomy and adenoidectomy, tonsillectomy and adenoidectomy withheld, and controls. The results were similar to those reported by McKee, in that there was a reduction in the incidence

of otitis media in the first year after tonsillectomy and adenoidectomy, but this difference was not maintained into the second year. However, in the second year of the trial, the total duration of episodes of otitis media in the tonsillectomy and adenoidectomy group lasted less than 60 percent as long as those that occurred before surgery. Roydhouse concluded that the operation not only reduced the incidence of otitis media quickly in the first year but also reduced the severity in both years. However, like the previous studies, patients whose main symptoms were aural were excluded, and there was no attempt to detect asymptomatic otitis media with effusion or impairment in hearing. In a second clinical trial, Roydhouse (1980) randomly divided 100 children with persistent otitis media into two groups, adenoidectomy with tympanostomy tube insertion and tympanostomy tube insertion alone. All had failed a nonsurgical treatment regimen. He compared these two groups with a third group of 69 other children who had had otitis media but had all been found to be free of middle ear effusion following the nonsurgical management and received no surgical treatment.

Table 8–20. **MEAN INCIDENCE PER YEAR OF OTITIS MEDIA IN CHILDREN RECEIVING TONSILLECTOMY AND ADENOIDECTOMY, COMPARED WITH TWO CONTROL GROUPS***

	Tonsillectomy and Adenoidectomy		Tonsillectomy and Adenoidectomy Withheld		Control	
	Mean Incidence	Number of Children	Mean Incidence	Number of Children	Mean Incidence	Number of Children
First year of trial	0.19	251	0.29	175	0.12	173
Second year of trial	0.09	204	0.07	122	0.08	173

*From Roydhouse, N.: A controlled study of adenotonsillectomy. Arch. Otolaryngol. 92:611–616, 1970.

The cure rate was similar in each of the operative groups, with a greater relapse rate in the nonadenoidectomy group, who required 9 percent more tympanostomy tube insertions. An estimation from radiographs of the size of the adenoids showed that the group cured without surgery had somewhat smaller adenoids. The relapse rate in the group who received tympanostomy tubes only was independent of the size of the adenoids. The study failed to show a favorable outcome following adenoidectomy.

In a recent study conducted in Bristol, England, of children with bilateral chronic otitis media with effusion, Maw (1984) randomly assigned subjects into (1) adenoidectomy, (2) adenoidectomy and tonsillectomy, and, (3) nonsurgical control. Tympanostomy tubes were inserted into only one ear of each child; the contralateral ear was not operated upon and was observed for one year. One third of the children in the nonsurgical control group had resolution of their middle ear effusion during the year, and one third of the two surgical groups had persistent or recurrent disease following adenoidectomy with or without tonsillectomy. Maw concluded that adenoidectomy conferred benefit in about one third of the subjects, but those children likely to benefit by the operation could not be identified prior to surgery. In addition, he reported that the addition of tonsillectomy to the adenoidectomy had no more beneficial effect than adenoidectomy alone.

Unfortunately, all of these prospective controlled studies had one or more of the following limitations in experimental design: (1) entry into the study was based on the occurrence of a sore throat and not on the presence of otitis media; (2) objective evidence of otitis media was not documented by tympanometry or audiometry; (3) other surgical procedures that may have been performed (myringotomy or tympanostomy tube insertions, for example) were not reported; (4) the technique of adenoidectomy (e.g., "midline sweep" or thorough removal of adenoid tissue from the fossa of Rosenmüller) was not described, nor was evidence of complete removal of the adenoids documented; and (5) nasal and eustachian tube function were not assessed objectively.

Children's Hospital of Pittsburgh Study

At the Children's Hospital of Pittsburgh randomized, controlled trials are currently in progress to determine the efficacy of tonsillectomy and adenoidectomy. The effect of adenoidectomy on otitis media is one of the primary research questions, and an attempt is being made to document and control those factors cited as lacking in the previous studies cited above. The criterion for entry into the study (to deal with the problem of performing adenoidectomies for otitis media with effusion) is documented episodes of recurrent acute otitis media or chronic otitis media with effusion in a child who has had a myringotomy and insertion of a tympanostomy tube at least once previously. Applying stringent surgical indications, of course, requires careful evaluation. After initial examination, each patient is examined every six weeks and at the time of any respiratory illness. Pneumatic otoscopy is always performed at every visit. A trained interviewer telephones each home every two weeks to determine whether there has been apparent or suspected illness, to make sure that any ill child is brought in promptly for examination, and to obtain routine information on school attendance, medication usage, and a number of minor symptoms.

Allergy screening is part of every child's work-up. A nasal smear is examined for eosinophils, and a battery of skin tests using common inhalant allergens is applied. Other regularly performed studies include lateral soft tissue radiographs of the nasopharynx, to assess adenoid size; sinus radiographs, when sinusitis is suspected; and audiometry and tympanometry, to evaluate hearing and middle ear status and tympanic membrane compliance.

The degree of middle ear disease developing in the adenoidectomy and nonadenoidectomy groups, respectively, is measured on the basis of three main parameters: (1) number of episodes per year of otitis media with effusion; (2) months of middle ear effusion; and (3) frequency with which myringotomy is carried out subsequent to the child's entering the clinical trial.

Data concerning subjects assigned randomly either to receive adenoidectomy or to enter the nonadenoidectomy control group are maintained separately from data concerning subjects whose parents decline randomization and opt for or against adenoidectomy.

Preliminary analyses of data currently available may be summarized by stating that, in study subjects: (1) adenoidectomy by no means eliminates the problem of recurrent otitis media in some children, whereas (2) adenoidectomy does somewhat reduce the rate, severity, or duration of recurrent episodes in others (Paradise et al., 1987). The following variables are being examined as potentially important in affecting the outcome of adenoidectomy for otitis media with effusion and in identifying which children might or might not benefit from surgery: age, sex, race, allergy, adenoid size, and eustachian tube function.

This study does not address the question of whether tonsillectomy and adenoidectomy is more effective in the prevention of otitis media with effusion than adenoidectomy alone, nor will it answer the question of the relative value of adenoidectomy with or without tonsillectomy for children who have not received myringotomy and insertion of tympanostomy tubes in the past. These questions are being addressed in a randomized clinical trial currently being conducted at the same institution.

Effect of Adenoidectomy on Eustachian Tube Function

In an attempt to improve criteria for the preoperative selection of patients for adenoidectomy, radiographic studies of the nasopharynx and eustachian tube prior to surgery and after adenoidectomy were reported (Bluestone et al., 1972). Of 27 patients who had preoperative obstruction of the nasopharyngeal end of the eustachian tube, adenoidectomy appeared to be helpful in 19 (70 percent). Results appeared to be quite poor in children with nasal allergy: only two out of 10 had good results. Furthermore, children who preoperatively showed reflux of contrast medium from the nasopharynx into the middle ear did not benefit from adenoidectomy. In this study, 20 of 33 children (60 percent) seemed to have a favorable response to adenoidectomy, but eight had worse middle ear disease after the operation than before. For example, a few of the children who had asymptomatic otitis media with effusion prior to adenoidectomy developed recurrent acute symptomatic otitis media with effusion following the procedure.

The ventilatory function of the eustachian tube has been studied using the inflation-deflation manometric technique both before and after adenoidectomy in a group of children with otitis media with effusion in whom a tympanostomy tube had been inserted (Bluestone et al., 1975). Inflation-deflation studies of the eustachian tube were obtained

in ears that remained intubated, aerated, and dry both before and eight weeks after adenoidectomy. Nasal pressures during swallowing were also determined in some. The results of this study indicated that, following adenoidectomy, eustachian tube ventilatory function improved in some, remained the same in others, and appeared to have been made worse in a few children. Improvement was related to a reduction of extrinsic mechanical obstruction of the eustachian tube (Fig. 8–11) or to nasal obstruction due to the adenoids (Fig. 8–12), whereas in those in whom the function was adjudged worse, the tube was considered to be more pliant after the adenoidectomy than before. This increase in compliance was attributed to loss of adenoid support of the eustachian tube in the fossa of Rosenmüller (Fig. 8–13). A comparable situation was described in the radiographic study in which several of the children demonstrated reflux of radiopaque liquid medium from the nasopharynx into the middle ear after the adenoidectomy but not before (Fig. 8–14).

However, neither of these studies included control subjects. In the current investigation of adenoidectomy conducted at the Children's Hospital of Pittsburgh, eustachian tube ventilatory function studies employing the inflation-deflation manometric technique are performed prior to and after randomized selection of children for the study and at any time an upper respiratory tract infection supervenes; the degree of nasal obstruction is also being assessed. Since eustachian tube ventilatory function has been shown to be affected adversely by an upper respiratory tract infection (Bluestone et al., 1977a), it is important to assess this function when an upper respiratory tract infection is present as well as when infection is absent in children both before and after randomization into either the adenoidectomy or control group. The goal of this study is to determine if adenoidectomy is efficacious in preventing otitis media with effusion in children, and if so, whether or not a simple eustachian tube function test may be helpful in determining who may be helped by the procedure. An additional question would be which type of adenoidectomy ("mid-line sweep" or also removing the adenoids from the fossa of Rosenmüller) is indicated for the individual child. It is hoped that some or all of these questions will be answered by the current studies.

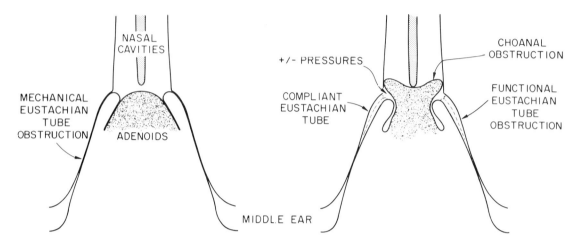

Figure 8–11. Two proposed mechanisms by which obstructive adenoids could alter eustachian tube function. The adenoids can cause extrinsic mechanical compression of the eustachian tube in the fossa of Rosenmüller (*left*). Obstruction of the posterior nasal choanae may result in abnormal nasopharyngeal pressures that develop during swallowing (Toynbee phenomenon). This can cause insufflation of nasopharyngeal secretions into the middle ear or prevent the tube from opening, or both (*right*).

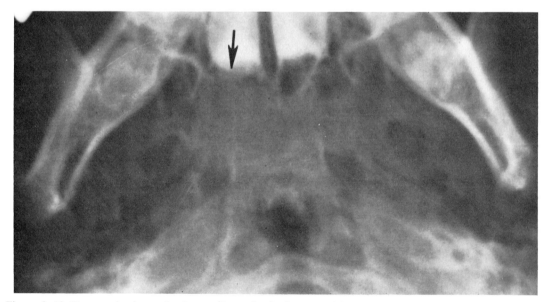

Figure 8–12. Retrograde obstruction in a radiograph of a five-year-old boy with otitis media. Radiopaque medium failed to enter the nasopharyngeal portion of the eustachian tube during both open-nose and closed-nose swallowing. Note enlarged adenoids (*arrow*).

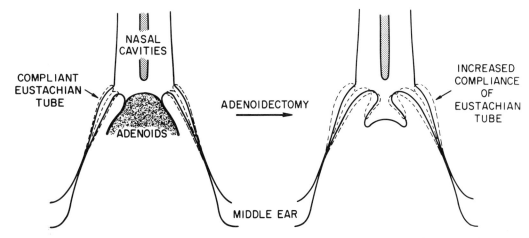

Figure 8–13. Proposed mechanism by which removal of adenoids can result in a more pliant eustachian tube after surgery than before. The increase in compliance following the surgery may be due to decrease in tubal support as a result of the adenoids' being removed from the fossa of Rosenmüller.

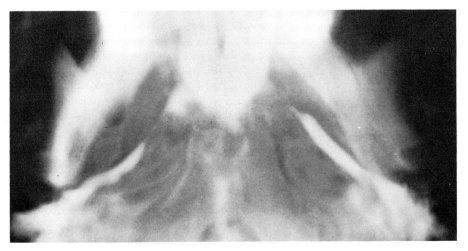

Figure 8–14. Postadenoidectomy radiograph of a child who demonstrated reflux of radiopaque medium from the nasopharynx into the middle ear. This did not occur during the preadenoidectomy radiographic study.

Conclusions

Prospective studies to determine the efficacy of tonsillectomy and adenoidectomy or adenoidectomy alone for otitis media have shown a modest reduction in the incidence of ear disease in some studies (McKee, 1963a, 1963b; Roydhouse, 1970) but no reduction in others (Kaiser, 1930; Mawson et al., 1967; Roydhouse, 1980) following surgery. However, all of these studies, unfortunately, suffered from shortcomings in design and method. The current studies of tonsillectomy and adenoidectomy being conducted in Pittsburgh are attempting to eliminate the problems of the earlier studies and to answer the questions of whether adenoidectomy is helpful in decreasing otitis media, so that children who stand to benefit can be helped, whereas those who may not can be spared the cost, discomfort, and risks of surgery.

Tympanoplasty for Atelectasis of the Tympanic Membrane

In selected cases in which severe atelectasis is present, a tympanoplastic procedure may be indicated. The most compelling indication for such a procedure would be the presence of a deep retraction pocket in the posterosuperior portion of the pars tensa that is unresponsive to nonsurgical and other surgical methods of management previously described for this defect. For example, if a tympanostomy tube had been inserted previously but the retraction pocket did not return to the neutral position after several months of equalization of the intratympanic pressure, tympanoplasty should be considered, since adhesive otitis media is most likely binding the drum to the ossicles and surrounding structures within the middle ear. Even though the natural history of such deep retraction pockets has not been formally studied, the risk of erosion necrosis of the incus or formation of a cholesteatoma, or both, appears to be quite high. It is frequently difficult to determine if there is only a retraction pocket present or if a cholesteatoma has already developed; therefore, a very thorough examination of the entire external canal and tympanic membrane should be performed with the otomicroscope. An examination under general anesthesia will be required for all infants and children in whom the examination is unsatisfactory without general anesthesia. At the time of the exam-

ination under anesthesia, a thorough examination of the retraction pocket, employing a curved, blunt probe, should be performed to determine the extent of the pocket. In addition, the continuity of the incus and stapes should be assessed, since erosion of the long process of the incus may require surgical correction. Frequently, when nitrous oxide is employed as one of the anesthetic agents, the retraction pocket can be seen to balloon laterally, as visualized through the otomicroscope. When this occurs, insertion of the tympanostomy tube will usually be sufficient to prevent recurrence of the retraction pocket. However, reinsertion of the tube may be needed if a retraction pocket recurs after spontaneous extubation.

There are many techniques advocated for repair of a severely atelectatic tympanic membrane, many of which have been shown to be quite successful (Goodhill, 1979; Sheehy, 1977). However, the surgeon should be cautioned that even though the graft "takes," the child will most likely have persistent eustachian tube dysfunction with sustained fluctuating or negative intratympanic pressure after the procedure, which could result in recurrence of the retraction pocket months or years later. Therefore, a tympanostomy tube should be inserted at the time of the tympanoplastic surgery and reinserted if atelectasis begins to recur after the tympanostomy tube is spontaneously extruded. Some surgeons prefer using tragal cartilage attached to its perichondrium to cover the area of the retraction pocket so that recurrence of an attic or posterosuperior retraction pocket can be prevented (Heermann et al., 1970).

All children who require tympanoplasty for severe atelectasis must be followed at relatively frequent intervals for the first year after the procedure and at appropriate intervals for several succeeding years, since recurrence of the atelectasis should always be anticipated.

Mastoidectomy and Middle Ear Surgery for Chronic Otitis Media with Effusion

On very rare occasions a child will require mastoidectomy and middle ear surgery to eliminate chronic otitis media with effusion when *all* other nonsurgical and surgical methods of management have failed. The operation, which has been advocated by Proctor (1971) and Paparella (1973) and described in detail by Proud and Duff (1976), should be reserved for only those children in whom a thorough search for an underlying origin of the chronic middle ear effusion has failed to uncover a cause, or, if a cause was found, appropriate management has failed to alleviate the problem (for example, the repair of a cleft palate). In addition, all attempts should have been made to maintain an aerated middle ear space by means of myringotomy and insertion of a tympanostomy tube, even though the procedure may have to be repeated many times for years. If, however, the myringotomy and thorough aspiration of the middle ear fluid is unsuccessful in eliminating the effusion and the insertion of a tympanostomy tube fails to provide an aerated middle ear space, the child may be considered a candidate for a mastoidectomy. Examination of the mastoid and middle ear space at the time of surgery may reveal a previously unsuspected mastoid osteitis, cholesterol granuloma, or cholesteatoma. However, even when these conditions are not present, the usual findings will be a cellular mastoid containing edematous, hyperplastic mucosa, with granulomatous tissue, polypoid tissue, and a very thick mucoid effusion. The condition is usually reversible with mastoid–middle ear surgery, but an aerated middle ear–mastoid air cell system should be maintained by the insertion of a tympanostomy tube at the time of the mastoid surgery; the tube should be reinserted if otitis media with effusion or atelectasis, or both, recurs.

It should be stressed that mastoidectomy and middle ear surgery is *rarely* indicated and should be performed only in those few children for whom other appropriate methods have been unsuccessful.

Hearing Aids

A management option recommended by some clinicians as an alternative to surgical intervention is fitting a hearing aid on a child who has conductive hearing loss due to chronic otitis media with effusion or chronic atelectasis of the tympanic membrane, or both. The rationale is that the hearing loss may interfere with normal development of speech, language, and learning, and the middle ear condition is self-limited and should improve as the child grows older. The fallacy

in this argument is that we do not know the natural history of chronic middle ear effusions and atelectasis. In some cases, these conditions can lead to middle ear damage. An excellent example is the population of children who have cleft palate, in whom cholesteatoma formation is a frequent sequela in spite of what apparently is aggressive medical, and even surgical, management of their ever-present chronic middle ear effusions and atelectasis. Therefore, the fitting of a hearing aid on such individuals could obscure the pathological complications and sequelae of otitis media in an effort to promote adequate hearing.

On the other hand, fitting a hearing aid on selected children should be considered and attempted when the hearing loss is interfering with the child's development and the middle ear disease cannot be reversed by medical or surgical methods. Insertion of tympanostomy tubes usually restores hearing to adequate levels when chronic otitis media with effusion is present. In some ears, especially those with severe atelectasis of the tympanic membrane, a tympanostomy tube either is difficult to insert or only remains in place for a short period. Fluctuating hearing loss in children so affected could be detrimental, and amplification of the hearing may be beneficial. Likewise, a child who already has damage to the ossicular chain and must wait to grow older before reconstructive middle ear surgery is performed may also be a good candidate for a hearing aid.

Therefore, the fitting of hearing aids should be considered in selected children, but close medical monitoring of such children is mandatory so that the possible development of complications and sequelae of otitis media and atelectasis are not masked.

Management of Special Populations

There are certain types of children who are known to be at high risk for developing otitis media and in whom continuing surveillance and more attentive management is necessary in order to prevent the complications and sequelae of the disease. In addition, children who have handicaps otherwise unrelated to middle ear disease may deserve special attention, since the occurrence of otitis media with its attendant conductive hearing loss may further compromise the pre-existing handicap and possibly interfere with the educational and social development of the child.

Infants and Children with Cleft Palate

Since otitis media with effusion is a universal finding in infants with an unrepaired cleft palate (Paradise et al., 1969; Stool and Randall, 1967), it seems reasonable to attempt to maintain the middle ears of these children free of effusion and with normal pressures. Since there is always a conductive hearing loss and usually discomfort associated with a middle ear effusion, elimination of otitis media as early in life as possible should be the goal of management. Medical treatment, such as a trial of antimicrobial therapy in young infants with an unrepaired cleft palate, has not been systematically tested; however, in older infants and children, the nonsurgical methods of management have usually been unsuccessful in eliminating middle ear effusion and restoring hearing. Therefore, the most reasonable method of management for young infants with an unrepaired cleft palate would be the insertion of a tympanostomy tube as early in life as feasible (Bluestone, 1971; Paradise and Bluestone, 1974). If a repair of a cleft lip is performed at two or three months of age, the tympanostomy tubes can be inserted at this time. In any event, a tympanostomy tube should probably be inserted sometime during the first six months of life. The overall reduction in middle ear disease that follows palate repair would appear to constitute a basis for consideration of earlier repair than might otherwise be undertaken (Paradise and Bluestone, 1974). Paradise, Bluestone, and Felder (1969) pointed out that the middle ear damage and hearing loss prevalent during later life in patients who had cleft palates probably originated with chronic middle ear effusion in infancy; they further suggest that the restrictions in language skill (McWilliams, 1966) and the psychological problems that also seem to be prevalent in these patients later in life may have the same origin, since the persistent middle ear effusion of infants with cleft palates is probably accompanied by variable degrees of hearing loss. When spontaneous extubation occurs in these children, the tubes should be reinserted if otitis media with effusion recurs.

Patients with a cleft palate and otitis media should be considered uncertain candidates for adenoidectomy, since there is a distinct possibility that the operation may worsen velopharyngeal function. In a retrospective study by Severeid (1972), adenoidectomy was not found to be effective in relieving otitis media in children with cleft palates.

Other Craniofacial Malformations

All children with craniofacial malformations who have an associated cleft palate will have a high incidence of otitis media early in life. Otitis media in these children should be managed as previously outlined for children with only cleft palates. Children in this category include those with Pierre Robin syndrome (glossoptosis, micrognathia, and cleft of the soft palate) and those with trisomy 21 (Down syndrome). The latter have an extremely high incidence of otitis media with effusion. Balkany and coworkers (1978, 1979) have reported that over 50 percent of such children will have a middle ear effusion and that more than three fourths have a conductive hearing loss. Antimicrobial therapy is usually not successful in eliminating the effusion, and most will require myringotomy and tympanostomy tube insertion to restore the hearing to normal. If a conductive hearing loss persists after successful placement of a tympanostomy tube (the middle ear appears to be aerated), then an ossicular malformation should be suspected, since this congenital anomaly is commonly found in association with these syndromes.

Even though the incidence of otitis media with effusion in many of the infants and children with craniofacial malformations has not been formally studied, children with some of the following malformations are considered to be at high risk for developing middle ear effusions: mandibulofacial dysostosis (Treacher Collins syndrome), craniofacial dysostosis (Crouzon disease), gonadal dysgenesis (Turner syndrome), and mucopolysaccharidosis (Hunter-Hurler syndrome) (see Table 8–21). However, any child with a congenital craniofacial malformation should be followed to detect the development of otitis media with effusion; a child acquiring this problem might most reasonably be managed by myringotomy with insertion of a tympanostomy tube.

Racial Groups

Certain racial groups are believed to have a high incidence of otitis media with effusion: American natives (Indians and Eskimos), the Maori of New Zealand, natives of Guam,

Table 8–21. CRANIOFACIAL MALFORMATIONS AND SYNDROMES ASSOCIATED WITH HIGH INCIDENCE OF OTITIS MEDIA WITH EFFUSION

Cleft palate, micrognathia, glossoptosis (Pierre Robin anomalad)
Trisomy 21 (Down syndrome)
Trisomy 13–15 (Patau syndrome)
Mandibulofacial dysostosis (Treacher Collins syndrome)
Oculoauriculovertebral dysplasia (Goldenhar syndrome)
Acrocephalosyndactyly (Apert syndrome)
Gonadal dysgenesis (Turner syndrome)
Craniometaphyseal dysplasia (Pyle disease)
Osteopetrosis (Albers-Schönberg disease)
Achondroplasia (Parrot disease)
Mucopolysaccharidosis (Hunter-Hurler syndrome)
Orofacial-digital syndrome (Mohr syndrome)
Craniofacial dysostosis (Crouzon disease)

Greenland Eskimos, Australian aborigines, and Laplanders. The prevalence and incidence of otitis media has not been systematically studied in these populations (or in other racial groups not listed that might also show such trends). However, early in life the children of these populations appear to develop recurrent acute otitis media, perforation of the tympanic membrane, otorrhea, and a propensity for chronic otitis media with discharge as a later sequela. When infants in these racial groups contract upper respiratory tract infections, which are so frequently associated with the ear disease, they should be aggressively treated by medical means, and antimicrobial therapy should be instituted for otitis media as early as possible. A perforation appears to be part of the natural history of ear disease in these children, and if it occurs, meticulous cleansing of the purulent material from the canal (aural toilet) should be performed frequently. In addition, an appropriate topical aural antibiotic, selected on the basis of the results of the culture, should be instilled. Antimicrobial prophylaxis is a reasonable treatment option for such children. Ensign, Ubanich, and Moran (1960) demonstrated a decreased incidence of otitis media in American Indians when prophylactic doses of a sulfonamide were administered. In a later study, Maynard, Fleshman, and Tschopp (1972) were able to decrease the incidence of otorrhea in about 50 percent of Alaskan Eskimos who were given a prophylactic daily dose of ampicillin over a one-year period. For those children in whom compliance was considered best, there was a two-thirds reduction in the incidence of ear discharge.

The insertion of tympanostomy tubes into the ears of such children has not been as successful in alleviating the recurrent otitis media as it has in children with cleft palates. This may be due to the basic differences in the origin and pathogenesis of the disease in these two groups of children: children with cleft palates usually have otitis media with effusion, whereas American natives more commonly have recurrent otitis media, followed by perforation and discharge.

If a perforation persists in infants and children who have a racial predilection for developing otitis media and tympanoplasty is not performed, a hearing aid should be fitted to help restore the child's hearing.

Immunocompromised Host

Infants and children who have congenital, acquired, or drug-induced compromise of their immune systems require special consideration when otitis media is present. Children with congenital conditions that compromise their defense systems are more susceptible to infections in general and may be more susceptible to otitis media in particular. When otitis media is present in patients with immune deficiency, the possibility of an unusual organism should be considered. Medications such as corticosteroids, antibiotics, and cytotoxic drugs may compromise the immune system. Lymphoproliferative disease states such as lymphoma or leukemia may also compromise the host.

For such children, the occurrence of acute signs and symptoms of otitis media warrants identification of the causative organism employing tympanocentesis and possibly drainage (i.e., myringotomy). Culture and sensitivity testing of the middle ear aspirate will be helpful in selecting the appropriate antimicrobial agent effective against the causative organism. In certain children who are immunocompromised, frequently recurrent and chronic otitis media are potentially life-threatening, and more permanent drainage may be required. Myringotomy and insertion of a tympanostomy tube should be considered to eliminate the middle ear effusion and prevent recurrence of suppurative disease, so as to prevent intracranial and intratemporal complications such as labyrinthitis and meningitis.

Immotile Cilia Syndrome

Infants and children with chronic otitis media with effusion, paranasal sinusitis, and bronchitis (and bronchiectasis) should be suspect of having a chronic respiratory tract infection secondary to abnormal cilia, which will significantly interfere with the mucociliary transport system (Eliasson et al., 1977). It is now appreciated that Kartagener syndrome (dextrocardia with situs inversus, bronchiectasis, sinusitis, or agenesis of the frontal sinuses) is associated with the immotile cilia syndrome. Patients with this condition should undergo bilateral myringotomy and tympanostomy tube insertion to eliminate the middle ear effusion, restore the hearing, and prevent the complications and sequelae of otitis media with effusion. Nonsurgical methods of management, such as antimicrobial prophylaxis, may be effective, but when a persistent effusion is present, myringotomy with insertion of a tympanostomy tube is indicated.

Concurrent Permanent Hearing Loss

Infants and children with pre-existing hearing losses who subsequently develop otitis media with effusion or abnormal negative middle ear pressure (atelectasis), or both, are at higher risk for impairment of language acquisition and learning than are those children whose hearing loss is only due to the middle ear effusion and negative pressure alone. Therefore, the former children should be observed at more frequent intervals than children without a concurrent permanent hearing loss and may require more aggressive management for the superimposed conductive hearing loss, since it is amenable to treatment. The pre-existing hearing loss may be conductive, sensorineural, or mixed. The child with a congenital malformation of the middle ear ossicles who has a conductive hearing loss may develop persistent or recurrent otitis media with effusion or high negative pressure, which would increase his hearing handicap. Likewise, children who have a pre-existing sensorineural hearing loss of some degree are often severely handicapped socially and educationally if they then acquire a middle ear effusion. These children should be managed in the same way as those without a concurrent hearing loss from another cause, but it is even more important to eliminate the middle ear effusion in these children rapidly and to prevent the development of any further hearing loss, if possible. If medical treatment does not eliminate the superimposed conductive hearing loss within a relatively short time, myringotomy and insertion of a tympanostomy tube should be considered at an earlier time than for children without a concurrent hearing loss. Middle ear effusion is common in all children but appears to have an even higher incidence in some children with a congenital middle ear malformation (e.g., Down syndrome) and those who have a sensorineural loss. For this reason, surgical intervention should be considered earlier in children who have recurrent middle ear effusion and persistent or fluctuating conductive hearing loss in order to prevent further impairment of hearing and, consequently, of development.

Today many children with moderate to severe permanent hearing losses attend regular schools ("mainstreaming"), and some may not even require a hearing aid. Regardless of their functional level of hearing, however, any child who has such a hearing loss should be evaluated more frequently for possible occurrence of otitis media with effusion than should the child without a permanent hearing loss. Children of all ages are of high risk, but infants, preschoolers, and young school-age children are at particular risk, since the incidence of otitis media is higher in these age groups. Examination of such infants and children twice a year would appear to be a reasonable goal if the child had no past history or evidence of the disease, but more frequent evaluation (three or four times per year) is desirable for those children who have had recurrent middle ear effusions. Since all infants and young children are at high risk for developing otitis media with effusion and high negative pressure, all infants identified as having a sensorineural hearing loss early in life should be more frequently examined for possible recurrence of otitis media. Even if such children show no objective evidence of middle ear effusion by otoscopy or tympanometry, or both, if there is a history of fluctuating hearing loss the child should be actively treated, since even the presence of transient high negative pressure may lead to a compounding of the educational handicap.

Schools or Programs for the Deaf

Children with severe to profound deafness who are enrolled in schools for the deaf or in special programs in regular schools ("mainstreamed") are at high risk for compounding their handicaps if they develop an added conductive hearing loss secondary to otitis media with effusion or high negative pressure, or both. Since the incidence of intercurrent middle ear problems appears to be high in such children, early identification employing a formal screening program such as the one proposed earlier is mandatory. Some children develop troublesome cerumen that obstructs the ear canal and may interfere with the function of a hearing aid. Such children should be examined frequently and cerumen periodically removed. As suggested earlier, otitis media with effusion or high negative pressure, or both, should be suspected during periods of upper respiratory tract infection, or when the children have signs and symptoms of otological disease such as otorrhea and otalgia, or when there has been a noticeable loss of hearing reported by the parents or teachers. Regular periodic screening employing otoscopy or tympanometry, or both, will identify those children with middle ear problems who might otherwise be overlooked because obvious signs and symptoms associated with hearing loss may be absent.

Treatment of such children would depend upon the type, severity, frequency, and duration of the middle ear problem. However, more aggressive treatment is indicated for this special population. Myringotomy and tympanostomy tube insertion should be considered earlier in such children when otitis media with effusion is frequently recurrent or chronic. Since sustained or transient high negative middle ear pressure without a middle ear effusion can cause a persistent or fluctuating conductive hearing loss, the insertion of tympanostomy tubes should also be considered at an earlier time than in nondeaf children. The presence of a hearing aid will not interfere with the function of tympanostomy tubes, since a small bore hole can be placed in the ear mold to provide ventilation. It is important when tympanostomy tubes are inserted in such children that a short tube be used so that the ear mold may be inserted.

Early identification and appropriate management of middle ear disease in a child with severe to profound deafness, especially those who utilize their residual hearing, are imperative so that maximum rehabilitation may be accomplished.

Immunoprophylaxis

S. pneumoniae is the most frequent bacterial organism isolated from middle ear fluids of children with acute otitis media (Klein, 1981). Relatively few serotypes are responsible for most infections; more than 90 percent of isolates of *S. pneumoniae* from middle ear fluids are among the 23 types present in the available pneumococcal vaccines (Klein, 1981). A 14-type pneumococcal polysaccharide vaccine was licensed for use in the United States in 1978. A 23-valent vaccine was licensed in 1983 and replaces the 14-type product. The vaccine contains purified polysaccharide antigens of types associated with otitis media in children. These types include Danish types 1, 2, 3, 4, 5, 6B, 7F, 8, 9N, 9V, 10A, 11A, 12F, 14, 15B, 17F, 18C, 19A, 19F, 20, 22F, 23F, and 33F. Each polysaccharide is extracted, separated, and combined into the final vaccine. A 0.5-ml dose contains 25 μg of each polysaccharide type dissolved in isotonic saline solution containing 0.25 percent phenol as a preservative; it is administered subcutaneously or intramuscularly. The vaccine is well tolerated. Children who receive the vaccine have some pain, erythema, and induration at the site of injection, and a small number have a minimal elevation in temperature. No significant reactions have been noted in children.

Each antigen produces an independent antibody response. In older children (more than two years of age) and adults, antibody develops in about two weeks. Studies in children indicate that, as with polysaccharide vaccines prepared from capsular materials of *H. influenzae* type b and *N. meningitidis* group C, children less than two years of age exhibit unsatisfactory serological responses to a single dose regimen. However, *N. meningitidis* group A (Gold et al., 1978) and *S. pneumoniae* type 3 (Makela et al., 1980) evoke significant antibody responses in infants as young as six months, suggesting that some polysaccharides are adequate immunogens in young infants.

Results of the Pneumococcal Vaccine Trials

Because of the frequency and morbidity of otitis media in young children, the importance of the pneumococcus as an etiological agent, and the limited number of serotypes responsible for most disease, investigations of 8- or 14-type pneumococcal vaccines for prevention of recurrent episodes of acute otitis media were initiated in 1975 in Boston, Massachusetts, and Huntsville, Alabama, and in 1977 in Oulu and Tampere, Finland.

The investigations were completed in 1980 (Karma et al., 1980; Makela et al., 1980, 1981; Sloyer et al., 1981; Teele et al., 1981). Results were evaluated by number of clinical episodes of acute otitis media and by bacteriological features of the infection, identified by aspiration of middle ear fluids.

Types of *S. pneumoniae* present in the vaccine were isolated less frequently from middle ear fluids of children in the vaccine group with acute episodes of otitis media following immunization than from children in the control group in each of the three studies. If the estimates of relative risk for the three studies are combined, the overall risk indicates a significant protective effect in children who received the vaccine.

The number of episodes of otitis media due to types not present in the vaccine and due to other pathogens (predominantly *H. influenzae*) was similar in the vaccine and control groups. Finnish children two to seven years of age who received pneumococcal vaccines had 50 percent fewer episodes of otitis media caused by types present in the vaccine. Acute otitis media was also reduced in a Swedish study of children between two and five years of age. Rosen and colleagues performed a double-blind trial of the 14-type vaccine; in contrast with the other vaccine studies, results were identified only by clinical evaluation (Rosen et al., 1983).

In spite of the decrease in middle ear infections due to pneumococcal types present in the vaccine, the clinical experience of children under two years of age in the vaccine groups was similar to that of children in the control groups. In general, the number of children who had one or more episodes of otitis media and the mean number of episodes of acute otitis media after immunization were similar in the vaccine and control groups. There were differences in some subsets; Huntsville children, six to 12 months of age, in the vaccine group had fewer episodes of otitis media than did children in the control group. The pneumococcal vaccine was effective in prevention of new clinical episodes of otitis media in black children six to 11 months of age in Huntsville, but the vaccine was ineffective in preventing otitis media in white infants of the same age (Howie et al., 1984). These data suggest racial differences in terms of preventing disease; prior studies had suggested genetic difference in response to polysaccharide vaccines (Ambrosino et al., 1986; Granoff et al., 1983).

The duration of middle ear effusion following an episode of pneumococcal otitis media was similar for the vaccine and the control groups (analyzed only by the Boston group).

Conclusions of the Vaccine Trials

There are both promise and disappointment in the results of the three pneumococcal vaccine trials for prevention of new episodes of acute otitis media. The vaccine *was* effective. Children who received either the 8- or 14-type vaccine had significantly fewer episodes of acute otitis media due to types of *S. pneumoniae* present in the vaccine. The disappointment occurred because the clinical experience with otitis media was not significantly altered; the reduction in pneumococcal type-specific infection in vaccinated children was of insufficient magnitude to affect the number of episodes of otitis media after immunization.

From the results of these studies, pneumococcal vaccine is not indicated for prevention of otitis media in children under two years of age but may be of value for children older than two years who still are suffering from recurrent episodes of acute otitis media.

Future Vaccines

New conjugate vaccines combining the polysaccharides of the pneumococcus or *H. influenzae* type b with a protein carrier such as diphtheria or tetanus toxoid are now in development and in clinical trial. These products are immunogenic in infants as young as three months of age (Eskola et al., 1985). It is conceivable that within a few years polysaccharide conjugate vaccines including four or more pneumococcal types, *H. influenzae* type b, and one or more meningococcal groups will be administered with diphtheria and tetanus toxoid and pertussis vaccine to children as young as two months of age.

Since nontypable *H. influenzae* lacks capsular materials, different techniques will be necessary to develop a vaccine. Current investigations focus on use of outer membrane proteins as candidate antigens for development of a vaccine (Gnehm et al., 1985).

Protective Effect of Immunoglobulins

Specific serum antibody is correlated with protection from homotypic infection, and prevention of disease may be achieved (albeit for limited duration) by administration of immunoglobulins. Since infants who have recurrent episodes of acute otitis media usually improve with age, it is possible that a program of passive immunization might be effective.

Diamont and colleagues suggested that patients with recurrent episodes of acute otitis media associated with hypo- or agammaglobulinemia are benefited by frequent administration of gammaglobulin. Children aged one to seven years were enrolled after the first visit to the Ear, Nose, and Throat Department in Halmstad, Sweden. Children born on an odd date were given gammaglobulin at their first visit and then once a month for six months. Children born on an even date received no gammaglobulin. Of the 113 children treated, 10 had one or more episodes of acute otitis media during the months of administration of the gammaglobulin; of 118 untreated children, 25 had one or more episodes of the disease during the same period of time. The protective effect of the gammaglobulin persisted during the eight months following cessation of administration; 25 episodes occurred in the treated group and 53 in the untreated group. In the untreated group, some patients had up to five episodes, whereas no patient in the treated group had more than two bouts of acute otitis media (Diamont et al., 1961). Investigations are now under way to evaluate the protective effect of hyperimmune globulins among American Indian children, who are highly susceptible to recurrent episodes of acute otitis media (Shurin, personal communication).

References

Alberti, P. W.: Myringotomy and ventilating tubes in the 19th century. Laryngoscope 84:805–815, 1974.

Ambrosino, D. M., Barrus, V. A., DeLange, G. G., and Siber, G. R.: Correlation of the Km(l) immunoglobulin allotypes with human anti-polysaccharide antibody concentrations. J. Clin. Invest. 78:361–365, 1986.

Applebaum, P. C., Bhamjee, A., Scragg, J. N., Hallett, A. F., Brown, A. J., and Cooper, R. C.: *Streptococcus pneumoniae* resistant to penicillin and chloramphenicol. Lancet 2:995–997, 1977.

Armstrong, B. W.: A new treatment for chronic secretory otitis media. Arch. Otolaryngol. 69:653, 1954.

Auritt, W. A., Hervada, A. R., and Fendrick, G.: Fatal pseudomembranous enterocolitis following oral ampicillin therapy. J. Pediatr. 93:882–883, 1978.

Balkany, T. J., Berman, S. A., Simmons, M. A., and Jafek, B. W.: Middle ear effusions in neonates. Laryngoscope 88:398–405, 1978.

Balkany, T. J., Downs, M .P., Jafek, B. W., and Krajicek, M. J.: Hearing loss in Down's syndrome. A treatable handicap more common than generally recognized. Clin. Pediatr. 18(2):116–118, 1979.

Barza, M.: The nephrotoxicity of cephalosporins: An overview. J. Infect. Dis. 137:S60–S73, 1978.

Bass, J. W., Steele, R. W., Wiebe, R. A., and Dierdorff, E. P.: Erythromycin concentrations in middle ear exudates. Pediatrics 48:417–422, 1971.

Beery, Q. C., Doyle, W. J., Cantekin, E. I., and Bluestone, C. D.: Longitudinal assessment of eustachian tube function in children. Laryngoscope 89:1446–1456, 1979.

Bergeson, P. S., Singer, S. A., and Kaplan, A. M.: Intramuscular injections in children. Pediatrics 70:944–948, 1982.

Berman, S., and Laver, B. A.: A controlled trial of cefaclor versus amoxicillin for treatment of acute otitis media in early infancy. Pediatr. Infect. Dis. 2:30–33, 1983.

Biedel, C. W.: Modification of recurrent otitis media by short-term sulfonamide therapy. Am. J. Dis. Child. 132:681–683, 1978.

Bland, R. D.: Otitis media in the first six weeks of life: Diagnosis, bacteriology, and management. Pediatrics 49:187–197, 1972.

Bluestone, C. D.: Eustachian tube obstruction in the infant with cleft palate. Ann. Otol. Rhinol. Laryngol. 80(Suppl. 2):1–30, 1971.

Bluestone, C. D.: Eustachian tube dysfunction. *In* Wiet, R. J., and Coulthard, S. W. (Eds.): *Proceedings of the Second National Conference on Otitis Media.* Columbus, Ohio, Ross Laboratories, 1979, pp. 50–58.

Bluestone, C. D.: Assessment of eustachian tube function. *In* Jerger, J., and Northern, J. (Eds.): *Clinical Impedance Audiometry.* Acton, Ma., American Electromedics Corporation, 1980, pp. 83–108.

Bluestone, C. D., Wittel, R. A., Paradise, J. L., et al.: Eustachian tube function as related to adenoidectomy for otitis media. Trans. Am. Acad. Ophthalmol. Otolaryngol. 76:1325–1339, 1972.

Bluestone, C. D., Beery, Q. C., and Andrus, W. S.: Mechanics of the eustachian tube as it influences susceptibility to and persistence of middle ear effusions in children. Ann. Otol. Rhinol. Laryngol. 83(Suppl. 11):27–34, 1974.

Bluestone, C. D., and Shurin, P. A.: Middle ear disease in children. Pediatr. Clin. North Am. 21:379–400, 1974.

Bluestone, C. D., Cantekin, E. I., and Beery, Q. C.: Certain effects of adenoidectomy on eustachian tube ventilatory function. Laryngoscope 85:113–127, 1975.

Bluestone, C. D., and Beery, Q. C.: Concepts in the pathogenesis of middle ear effusions. Ann. Otol. Rhinol. Laryngol. 85(Suppl. 25):182–186, 1976.

Bluestone, C. D., Cantekin, E. I., and Beery, Q. C.: Effect of inflammation on the ventilatory function of the eustachian tube. Laryngoscope 87:493–507, 1977a.

Bluestone, C. D., Cantekin, E. I., Beery, Q. C., Douglas, G. S., Stool, S. E., and Doyle, W. J.: Functional eustachian tube obstruction in acquired cholesteatoma and related conditions. *In* McCabe, B. F., Sade, J., and Abramson, M. (Eds.): *Cholesteatoma: First International Congress.* Birmingham, Ala., Aesculapius Pub. Co., 1977b, p. 325–335.

Bluestone, C. D., Cantekin, E. I., Beery, Q. C., and Stool, S. E.: Function of the eustachian tube related to surgical management of acquired aural cholesteatoma in children. Laryngoscope 88:1155–1163, 1978.

Bluestone, C. D., Cantekin, E. I., and Douglas, G. S.: Eustachian tube function related to the results of tympanoplasty in children. Laryngoscope 89:450–458, 1979.

Bluestone, C. D., and Cantekin, E. I.: Management of the patulous eustachian tube. Laryngoscope 91:149–152, 1981.

Bluestone, C. D., Gellis, S. S., Rundkrantz, H., Nelson, J. D., Paradise, J. L., Thomsen, J., and Van Buchem, F. L.: Panel Discussion: Controversies in antimicrobial therapy for otitis media. In Lim, D. J., Bluestone, C. D., Klein, J. O., and Nelson, J. D. (Eds.): *Recent Advances in Otitis Media with Effusion.* Burlington, Ont., B. C. Decker, Inc., 1984, pp. 290–292.

Blumer, J. L., Bertino, J. S., and Husak, M. P.: Comparison of cefaclor and trimethoprim-sulfamethoxazole in the treatment of acute otitis media. Pediatr. Infect. Dis. 3:25–29, 1984.

Braun, P.: Hepatotoxicity of erythromycin. J. Infect. Dis. 119:300–306, 1969.

Campos, J., Garcia-Tornel, S., and Sanfeliu, I.: Susceptibility studies of multiply resistant *Haemophilus influenzae* isolated from pediatric patients and contacts. Antimicrob. Agents Chemother. 25:706–709, 1984.

Cantekin, E. I., and Bluestone, C. D.: A membrane ventilating tube for the middle ear. Ann. Otol. Rhinol. Laryngol. 85(Suppl. 25):270–276, 1976.

Cantekin, E. I., Bluestone, C. D., Rockette, H. E., and Beery, Q. C.: Effect of oral decongestant with and without antihistamine on eustachian tube function. Ann. Otol. Rhinol. Laryngol. 89(Suppl. 68):290–295, 1980a.

Cantekin, E. I., Doyle, W. J., Phillips, C. D., and Bluestone, C. D.: Gas absorption in the middle ear. Ann. Otol. Rhinol. Laryngol. 89(68):71–75, 1980b.

Cantekin, E. I., Phillips, D. C., Doyle, W. J., Bluestone, C. D., and Kimes, K. K.: Effect of surgical alterations of the tensor veli palatini muscle on eustachian tube function. Ann. Otol. Rhinol. Laryngol. 89(Suppl. 68):47–53, 1980c.

Cantekin, E. I., Mandel, E. M., Bluestone, C. D., Rockette, H. E., Paradise, J. L., Stool, S. E., Fria, T. J., and Rogers, K. D.: Lack of efficacy of a decongestant-antihistamine combination for otitis media with effusion ("secretory" otitis media) in children. N. Engl. J. Med. 308:297–301, 1983.

Casselbrant, M. L., Okeowo, P. A., Flaherty, M. R., Feldman, R. M., Doyle, W. J., Bluestone, C. D., Rogers, K. D., and Hanley, T.: Prevalence and incidence of otitis media in a group of preschool children in the United States. In Lim, D. J., Bluestone, C. D., Klein, J. O., and Nelson, J. D. (Eds.): *Recent Advances in Otitis Media with Effusion.* Burlington, Ont., B.C. Decker, Inc., 1984, pp. 16–19.

Cates, K. L., Gerrard, J. M., Giebink, G. S., Lund, M. E., Bleeker, E. Z., O'Leary, M. C., Krivit, W., and Quie, P. G.: A penicillin-resistant pneumococcus. J. Pediatr. 93:624–626, 1978.

Chaput de Saintonge, D. M., Levine, D. F., Templae Savage, I., et al.: Trial of three-day and ten-day courses of amoxycillin in otitis media. Br. Med. J. 284:1078–1081, 1982.

Clemis, J. D.: Allergic factors in management of middle ear effusions. Recent advances in middle ear effusions. Ann. Otol. Rhinol. Laryngol. 85(Suppl. 25):259–262, 1976.

Coffey, J. D., Jr.: Concentration of ampicillin in exudate from acute otitis media. J. Pediatr. 72:693–695, 1968.

Collipp, P. J.: Evaluation of nose drops for otitis media in children. Northwest Medicine 60:999–1000, 1961.

Craig, W. A., and Kirby, W. M. M. (Eds.): Pulse dosing of antimicrobial drugs with special reference to bacampicillin. Rev. Infect. Dis. 3:1, 1981.

Danon, J.: Cefotaxime concentrations in otitis media effusion. J. Antimicrob. Chemother. 6(Suppl. A):131–132, 1980.

Diamant, M., and Diamant, B.: Abuse and timing of use of antibiotics in acute otitis media. Arch. Otolaryngol. 100:226–232, 1974.

Domagk, G.: Ein beitrag zur Chemotherapie der bakteriellen Infektionen. Dtsch. Med. Wochenschr. 61:250–253, 1935.

Domart, A., Hazard, J., and Husson, R.: Fatal bone marrow aplasia after intramuscular chloramphenicol administration in two adults. Sem. Hop. Paris 37:2256–2258, 1961.

Douglas, R. M., Moore, B. W., Miles, H. B., Davies, L. M., Graham, N. M., Ryan, P. Worswick, D. A., and Albrecht, J. K.: Prophylactic efficacy of intranasal alpha 2-interferon against rhinovirus infections in the family setting. N. Engl. J. Med. 314:65–70, 1986.

Draper, W. L.: Secretory otitis media in children. Laryngoscope 67:636–653, 1967.

Draper, W. L.: Allergy in relationship to the eustachian tube and middle ear. Otolaryngol. Clin. North Am. 7:749, 1974.

Eliasson, R., Mossberg, B., Camner, P., and Afzelius, B. A.: The immotile cilia syndrome: A congenital ciliary abnormality as an etiologic factor in chronic airway infections and male sterility. N. Engl. J. Med. 297:1–6, 1977.

Ensign, R. R., Ubanich, E. M., and Moran, J.: Prophylaxis for otitis media in an Indian population. Am. J. Publ. Health 50:195–199, 1960.

Evans, W. E., Feldman, S., Barker, L. F., Ossi, M., and Chaudhary, S.: Use of gentamicin serum levels to individualize therapy in children. J. Pediatr. 93:133–137, 1978.

Feder, H. M., Jr.: Comparative tolerability of ampicillin, amoxicillin, and trimethoprim-sulfamethoxazole suspension in children with otitis media. Antimicrob. Agents Chemother. 121:426–427, 1982.

Feigin, R. D., Kenney, R. E., Nusrala, J., Shakelford, P. G., and Lins, R. D.: Efficacy of clindamycin therapy for otitis media. Arch. Otolaryngol. 98:27–31, 1973.

Fernandez, A. A., and McGovern, J. P.: Secretory otitis media in allergic infants and children. South. Med. J. 58:581, 1965.

Finegold, S. M.: Anerobic infections in otolaryngology. Ann. Otol. Rhinol. Laryngol. 90(84):13–16, 1981.

Finland, M., and Hewitt, W. L. (Guest Eds.): Second international symposium on gentamicin, an aminoglycoside antibiotic. J. Infect. Dis. 124:S1–S300, 1971.

Finland, M., Brumfitt, W., and Kass, E. H. (Guest Eds.): Advances in aminoglycoside therapy: Amikacin. J. Infect. Dis. 134:S235–S460, 1976.

Finland, M., and Neu, H. C. (Guest Eds.): Tobramycin. Symposium of the ninth international congress of chemotherapy in London, England. J. Infect. Dis. 134:S1–S234, 1976.

Fraser, J. G., Mehta, M., and Fraser, P. M.: The medical treatment of secretory otitis media: A clinical trial of three commonly used regimens. J. Laryngol. Otol. 91:757–765, 1977.

Friedman, C. A., Lovejoy, F. C., and Smith, A. L.: Chloramphenicol disposition in infants and children. J. Pediatr. 95:1071, 1979.

Friedman, P. A., Doyle, W. J., Casselbrant, M. L., Bluestone, C. D., and Fierman, P.: Immunologic-mediated eustachian tube obstruction: A double-blind crossover study. J. Allergy Clin. Immunol. 71:442–447, 1983.

Fuchs, P. C., Gavan, T. L., Gerlach, E. H., Jones, R. N.,

Barry, A. L., and Thornsberry, C.: Ticarcillin: A collaborative *in vitro* comparison with carbenicillin against over 9,000 clinical bacterial isolates. Am. J. Med. Sci. 274:255–263, 1977.

Gebhart, D. E.: Tympanostomy tubes in the otitis media–prone child. Laryngoscope 91:849–866, 1981.

Ginsburg, C. M., McCracken, G. H., and Nelson, J. D.: Pharmacology of oral antibiotics used for treatment of otitis media and tonsillopharyngitis in infants and children. Ann. Otol. Rhinol. Laryngol. 90:37–43, 1981.

Gnehm, H. E., Pelton, S. I., Gulati, S., and Rice, P. A.: Characterization of antigens from nontypable *Haemophilus influenzae* recognized by human bactericidal antibodies. Role of Haemophilus outer membrane proteins. J. Clin. Invest. 75:1645–1658, 1985.

Gold, R., Lepow, M. L., Goldschneider, I., Draper, T. S., and Gotschlick, E. C.: Antibody responses of human infants to three doses of Group A *Neisseria meningitidis* polysaccharide vaccine administered at two, four, and six months of age. J. Infect. Dis. 138:731–735, 1978.

Goodhill, V.: Ear Diseases, Deafness, and Dizziness. Hagerstown, Md., Harper & Row, 1979, pp. 356–379.

Gorbach, S. L., and Bartlett, J. G.: Pseudomembranous enterocolitis: A review of its diverse forms. J. Infect. Dis. 135:S89–S94, 1977.

Gottschalk, H. G.: Further experience with controlled middle ear inflation in treatment of serous otitis. EENT Monthly 45:49, 1966.

Granoff, D. M., Squires, J. E., Munson, R. S., Jr., and Suarez, B.: Siblings of patients with Haemophilus meningitis have impaired anticapsular antibody responses to Haemophilus vaccine. J. Pediatr. 103:185–191, 1983.

Green, G. R., Rosenblum, A. H., and Sweet, L. C.: Evaluation of penicillin hypersensitivity: Value of clinical history and skin testing with penicilloylpolysine and penicillin G. A cooperative prospective study of the penicillin study group of the American Academy of Allergy. J. Allergy Clin. Immunol. 60:339–345, 1977.

Grilliat, J. P., Streiff, F., and Hua, G.: Fatal cytopenia after chloramphenicol hemisuccinate therapy. Ann. Med. (Nancy) 5:754–762, 1966.

Halstead, C., Lepow, M. L., Balassanian, N., Emmerich, J., and Wolinsky, E.: Otitis media: Clinical observations, microbiology and evaluation of therapy. Am. J. Dis. Child. 115:542–551, 1968.

Hanson, D. G., and Ulvestad, R. F.: Otitis media and child development: Speech, language and education. Ann. Otol. Rhinol. Laryngol. 88(Suppl. 60):13–28, 1979.

Haverkos, H. W., Caparosa, R., Ya, V. L., and Kamerer, D.: Moxalactam therapy. Its use in chronic suppurative otitis media and malignant external otitis. Arch. Otolaryngol. 108:329–333, 1982.

Hayden, F. G., Albrecht, J. K., Kaiser, D. L., and Gwaltney, J. M., Jr.: Prevention of natural colds by contact prophylaxis with intranasal alpha 2-interferon. N. Engl. J. Med. 314:71–75, 1986.

Healty, G. B.: Antimicrobial therapy of chronic otitis media with effusion. Int. J. Pediatr. Otorhinolaryngol. 8:13–17, 1984.

Healy, G. B., and Teele, D. W.: The microbiology of chronic middle ear effusions in young children. Laryngoscope 87:1472–1478, 1977.

Heermann, J., Jr., Heermann, H., and Kopstein, E.: Fascia and cartilage palisade tympanoplasty: Nine years' experience. Arch. Otolaryngol. 91:228–241, 1970.

Heisse, J. W.: Secretory otitis media: Treatment with depomethylprednisone. Laryngoscope 73:54–59, 1963.

Herberts, G., Jeppson, P. H., Nylen, O., and Branesfors-Helander, P.: Acute otitis media: Etiological and therapeutical aspects of acute otitis media. Prac. Otol. Rhinol. Laryngol. 33:191–202, 1971.

Higham, M., Cunningham, F. M., and Teele, D. W.: Ceftriaxone administered once or twice a day for treatment of bacterial infections of childhood. Pediatr. Infect. Dis. 4:22–26, 1985.

Holmquist, J.: Medical treatment in ears with eustachian tube dysfunction. Presented at the Symposium on Physiology and Pathophysiology of the Eustachian Tube and Middle Ear, September 28, 1977, Freiburg, West Germany.

Howard, J. E., Nelson, J. D., Clashen, J., and Jackson, L. H.: Otitis media of infancy and early childhood: A double-blind study of four treatment regimens. Am. J. Dis. Child. 130:965–970, 1976.

Howie, V. M., Ploussard, J., Sloyer, J. L., and Hill, J. C.: Use of pneumococcal polysaccharide vaccine in preventing otitis media in infants: Different results between racial groups. Pediatrics 73:79–81, 1984.

Howie, V. M., and Ploussard, J. H.: The *"in vivo* sensitivity test"*: Bacteriology of middle ear exudate during antimicrobial therapy in otitis media. Pediatrics 44:940–944, 1969.

Howie, V. M., and Ploussard, J. H.: Efficacy of fixed combination antibiotics versus separate components in otitis media. Clin. Pediatr. (Phila.) 11:205–214, 1972.

Howie, V. M., Ploussard, J. H., and Sloyer, J.: Comparison of ampicillin and amoxicillin in the treatment of otitis media in children. J. Infect. Dis. 129:S818–S184, 1974.

Ingvarsson, L., and Lundgren, K.: The duration of penicillin treatment of acute otitis media children. Acta Otolaryngol. (Stockh.) Suppl. 386:112–114, 1982.

Jacobs, M. R., Koornhof, H. J., Robins-Browne, R. M., Stevenson, C. M., Vermaak, Z. A., Freiman, I., Miller, G. B., Witcomb, M. A., Issacson, M., Ward, J. I., and Austrian, R.: Emergence of multiply resistant pneumococci. N. Engl. J. Med. 299:735–740, 1978.

Jokipii, L., Karma, P., and Jokipii, A. M.: Access of metronidazole into the chronically inflamed middle ear with reference to anaerobic bacterial infection. Arch. Otolaryngol. 220:167–174, 1978.

Kaiser, A. D.: Results on tonsillectomy: A comparative study of 2,200 tonsillectomized children with an equal number of controls three and ten years after operation. JAMA 95:837–842, 1930.

Kamme, C.: Evaluation of the *in vitro* sensitivity of *Neisseria catarrhalis* to antibiotics with respect to acute otitis media. Scand. J. Infect. Dis. 2:117–120, 1970.

Kamme, C.: Penicillin-resistant *Branhamella catarrhalis*. Lakartidningen 77:4858–4859, 1980.

Kamme, C., Lundgren, K., and Rundkrantz, H.: The concentration of penicillin V in serum and middle ear exudate in acute otitis media in children. Scand. J. Infect. Dis. 1:77–83, 1969.

Kaplan, S. L., Mason, E. O., Jr., Mason, S. K., et al.: Prospective comparative trial of moxalactam versus ampicillin or chloramphenicol for treatment of *Haemophilus influenzae* type b meningitis in children. J. Pediatr. 104:447–453, 1984.

Karma, P., Luotonen, J., Timonen, M., Pontynen, S., et al.: Efficacy of pneumococcal vaccination against recurrent otitis media. Preliminary results of a field trial in Finland. Ann. Otol. Rhinol. Laryngol. 89(68):357–362, 1980.

Kenna, M. A., Bluestone, C. D., Reilly, J. S., and Lusk,

R. P.: Medical management of chronic suppurative otitis media without cholesteatoma in children. Laryngoscope 96:146–151, 1986.

Khanna, S. M., and Tonndorf, J.: Tympanic membrane vibrations in cats studied by time-averaged holography. J. Acoust. Soc. Am. 51:1904, 1972.

Kilby, D., Richards, S. H., and Hart, G.: Grommets and glue ears. Two year results. J. Laryngol. Otol. 86:881–886, 1972.

Kinmonth, A. L., Storrs, C. N., and Mitchell, R. G.: Meningitis due to chloramphenicol-resistant *Haemophilus influenzae* type b. Br. Med. J. 1:694, 1978.

Kirby, W. M. M. (Chrmn.): Symposium on carbenicillin. A clinical profile. J. Infect. Dis. 122:S1–S116, 1970.

Kjellman, N. I., Synnerstad, B., and Hansson, L. O.: Atopic allergy and immunoglobulins in children with adenoids and recurrent otitis media. Acta Paediatr. Scand. 65:593–600, 1976.

Klein, J. O.: Epidemiology of pneumococcal disorders in infants and children. Rev. Infect. Dis. 3:246–253, 1981.

Klein, J. O. (Ed.): Symposium on long-acting penicillins. Pediatr. Infect. Dis., 4:569–605, 1985.

Klimek, J. J., Nightingale, C., Lehmann, W. B., and Quintiliani, R.: Comparison of concentrations of amoxicillin and ampicillin in serum and middle ear fluid of children with chronic otitis media. J. Infect. Dis. 135:999–1002, 1977.

Klimek, J. J., Bates, T. R., Nightingale, C., Lehmann, W. B., Ziemniak, J. A., and Quintiliani, R.: Penetration characteristics of trimethoprim-sulfamethoxazole in middle ear fluid of patients with chronic serous otitis media. J. Pediatr. 96:1087–1089, 1980.

Kokko, E.: Chronic secretory otitis media in children: A clinical study. Acta Otolaryngol. Suppl. 327:7–44, 1974.

Krasinski, K., Kusmeisz, H., and Nelson, J. D.: Pharmacologic interactions among chloramphenicol, phenytoin and phenobarbital. Pediatr. Infect. Dis. 1:232, 1982.

Krause, P. J., Owens, N. G., Nightingale, C. H., Klimek, J. J., Lehmann, W. B., Quintiliani, R.: Penetration of amoxicillin, cefaclor, erythromycin-sulfisoxazole, and trimethoprim-sulfamethoxazole into the middle ear fluid of patients with chronic serous otitis media. J. Infect. Dis. 145:815–821, 1982.

Lahikainen, E. A.: Clinico-bacteriologic studies on acute otitis media: Aspiration of tympanum as diagnostic and therapeutic method. Acta Otolaryngol. (Stockh.) 107(Suppl.):1–82, 1953.

Lahikainen, E. A.: Penicillin concentration in middle ear secretion in otitis. Acta Otolaryngol. (Stockh.) 70:358–362, 1970.

Lahikainen, E. A., Vuori, M., and Virtanen, S.: Azidocillin and ampicillin concentrations in middle ear effusion. Acta Otolaryngol. (Stockh.) 84:227–232, 1977.

Laxdal, O. E., Merida, J., and Trefor Jones, R. H.: Treatment of acute otitis media: A controlled study of 142 children. Can. Med. Assoc. J. 102:263–268, 1970.

Levine, B. B., Redmond, A. P., Fellner, M. J., Voss, H. E., and Levytska, V.: Penicillin allergy and the heterogeneous immune responses of man to benzylpenicillin. J. Clin. Invest. 45:1895–1906, 1966.

Lildholdt, T., Cantekin, E. I., Bluestone, C. D., and Rockette, H. E.: Effect of topical nasal decongestant on eustachian tube function in children with tympanostomy tubes. Acta Otolaryngol. (Stockh.), 94:93–97, 1982.

Lildholdt, T., Cantekin, E. I., Marshak, G., Bluestone, C. D., Rohn, D. C., and Schuit, K. E.: Pharmacokinet-

ics of cefaclor in chronic middle ear effusions. Ann. Otol. Rhinol. Laryngol. 90(84):44–47, 1981.

Liston, T. E., Foshee, W. S., and Pierson, W. D.: Sulfisoxazole chemoprophylaxis for frequent otitis media. Pediatrics 71:524–530, 1983.

Liu, Y. S., Lim, D. S., and Lang, R. W.: Chronic middle ear effusions: Immunological and bacteriological investigations. Arch. Otolaryngol. 101:278–286, 1975.

Liu, Y. S., Lim, D. J., Lang, R., and Birck, H. G.: Microorganisms in chronic otitis media with effusion. Ann. Otol. Rhinol. Laryngol. 85(25):245–249, 1976.

Lorentzen, P., and Haugsten, P.: Treatment of acute suppurative otitis media. J. Laryngol. Otol. 91:331–340, 1977.

Lundgren, K., Ingvarsson, L., and Rudcrantz, H.: The concentration of penicillin V in middle ear exudate. Int. J. Pediatr. Otorhinolaryngol. 1:93–96, 1979.

Mace, J. W., Janik, D. S., Sauer, R. L., and Quilligan, J. J.: Penicillin-resistant pneumococcal meningitis in an immunocompromised infant. J. Pediatr. 91:506–507, 1977.

Makela, P. H., Sibakov, M., Herva, E., and Henricksen, J.: Pneumococcal vaccine and otitis media. Lancet 2:547–551, 1980.

Makela, P. H., Leinonen, M., Tukander, J., and Karma, P.: A study of the pneumococcal vaccine in prevention of clinically acute attacks of recurrent otitis media. Rev. Infect. Dis. 3:S124–S130, 1981.

Maknin, M. L., and Jones, P. K.: Oral dexamethasone for treatment of persistent middle ear effusion. Pediatrics 75:329–335, 1985.

Mandel, E. M., Bluestone, C. D., Rockette, H. E., Blatter, M. M., Resinger, K. S., Wucher, F. R., and Harper, J.: Duration of effusion after antibiotic treatment for acute otitis media: Comparison of cefaclor and amoxicillin. Pediatr. Infect. Dis. 1:310–316, 1982.

Mandel, E. M., Bluestone, C. D., Paradise, J. L., Cantekin, E. I., Rockette, H. E., Fria, T. J., Stool, S. E., and Marshak, G.: Efficacy of myringotomy with and without tympanostomy tube insertion in the treatment of chronic otitis media with effusion in infants and children: Results for the first year of a randomized clinical trial. *In* Lim, D. J., Bluestone, C. D., Klein, J. O., and Nelson, J. D. (Eds.): *Recent Advances in Otitis Media with Effusion.* Toronto, B. C. Decker Inc., 1984, pp. 308–311.

Mandel, E. M., Rockette, H. E., Bluestone, C. D., Paradise, J. L., and Nozza, R. J.: Efficacy of amoxicillin with and without decongestant-antihistamine for otitis media with effusion in children: Results of a double-blind, randomized trial. NEJM, 316:432–437, 1987.

Marchant, C. D., Shurin, P. A., Turczyk, V. A., et al.: A randomized controlled trial of cefaclor compared with trimethoprim-sulfamethoxazole for treatment of acute otitis media. J. Pediatr. 105:633–638, 1984.

Marshak, G., and Neriah, Z. B.: Adenoidectomy vs tympanostomy in chronic secretory otitis media. Ann. Otol. Rhinol. Laryngol. 89(Suppl. 68):316–318, 1981.

Mattar, M. E., Markello, J., and Yaffe, S. J.: Pharmaceutic factors affecting pediatric compliance. Pediatrics 55:101–108, 1975.

Maw, A. R.: Chronic otitis media with effusion and adenotonsillectomy: A prospective randomized controlled study. *In* Lim, D. J., Bluestone, C. D., Klein, J. O., and Nelson, J. D. (Eds.): *Recent Advances in Otitis Media with Effusion.* Toronto, B. C. Decker Inc., 1984, pp. 299–302.

Mawson, S. R.: The eustachian tube. *In* Mawson, S. R. (Ed.): *Disease of the Ear.* Baltimore, The Williams & Wilkins Co., 1974.

Mawson, S. R., Adlington, R., and Evans, M.: A controlled study evaluation of adeno-tonsillectomy in children. J. Laryngol. Otol. 81:777–790, 1967.

Mawson, S. R., and Fagan, P.: Tympanic effusions in children: Long-term results of treatment by myringotomy, aspiration and indwelling tubes (grommets). J. Laryngol. Otol. 86:105–119, 1972.

Maynard, J. E., Fleshman, J. K., and Tschopp, C. F.: Otitis media in Alaskan Eskimo children: Prospective evaluation of chemoprophylaxis. JAMA 219:597, 1972.

McCracken, G. H., Jr., and Nelson, J. D.: *Antimicrobial Therapy for Newborns*. 2nd Ed. New York, Grune & Stratton, 1983.

McCracken, G. H., Jr., Threlkeld, N., Mize, S., et al.: Moxalactam therapy for neonatal meningitis due to gram-negative enteric bacilli. A prospective controlled evaluation. JAMA 252:1427–1432, 1984.

McKee, W. J. E.: A controlled study of the effects of tonsillectomy and adenoidectomy in children. Br. J. Prev. Soc. Med. 17:46–49, 1963a.

McKee, W. J. E.: The part played by adenoidectomy in the combined operation of tonsillectomy with adenoidectomy: Second part of a controlled study in children. Br. J. Prev. Soc. Med. 17:133–140, 1963b.

McLinn, S. E.: Cefaclor in treatment of otitis media and pharyngitis in children. Am. J. Dis. Child. 134:560–563, 1980.

McLinn, S. E., Goldberg, F., Kramer, R., et al.: Double-blind multicenter comparison of cyclacillin and amoxicillin for the treatment of acute otitis media. J. Pediatr. 101:607–621, 1982.

McLinn, S. E., and Serlin, S.: Cyclacillin versus amoxicillin as treatment for acute otitis media. Pediatrics 71:196–199, 1983.

McWilliams, B. J.: Speech and hearing problems in children with cleft palate. J. Am. Med. Wom. Assoc. 21:1005, 1966.

Meistrup-Larsen, K.-I., Sorensen, H., Johnson, N.-J., Thomsen, J., Mygind, N., and Sederberg-Olsen, D.: Two versus seven days penicillin treatment for acute otitis media. A placebo controlled trial in children. Acta Otolaryngol. (Stockh.), 96:99–104, 1983.

Miller, G. F.: Influence of an oral decongestant on Eustachian tube function in children. J. Allergy 45:187–193, 1970.

Moellering, R. C., Jr., and Swartz, M. N.: Drug therapy. The newer cephalosporins. N. Engl. J. Med. 294:24–28, 1976.

Muenker, G.: Results after treatment of otitis media with effusion. Ann. Otol. Rhinol. Laryngol. 89(Suppl. 68): 308–311, 1980.

Murray, D. L., Singer, D. A., and Singer, A. B.: Cefaclor: A cluster of adverse reactions. N. Engl. J. Med. 303:1003, 1980.

Mygind, N., Meistrup-Larsen, K.-I., Thomsen, J., Thomsen, V. F., Josefsson, K., and Sorenson, H.: Penicillin in acute otitis media: A double-blind placebo-controlled trial. Clin. Otolaryngol. 6:5–13, 1981.

National Center for Health Statistics: Surgical Operations In Short-Stay Hospitals: United States—1971. (DHEW Publication No. HRA-75-1769) Rockville, Md., United States Department of Health, Education and Welfare, 1974.

Nelson, J. D., and McCracken, G. H.: The drug of choice for otitis media? J. Pediatr. Infect. Dis. 6:5, 1980.

Nelson, J. D., Ginsburg, C. M., McLeland, O., Clahsen, J., Culbertson, M. C., Jr., and Carder, H.: Concentrations of antimicrobial agents in middle ear fluid, saliva, and tears. Int. J. Pediatr. Otorhinolaryngol. 3:327–334, 1981.

Neu, H. C.: A symposium on the tetracyclines: A major appraisal. Introduction. Bull. N.Y. Acad. Med. 54:141–155, 1978.

Neu, H. C., McCracken, G. H., Jr.: Proceedings of a conference: Clinical pharmacology and efficacy of cefixime. Pediatr. Infect. Dis. J. 6:951–1009, 1987.

Nilson, B. W., Poland, R. L., Thompson, R. S., Morehead, D., Baghdassarian, A., and Carver, D. H.: Acute otitis media: Treatment results in relation to bacterial etiology. Pediatrics 43:351–358, 1969.

Odio, C. M., Kusmiesz, R. N., Shelton, S., and Nelson, J. D.: Comparative treatment trial of Augmentin versus cefaclor for acute otitis media with effusion. Pediatrics 75:819–826, 1985.

Ogawa, S., Satoh, I., Tanaka, H.: Patulous eustachian tube. A new treatment with infusion of absorable gelatin sponge solution. Arch. Otolaryngol. 102:276–280, 1976.

Olson, A. L., Klein, S. W., Charney, E., MacWhinney, J. B., McInerny, T. K., Miller, R. L., Nazarian, L. F., and Cunningham, D.: Prevention and therapy of serous otitis media by oral decongestant: A double-blind study in pediatric practice. Pediatrics 61:679–684, 1978.

Oppenheimer, P.: Short-term steroid therapy—treatment of serous otitis media in children. Arch. Otolaryngol. 88:38, 1968.

Oppenheimer, R. P.: Serous otitis: Review of 992 patients. EENT Monthly 54:37–40, 1975.

Paparella, M. M.: The middle ear effusions. *In* Paparella, M. M., and Shumrick, D. A. (Eds.): Otolaryngology, Vol. 1. Philadelphia, W. B. Saunders Co., 1973, pp. 93–112.

Paradise, J. L.: On tympanostomy tubes, rationale, results, reservations, and recommendations. Pediatrics 60:86–90, 1977.

Paradise, J. L.: Otitis media in infants and children: Review article. Pediatrics 65:917–943, 1980.

Paradise, J. L., Bluestone, C. D., and Felder, H.: The universality of otitis media in fifty infants with cleft palate. Pediatrics 44:35–42, 1969.

Paradise, J. L., and Bluestone, C. D.: Early treatment of the universal otitis media in infants with cleft palate. Pediatrics 53:48–54, 1974.

Paradise, J. L., Bluestone, C. D., Rogers, K. D., Taylor, F. H., Colborn, D. K., Bachman, R. Z., Bernard, B. S., Smith, C. G., Stool, S. E., and Schwarzbach, R. H.: Efficacy of adenoidectomy for recurrent otitis media: Results from parallel random and nonrandom trials. Pediatr. Res. 21:286A, 1987.

Paredes, A., Taber, L. H., Yow, M. D., Clark, D., and Nathan, W.: Prolonged pneumococcal meningitis due to an organism with increased resistance to penicillin. Pediatrics 58:378–381, 1976.

Parker, C. W.: Allergic drug responses—mechanisms and unsolved problems. CRC Crit. Rev. Toxicol. 1:261–281, 1972.

Perlman, H. B.: The eustachian tube: Abnormal patency and normal physiologic state. Arch. Otolaryngol. 30:212–238, 1939.

Perrin, J. M., Charney, E., MacWhinney, J. B., Jr., McInerny, T. K., Miller, R. L., and Nazarian, L. F.: Sulfisoxazole as chemoprophylaxis for recurrent otitis media: a double-blind crossover study in pediatric practice. N. Engl. J. Med. 291:664–667, 1974.

Persico, M., Podoshin, L., and Fradis, M.: Otitis media with effusion. Ann. Otol. Rhinol. Laryngol. 87:191, 1978.

Petz, L. D.: Immunologic cross-reactivity between penicillins and cephalosporins: A review. J. Infect. Dis. 137:S74–S79, 1978.

Petz, L. D., and Fudenberg, H. H.: Coombs-positive hemolytic anemia caused by penicillin administration. N. Engl. J. Med. 274:171–181, 1966.

Phillips, M. J., Manning, H., Knight, N. J., et al.: Secretory otitis media. Lancet 2:1176–1178, 1974.

Physicians' Desk Reference. Oradell, NJ: Medical Economics Inc., 1988, pp. 826, 1713.

Politzer, A.: *Disease of the Ear.* Philadelphia, Lea & Febiger, 1909.

Prince, R. A., Wing, D. S., Weinberger, M. M., et al.: Effect of erythromycin on theophylline kinetics. J. Allergy Clin. Immunol. 68:427–431, 1981.

Proctor, B.: Attic-aditus block and the tympanic diaphragm. Ann. Otol. Rhinol. Laryngol. 80:371–375, 1971.

Proud, G. O., and Duff, W. E.: Mastoidectomy and epitympanotomy. Ann. Otol. Rhinol. Laryngol. 85(25):289–292, 1976.

Puhakka, H., Virolainen, E., Aantaa, E., Tuohimaa, P., Eskola, J., and Ruuskanen, O.: Myringotomy in the treatment of acute otitis media in children. Acta Otolaryngol. (Stockh.) 88:122–126, 1979.

Pulec, J. L.: Abnormally patent eustachian tubes: Treatment with injection of polytetrafluoroethylene (Teflon) paste. Laryngoscope 77:1543–1554, 1967.

Qvarnberg, Y., and Palva, T.: Active and conservative treatment of acute otitis media: Prospective studies. Ann. Otol. Rhinol. Laryngol. 89(68):269–270, 1980.

Rapp, D. J., and Fahey, D.: Review of chronic secretory otitis and allergy. J. Asthma Res. 10:193–218, 1973.

Restrepo, M. A., and Zambrano, F.: II. Late onset aplastic anemia secondary to chloramphenicol. Report of ten cases. Antioquia Medica 18:593–606, 1968.

Riding, K. H., Bluestone, C. D., Michaels, R. H., Cantekin, E. I., Doyle, W. J., and Poziviak, C.: Microbiology of recurrent and chronic otitis media with effusion. J. Pediatr. 93:739–743, 1978.

Rinkle, H. J.: The management of clinical allergy. Arch. Otolaryngol. Part I—76:491, 1962; Part II—77:42, 1963; Part III—77:205, 1963; Part IV—77:302, 1963.

Roddey, O. F., Jr., Earle, R., Jr., and Haggerty, R.: Myringotomy in acute otitis media: A controlled study. JAMA 197:849, 1966.

Rodriguez, W. J., Schwartz, R. H., Sait, T., Kahn, W. N., Chhabra, O. P., Chang, M. J., Reddy, S., Marks, L. A., and Gold, J. A.: Erythromycin-sulfamethoxazole vs. amoxicillin in the treatment of acute otitis media in children: A double-blind, multiple-dose comparative study. Am. J. Dis. Child. 139:766–770, 1985.

Rosen, C., Christensen, P., Hovelius, B., and Prellner, K.: Effect of pneumococcal vaccination on upper respiratory tract infections in children. Design of a follow-up study. Scand. J. Infect. Dis. (Suppl.) 39:39–44, 1983.

Roth, R. P., Cantekin, E. I., Bluestone, D. C., Welch, R. M., and Cho, Y. W.: Nasal decongestant activity of pseudoephedrine. Ann. Otol. Rhinol. Laryngol. 86:235–242, 1977.

Roydhouse, N.: A controlled study of adenotonsillectomy. Arch. Otolaryngol. 92:611–616, 1970.

Roydhouse, N.: Adenoidectomy for otitis media with effusion. Ann. Otol. Rhinol. Laryngol. 89(Suppl. 68):312–315, 1980.

Rubenstein, M. M., McBean, J. B., Hedgecock, L. D., and Stickler, G. B.: The treatment of acute otitis media in children: III. A third clinical trial. Am. J. Dis. Child. 109:308–313, 1965.

Rudberg, R. D.: Acute otitis media: Comparative therapeutic results of sulfonamide and penicillin administered in various forms. Acta Otolaryngol. 113:1–79, 1954.

Saah, A. J., Blackwelder, W. C., and Kaslow, R. A.: Commentary: Treatment of acute otitis media. JAMA 248:1071–1072, 1982.

Schuller, D. E.: Prophylaxis of otitis media in asthmatic children. Pediatr. Infect. Dis. 2:280–283, 1983.

Schwartz, D. M., Schwartz, R. H., and Redfield, N. P.: Treatment of negative middle ear pressure and serous otitis media with Politzer's technique: An old procedure revised. Arch. Otolaryngol. 104:487–490, 1978.

Schwartz, R., Barsanti, R. G., and Rodriguez, W. J.: Private practice view of otitis media. Pediatrics 61:937–938, 1978.

Schwartz, R. H., Puglese, J., and Rodriguez, W. J.: Sulfamethoxazole prophylaxis in the otitis-prone child. Arch. Dis. Child. 57:590–593, 1982.

Schwartz, R. H., Puglese, J., and Schwartz, D. M.: Use of a short course of prednisone for treating middle ear effusion: A double-blind cross-over study. Ann. Otol. Rhinol. Laryngol. 89(Suppl. 68):296–300, 1980.

Schwartz, R. H., Rodriguez, W. G., and Schwartz, D. M.: Office myringotomy for acute otitis media: Its value in preventing middle ear effusion. Laryngoscope 91:616–619, 1981.

Schwartz, R. H., and Schwartz, D. M.: Acute otitis media: Diagnosis and drug therapy. Drugs 19:107–118, 1980.

Scott, J. L., Finegold, S. M., Belkin, G. A., and Lawrence, J. S.: A controlled double-blind study of the hematologic toxicity of chloramphenicol. N. Engl. J. Med. 272:1137–1142, 1965.

Senturia, B. H., Gessert, C. F., Carr, C. D., and Bauman, E. S.: Studies concerned with tubotympanitis. Ann. Otol. Rhinol. Laryngol. 67:440–467, 1958.

Severeid, L.: A longitudinal study of the efficacy of adenoidectomy in children with cleft palate and secondary otitis media. TAA00, 876:1319–1324, 1972.

Shah, N.: Use of grommets in "glue" ears. J. Laryngol. Otol. 85:283–287, 1971.

Shea, J. J.: Autoinflation treatment of serous otitis media in children. J. Laryngol. Otol. 85:1254–1258, 1971.

Sheehy, J. L.: Surgery of chronic otitis media. *In* English, G. (Ed.): Otolaryngology, Vol. 1. Hagerstown, Md., Harper & Row, 1977.

Shurin, P. A., Howie, V. M., Pelton, S. I., Ploussard, J. H., and Klein, J. O.: Bacterial etiology of otitis media during the first six weeks of life. J. Pediatr. 92:893–896, 1978.

Shurin, P. A., Pelton, S. I., and Klein, J. O.: Otitis media in the newborn infant. Ann. Otol. Rhinol. Laryngol. 85(25):216–222, 1976.

Silverstein, H., Bernstein, J. M., and Lerner, P. I.: Antibiotic concentrations in middle ear effusion. Pediatrics 38:33–39, 1966.

Sloyer, J. L., Jr., Ploussard, J. H., and Howie, V. M.: Efficacy of pneumococcal polysaccharide vaccine in preventing acute otitis media in infants in Huntsville, Alabama. Rev. Infect. Dis. 3:S119–S123, 1981.

Smith, H., and Aronson, S. S.: Organizational approach to medication administration in day care. Rev. Inf. Dis. 8:657–659, 1986.

Sorenson, H.: Antibiotics in suppurative otitis media. Otolaryngol. Clin. North Am. 10:45–50, 1977.

Stanievich, J. F., Bluestone, C. D., Lima, J. A., Michaels, R. H., Rohn, D., and Effron, M. Z.: Microbiology of chronic and recurrent otitis media with effusion in young infants. Int. J. Pediatr. Otorhinolaryngol. 3:137–143, 1981.

Stechenberg, B. W., Anderson, D., Chang, M. J., Dunkle, L., Wong, M., vanReken, D., Pickering, L. K., and Feigin, R. D.: Cephalexin compared to ampicillin treatment of otitis media. Pediatrics 58:532–536, 1976.

Stickler, G. B., and McBean, J. B.: The treatment of acute otitis media in children: A second clinical trial. JAMA 187:85–89, 1964.

Stickler, G. B., Rubenstein, M. M., McBean, J. B., Hedgecock, L. D., Hugstad, B. A., and Griffing, T.: Treatment of acute otitis media in children: IV. A fourth clinical trial. Am. J. Dis. Child. 114:123–130, 1967.

Stool, S. E., and Randall, P.: Unexpected ear disease in infants with cleft palate. Cleft Palate J. 4:99, 1967.

Stroud, M. H., Spector, G. J., and Maisel, R. H.: Patulous eustachian tube syndrome: a preliminary report of the use of the tensor veli palatini transposition procedure. Arch. Otolaryngol 99:419–421, 1974.

Sundberg, L., Eden, T., Ernstson, S., and Pahlitzsch, R.: Penetration of erythromycin through respiratory mucosa. Acta. Otolaryngol. (Stockh.) Suppl. 365:1–17, 1979.

Teele, D. W., Pelton, S. I., and Klein, J. O.: Bacteriology of acute otitis media unresponsive to initial antimicrobial therapy. J. Pediatr. 98:537–539, 1981.

Tetzlaff, T. R., Ashworth, C., and Nelson, J. D.: Otitis media in children less than 12 weeks of age. Pediatrics 59:827–832, 1977.

Tos, M., and Poulsen, G.: Secretory otitis media: Late results of treatment with grommets. Arch. Otolaryngol. 102:672–675, 1976.

Valsalva, A.: Tractus de aure humana. In Stevenson, R. S., and Guthrie, D. (Eds.): A History of Otolaryngology. Edinburgh, E. and S. Livingstone Ltd., 1949.

van Buchem, F. L., Dunk, J. H. M., and van't Hof, M. A.: Therapy of acute otitis media: Myringotomy, antibiotics, or neither? A double-blind study in children. Lancet 2:883–887, 1981.

van Buchem, F. L., Peeters, M. F., and van't Hof, M. A.: Acute otitis media: A new treatment strategy. Par. Med. J. [Clin. Res.] 290:1033–1037, 1985.

Van Dishoeck, H. A. E., Derks, A. C. W., and Voorhorst, R.: Bacteriology and treatment of acute otitis media in children. Acta Otolaryngol. (Stockh.) 50:250–262, 1959.

Virtanen, S., and Lahikainen, E. A.: Ampicillin concentrations in middle ear effusions in acute otitis media after administration of bacampicillin. Infection 7(5):472–474, 1979.

Waickman, F. J.: Allergic management of otitis media. Transactions of the Second National Conference on Otitis Media. Columbus, Ohio, Ross Laboratories, 1979, pp. 109–114.

Wallerstein, R. O., Condit, P. K., Kasper, C. K., Brown, J. W., and Morrison, F. R.: Statewide study of chloramphenicol therapy and fatal aplastic anemia. JAMA 208:2045–2050, 1969.

Ward, J.: Antibiotic-resistant Streptococcus pneumoniae: Clinical and epidemiological aspects. Rev. Infect. Dis. 3:254–266, 1981.

Ward, J. I., Tsai, T. F., Filice, G. A., and Fraser, D. W.: Prevalence of ampicillin- and chloramphenicol-resistant strains of Haemophilus influenzae causing meningitis and bacteremia: National survey of hospital laboratories. J. Infect. Dis. 138:421–424, 1978.

Whitcomb, N. J.: Allergy therapy in serous otitis media associated with allergic rhinitis. Clin. Allergy 23:232–236, 1965.

Yagi, H. I. A.: The surgical treatment of secretory otitis media in children. J. Laryngol. Otol. 91:267–270, 1977.

Zanga, J., Donland, M. A., Newton, J., et al.: Administration of medication in school. Pediatrics 74:433–438, 1984.

9

Complications and Sequelae: Intratemporal

Intracranial suppurative complications of otitis media, including meningitis, brain abscess, and lateral sinus thrombosis, are relatively uncommon today. Intratemporal complications, those that occur within the aural cavity and adjacent structures of the temporal bone, are more common. These include acute and chronic perforation of the tympanic membrane, chronic suppurative otitis media, mastoiditis, cholesteatoma and retraction pocket, adhesive otitis media, tympanosclerosis, and ossicular discontinuity and fixation (Fig. 9–1). The most frequent complication or sequela of otitis media is hearing loss that accompanies most episodes of otitis media. Recent studies indicate that children who had recurrent episodes of otitis media or persistent middle ear effusion perform less well on tests of speech and language than do their disease-free peers. These data suggest that delay or impairment of development may be an important sequela of otitis media. In this chapter we discuss the epidemiology, pathogenesis, microbiology, and management of intratemporal complications and sequelae of otitis media. In the next chapter, similar information is presented for intracranial complications and sequelae.

For many of the aural and intratemporal complications and sequelae of otitis media, surgery is indicated. The concepts of the surgical procedures are described in *Pediatric Otolaryngology* (Bluestone and Stool, 1983).

HEARING LOSS

Fluctuating or persisting loss of hearing is present in most children who have middle ear effusion; impairment of hearing is the most prevalent complication of otitis media with effusion.

Conductive Hearing Loss

Audiograms of children with middle ear effusion usually reveal a mild to moderate conductive loss in the range of 15 to 40 dB. With such deficits, the softer speech sounds and voiceless consonants may be missed. The average audiogram of a child with otitis media with effusion is presented in Figure 9–2. The hearing loss is not influenced by the quality of fluid in the middle ear; ears with thin fluids are not impaired to the same degree as those with fluids of glue-like consistency (Brown et al., 1983; Weiderhold et al., 1980). Ears that are partially filled with fluid (identified otoscopically by the presence of bubbles or an air-fluid level) have lesser hearing impairment than ears that are completely filled with fluid (Fria et al., 1985). The hearing impairment is usually reversed with resolution of the effusion. On occasion, permanent conductive hearing loss occurs owing to irreversible changes resulting from recurrent acute or chronic inflammation (e.g., ad-

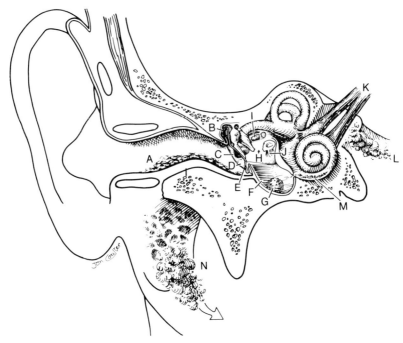

Figure 9–1. Intratemporal complications and sequelae of otitis media include: *A*, infectious eczematoid dermatitis; *B*, cholesteatoma; *C*, retraction pocket of tympanic membrane; *D*, tympanosclerosis; *E*, perforation of tympanic membrane; *F*, chronic suppurative otitis media; *G*, cholesterol granuloma; *H*, ossicular discontinuity; *I*, facial paralysis; *J*, adhesive otitis media with fixation of the ossicles; *K*, hearing loss; *L*, petrositis; *M*, labyrinthitis; and *N*, mastoiditis with extension into the neck (Bezold's abscess). (From Teele, D. W., Klein, J. O., Rosner, B. A., and the Greater Boston Otitis Media Study Group: Otitis media with effusion during the first three years of life and development of speech and language. Pediatrics 74:282–287, 1984.)

hesive otitis media or ossicular discontinuity). High negative pressure in the ear, or atelectasis, in the absence of effusion is another cause of conductive loss.

Sensorineural Hearing Loss

Sensorineural hearing loss may also result from acute otitis media or otitis media with effusion. A reversible hearing impairment is generally attributed to the effect of increased tension and stiffness of the round window membrane. A permanent sensorineural loss may occur, presumably as a result of spread of infection or products of inflammation through the round window membrane (Morizono et al., 1985; Paparella et al., 1972), development of a perilymphatic fistula in the oval round window (Grundfast and Bluestone, 1978; Supance and Bluestone, 1983), or a suppurative complication such as labyrinthitis.

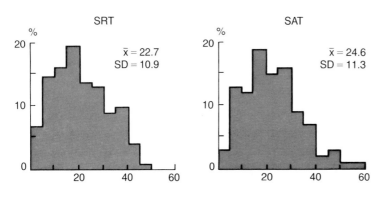

Figure 9–2. Frequency distribution of thresholds for speech stimuli associated with otitis media with effusion. *Left,* speech reception threshold (SRT) of 540 children; *right,* speech awareness threshold (SAT) of 222 infants. HL indicates hearing level. (From Fria T. J., Cantekin, E. I., and Eichler, J. A.: Hearing acuity of children with otitis media with effusion. Arch. Otolaryngol. 111:10–16, 1985.)

Studies of Hearing Loss with Acute Otitis Media

Few studies of hearing have been performed during acute episodes of otitis media. Olmstead and coworkers (1964) studied children two-and-one-half to 12 years of age with a diagnosis of acute otitis media who were seen in the Outpatient Department of St. Christopher's Hospital in Philadelphia. Of 82 children enrolled in the study, 33 percent had no loss of hearing on the initial audiometric test following acute infection; 40 percent had loss of hearing (up to 15 dB) initially, which disappeared in one to six months; 12 percent had loss of hearing throughout the six-month period of observation; and 15 percent had loss of hearing initially but were lost to the study between one and four months after the acute episode of otitis media. The children had no prior history of hearing difficulty or chronic ear infection. Otoscopic examinations were not performed after initial diagnosis, and data were not presented concerning duration of fluid in the middle ear. These data indicate that after a single episode of acute otitis media, many children have prolonged impairment of hearing.

Hearing loss has also been identified in children who have apparently recovered from acute otitis media. A longitudinal study of Alaskan Eskimo children showed a statistically significant association between the frequency of episodes of otitis media and hearing loss of greater than 26 dB. Of children who had one or more attacks of otitis media per year, 49 percent had hearing loss; hearing loss was evident in 15 percent of children with no diagnosed episodes of otitis media (Reed et al., 1967). Other studies with differing criteria have found the incidence of hearing loss associated with acute otitis media to vary between 6 and 30 percent (Lowe et al., 1963; Neil et al., 1966).

Studies of Hearing Loss with Otitis Media with Effusion

Hearing loss is a frequent accompaniment of persistent middle ear effusion (documented at the time of surgery) (Bluestone et al., 1973; Kokko, 1974). Fria and colleagues (1985) evaluated hearing in 222 infants (aged seven to 24 months) and 540 older children (aged two to 12 years). Both the younger and older children had, on average, thresholds for speech reception and speech awareness of 24.6 and 22.7 dB, respectively (Fig. 9–2). Not all children with middle ear effusion have apparent hearing impairment. About one third of the children had air conduction thresholds of 15 dB, but approximately 25 percent of children with middle ear effusion had thresholds of up to 30 dB. The cumulative frequency curves were similar for children of various ages and for duration of effusion. This large study provides a very complete picture of the number of children affected and the extent of the hearing loss when middle ear effusion is present.

Audiometric techniques for children of various ages are discussed in Chapter Seven, Otitis Media.

EFFECTS OF OTITIS MEDIA ON DEVELOPMENT OF THE CHILD

Do children suffer long-term sequelae due to the acute otitis media or persistent effusions of the middle ear because of impairment of hearing? Much has been written about the handicap imposed on the severely hearing impaired child, but less is known about the effects on the young child of the mild and fluctuating hearing loss associated with otitis media.

Sensorineural hearing loss has been associated with impairment in the cognitive, language, and emotional development of children. Children with sensorineural hearing impairment, when compared with peers who have normal hearing, are significantly retarded in development of vocabulary (Young and McConnell, 1957), are placed below their grade level in school (Kodman, 1963), have poorer articulation and auditory discriminatory abilities (Goetzinger et al., 1964), and have a high rate of maladjusted behavior patterns (Fisher, 1966) and disturbances in psychosocial adjustment (Peckham et al., 1972).

The first months of life are important in language acquisition. The infant is capable of speech sound discrimination as early as one month of age. By six weeks of age, the infant is attracted to human voices more than to environmental sounds and to female more than to male voices. At five to six months the infant enters the babble phase and plays with sound-making. The child is putting words together in sentences by 18 months of age,

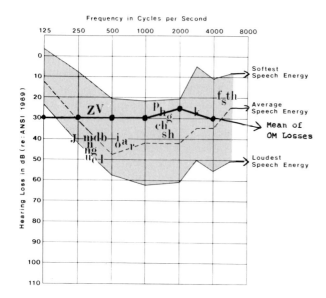

Figure 9–3. Range of speech energy related to standard audiogram. Shaded area shows range of sound energy present in normal speech, and dashed line indicates average of speech energy (adapted from Skinner, 1978). Line connected by solid circles shows mean of hearing losses from otitis media. It can be seen that softer speech sounds may not be heard when otitis media is present.

and by four years the child produces all the basic syntactic structures that he or she will ever use (Menyuk, 1977).

Since so much progress in language acquisition is made during infancy, any problems in receiving or interpreting sound signals might have a significant effect on development of speech and language. Softer speech sounds and voiceless consonants, in particular, may be missed or confused when effusion is present in the middle ear (Fig. 9–3) (Downs, 1983). Important differences have been identified in the early patterns of vocalization of the hearing-impaired infant when compared with hearing infants. How these data about differences in infant babble relate to ultimate development of speech and language when the hearing impairment is mild and fluctuating is unknown.

The current hypothesis for the effects of otitis media on development of the child is presented in Figure 9–4. Children with severe or recurrent otitis media have prolonged time spent with middle ear effusion. Hearing impairment (average loss approximately 25 dB) accompanies the effusion in most children, and if the hearing impairment occurs at a time of rapid intellectual growth, the result may be impaired development of speech, language, and cognitive abilities.

Recent Studies

The results of more than a dozen studies suggest that children with histories of recurrent episodes of acute otitis media score lower in tests of speech and language than do disease-free peers. A brief resume of the results of selected studies follows:

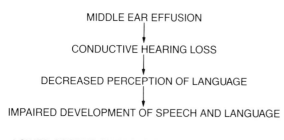

Figure 9–4. Long-term sequelae of middle ear effusion.

1. One of the earliest and most widely cited studies is that of Holm and Kunze of Seattle (1969). Children aged five to nine years who had a history of chronic otitis media with onset before two years of age were compared with children in a control group matched for age, sex, and socioeconomic background. Children with a history of ear disease were delayed in all language skills requiring the receiving or processing of auditory stimuli, but the groups were similar in tests measuring visual and motor skills (Fig. 9–5). Diagnosis of otitis media was made on the basis of history; otoscopic and audiometric examinations were not performed, and the sample size was small (16 children in each group).

2. Eskimo children were observed prospectively during the first four years of life and had tests of hearing, intelligence, and assessment of school performance at age 10 years (Kaplan et al., 1973). Children with recurrent episodes of otitis media (defined as the presence of a draining ear) during the first two years of life and with loss of hearing of 26 dB or more had lower scores in tests

of reading, mathematics, and language than did children who had little or no disease in infancy. Otorrhea was the sole criterion for otitis media; data were not available about the presence or duration of middle ear effusions or episodes of acute otitis media that did not result in otorrhea.

3. Aboriginal children from Brisbane, Australia, were studied by Lewis (1976). Children aged seven to nine years of age who "failed otoscopic examinations" and had hearing deficits measured by audiometry or tympanometry over a four-year period were compared with age-matched control children who had consistently passed the audiometric tests and were assumed to be disease-free. Children with ear disease had mean scores for speech and language development that were significantly lower than those of the children without ear disease. The sample size was small—14 children with disease and 18 controls.

4. Needleman (1977) evaluated 20 children three to eight years of age with a history of recurrent otitis media and first episode before age 18 months. Twenty control sub-

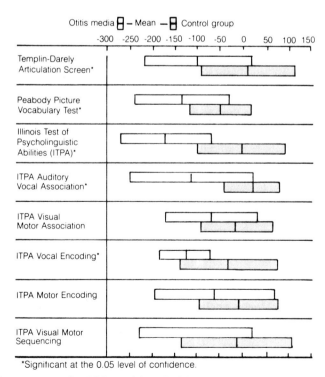

*Significant at the 0.05 level of confidence.

Figure 9–5. Results of language tests in children with and without otitis media (standard score mean and standard deviation). (From Holm, V. A., and Kunze, L. H.: Effects of chronic otitis media on language and speech development. Pediatrics 43:833–839, 1969.)

jects who had no history of hearing problems or recurrent ear infections were matched with the patients for age, grade, and socioeconomic status. The children were evaluated for their ability to use speech sounds expressively and receptively. Children with a history of ear disease had poorer phonological abilities than did matched-control children. Diagnosis of ear disease was based on history alone.

5. Sak and Ruben (1982) used a sibling control for children with histories of otitis media. Children received tests of speech and language between eight and 11 years of age. One sibling of each pair had had a documented history of persistent otitis media beginning before five years of age, whereas the other sibling had had no middle ear problem. The children who had had otitis media showed a lower verbal IQ, poorer auditory reception, and lower spelling achievement than their matched sibling controls.

More of the siblings with otitis were boys than were the control siblings, and more minor middle ear abnormalities identified by audiometry or tympanometry were prevalent among the otitis media siblings than among the control siblings, suggesting the possibility that deficits were associated with recent, rather than earlier, middle ear disease.

6. Friel-Patti and coworkers (1982) examined the association of otitis media early in life with language development at 12, 18, and 24 months. The infants had been selected from intensive care units of low-birthweight nurseries and were predominantly from low socioeconomic groups. Frequent episodes of otitis media were correlated with a higher prevalence of language delay, but no correlation was found between hearing impairment measured by auditory brain stem response testing and language delay.

7. To determine the association between time spent with middle ear effusion and development of speech, language, and cognitive abilities, Teele and colleagues studied 190 white children of varying socioeconomic strata from Greater Boston. The children were selected from a cohort of children in five health centers who were followed from birth with regular examinations of the middle ear at each visit to office or clinic, whether for illness or for routine care. The study was prospective, used uniform criteria for diagnosis of otitis media and middle ear effusion, and tested children from all socioeconomic strata (Teele et al., 1984).

Tests of speech and language administered at the third birthday included the Peabody Picture Vocabulary Test (a test of both early receptive and expressive language), the Fisher-Logemann and Goldman-Fristoe Tests of Articulation (tests of production of speech sound), and other measurements of complexity of language structure and estimates of intelligibility.

Children who had spent fewer than 30 days with middle ear effusion during the first three years of life were compared with those who had spent 30 to 129 days with middle ear effusion during the first three years of life and with those who had spent 130 or more days with middle ear effusion from birth to age three years. In summary, the results identified (1) Lower scores on tests for the total number of children tested, but significant differences were present only in the scores of children from the high socioeconomic group. No significant differences were found for children from low socioeconomic groups (Table 9–1). The basis for the difference in results for children in lower and upper socioeconomic strata is unclear but might be accounted for by the lower scores of children in the low socioeconomic group. The tests used may have been insensitive to differences in performance by these children at three years of age. (2) Increased time with middle ear effusion during the first year of life was most significantly associated with lower scores in children tested at three years of age. Confounding variables such as race and birth order were either controlled for or excluded.

Table 9–1. **OTITIS MEDIA WITH EFFUSION AND SCORES OF TESTS OF SPEECH AND LANGUAGE AT AGE THREE YEARS, PEABODY PICTURE VOCABULARY TEST***

Time with Middle Ear Effusion	All Children	High Socioeconomic Status	Low Socioeconomic Status
Less than 30 days	101.4	104.8	96.6
More than 130 days	96.4	99.6	92.5
	p = 0.002	p = 0.0001	p = nonsignificant

*Total sample, 190 children: 106, high socioeconomic status; 84, low socioeconomic status.

8. Hubbard and colleagues in Pittsburgh (Hubbard et al., 1985) evaluated two matched pairs of children with repaired palatal clefts. The treatment of the children had been equivalent, with the exception that one group had undergone early myringotomy with placement of tympanostomy tubes (mean age, three months), and the other group had undergone initial myringotomy later (mean age, 30.8 months) or not at all. Hearing acuity and consonant articulation were significantly less impaired in the group undergoing early myringotomy. Mean verbal performance and full scale IQs and scores on psychosocial indices were normal in both groups and did not differ significantly between the groups.

9. Watanabe and colleagues (1985) studied total speaking time in infants and children with and without middle ear effusion. To support the premise that improvements in the child's performance occurred when hearing improved with resolution of middle ear effusion, the authors developed a technique to identify time of vibration of the vocal cords. Duration of speaking time was measured in children with otitis media with effusion before and after placement of tympanostomy tubes. Preoperative speaking time was found to be eight minutes and two seconds per measured hour when middle ear effusion was present and 10 minutes per hour when the effusion cleared following placement of tympanostomy tubes. The implications of this innovative study are uncertain but suggest that hearing improvement increases speaking time and causes the child's ordinary behavior to be more animate.

Other recent studies of otitis media and language performance include a study of Montreal children, aged three to five years, that identified significant differences among the children with histories of otitis media and matched controls (Schlieper et al., 1985), a study of Danish children three to nine years of age that did not show an effect of otitis media with effusion early in life on reading achievement (Lous and Fiellau-Nikolajsen, 1984), and evaluation of Apache Indian children six to eight years of age who had contrasting histories of otitis media but no significant difference in language performance (Fischler et al., 1985).

These reports are disturbing but most have one or more flaws in design: (1) reliance on retrospective history of acute otitis media, (2) uncertain validity of diagnosis of otitis media, (3) lack of information about middle ear effusion, (4) presence of significant hearing impairment in subjects at time of tests of speech and language, (5) small numbers of subjects, (6) special populations tested (Australian aborigines or Alaskan Eskimos, or children with cleft palate, for example), and (7) inadequate criteria for selection of children without disease used for comparison. Hignett summarized the study design issues and evaluated the effectiveness of 10 early studies of otitis media and speech, language, and behavior (Hignett, 1983). The recent studies of Teele and coworkers (1984) and Hubbard and associates (1985) represent significant advances in study design when compared with prior investigations. But each of these studies have been subject to criticism (Leviton and Bellinger, 1985; Paradise and Rogers, 1986) because of perceived limitations and deficiencies. These inadequacies of study design prevent general application of these results to planning care for young children, but they do not prevent concern that many children may suffer from the sequelae of otitis media with persistent middle ear effusion in infancy.

Factors of Importance in Analysis of Studies of Otitis Media and Development of Speech, Language, and Cognitive Abilities

Quality of Parenting. Language development is an interactive process in which the quality of parent-child interaction is an important factor. The quality of parenting is difficult to measure but undoubtedly plays a significant role in the development of language for the child.

Family Stress. The parents and siblings of a child with recurrent otitis media must contend with earaches in the middle of the night, irritability and inattentiveness of the child, and the expense and inconvenience of frequent visits to the physician. Although some families can accept and cope with the stress of a child's recurrent illnesses, other families cannot. A constellation of disturbances in psychosocial development may result.

Recurrent and Persistent Otitis Media as a Chronic Disease. The systemic effects of illness, including irritability, malaise, lethargy, and local or generalized pain, may be sufficiently distracting to affect development. These effects of a chronic illness must be distinguished from the specific effects of otitis media (i.e., hearing loss) in the interpretation of the sequelae of the disease. Is the child treated differently by the parents, siblings, peers, or teachers because of the recurrent illnesses? Is the child vulnerable to effects unassociated with the specific morbidity of the disease (kept indoors, away from peers, or out of exercise and athletic programs)?

Critical Ages for Effects of Otitis Media. Otitis media of similar duration may affect children differently at different ages. There may be critical periods of perception of language when the child is most vulnerable to mild, fluctuating, or persistent hearing loss. The results of the Boston study suggested that the children were most affected by middle ear effusion when disease occurred during the first year of life (Teele et al., 1984). During early stages of language development, the child learns the sounds of the language; different or changing auditory signals resulting from persistent or fluctuating hearing deficits may impede the child's abilities to form linguistic categories (Berko-Gleason, 1983).

Auditory Deprivation. Studies in birds and rodents indicate that deprivation of sound early in life leads to identifiable changes in auditory sectors of the brain. A decrease in the size and number of neurons in the auditory nuclei of mice occurred when the animals were deprived of auditory stimuli during early development (Webster, 1983). In normal postnatal development of the mouse, the neurons of the auditory brain stem reach adult size by age 12 days, the time of onset of hearing. Mice that underwent auditory deprivation by experimentally produced conductive hearing loss from four to 45 days after birth had auditory brain stem neurons that were significantly smaller than normal. If the mice who underwent induced hearing loss early in life were returned to normal hearing after 45 days, the smaller-than-normal neurons were retained. The size of the neurons was not altered in mice raised in a normal sound environment until 45 days and then deprived of sound until 90 days of age.

These data demonstrate that a period exists in the development of mice during which adequate sound stimulation is needed to establish the normal size of neuronal cells in the auditory brain stem. These experimental data in animals raise concerns about irreparable damage from temporary conductive hearing loss in infants. However, Webster points out that the factors in the experimental model differ from the mild to moderate hearing losses of otitis media with effusion in humans; in the experimental model the conductive loss is approximately 50 dB, greater than the loss in most cases of otitis media with effusion. The loss is persistent rather than fluctuating, and the impairment starts at the inception of hearing in the mouse, whereas inception of sound occurs prenatally in the human. The author concludes that although the restrictions of the animal model must be kept in mind, "the fact that early auditory restriction has a profound effect on the central nervous system in one mammal must arouse concern about possible related effects in humans."

Unilateral Hearing Loss. Unilateral hearing loss has not been considered a handicap for children. Recent data indicate, however, that children with unilateral hearing impairment score less well on auditory, linguistic, and behavioral tests than do children without hearing impairment (Bess and Tharpe, 1984). Although the children studied had sensorineural hearing deficits, the data suggest that we should no longer accept as benign a unilateral hearing loss. Children with unilateral conductive loss may also suffer during critical periods of language perception by confused speech signals.

Effects of Group Day Care. Respiratory infections are readily spread among children in day care, and children in day care are likely to have more episodes of otitis media than will children in home care. In relation to development of language, the quantity and quality of the speech sounds around the infants in group care differ from those presented to the child in home care. The factors of increased number of infections and differences in the speech environment in group day care will need to be considered in future studies.

Psychosocial Effects of Otitis Media. Does otitis media with mild and fluctuating hearing loss affect the child's motivation and perception of others? Gray (1983) suggested that inconsistencies in the child's ability to hear may have a lasting effect on the child's motivation to achieve and may cause strain in relationships with teachers and parents.

Other Primary Variables That May Relate to Early Childhood Language Development. Future study designs must also consider these additional factors: visual status, physical and motor development, social and emotional development, nutritional status and history of medications, dialect exposure, birth order, and number of siblings.

Test Results and Functional Significance. Do a few percentage points of one or more standard tests of speech, language, or cognitive abilities affect the child's capability to function in the school, play, and home settings? Some investigators question whether these are statistical differences of limited importance to child development. But there are reasons for concern. Since the data are expressed here in terms of mean differences, some children will be close to or better than the norm, but others will have scores that are much lower. Otitis media is so common in early childhood that even if a small percentage of children are adversely affected in terms of development, the number of children who suffer is large. Of the 3.7 million children born in the United States each year, more than one third will have recurrent episodes of otitis media (three or more) by three years of age. If only 10 percent of the children with recurrent episodes are affected adversely, the national impact is greater: more than 100,000 of each year's newborn infants would be involved.

Since the tests measure the child's potential for achievement, it is possible that the loss suffered by the child with frequent and recurrent episodes of otitis media accompanied by hearing loss in early infancy is never perceived by the parents, teachers, or physicians. The child is not obviously slow or behind his peers. The failure of the child to reach his or her potential is a loss for the child and the family, and because the number of children is large each year, it must be considered a national concern.

Summary: Role of Otitis Media in Infant Development

The accumulated results of the various studies of otitis media and development of speech, language, and cognitive abilities suggest that children do suffer long-term effects from otitis media early in life. The scientific evidence, however, remains incomplete. Some experts are skeptical about available data (Paradise, 1983; Ventry, 1983). Ventry concluded that no causal link had been established (by 1982) between early recurrent middle ear effusion and language delay or learning problems. Rapin (1979) noted that no studies published by 1977 "met the standards

of rigor needed to provide a definitive answer to this question, although the burden of the evidence is that a persistent and mild hearing loss, especially if present since infancy, probably has a measurably deleterious effect on the language of most, but not all, children." The authors believe that Dr. Rapin's statement is as applicable today as it was in 1977.

The difficulties in study design needed to resolve the issues and account for many of the variables are formidable. The optimal design will need to include frequent otoscopic observations beginning soon after birth to develop a chronology of time spent with middle ear effusion. Assessments of hearing will need to be performed in infants when they have effusion and are free of effusion to measure the duration and severity of hearing deficits. All of this will need to be done in the first years of life when hearing assessments are more difficult and less precise than in the older child. The study will need to be cross-sectional and prospective from birth and should be performed by validated otoscopists. Tests of speech, language, and cognitive abilities will need to be selected that are accurate and standardized for the populations to be tested. The tests should be performed at least annually to define the time of onset or the effect of otitis media on development. The previous section identified the other variables that will need to be considered, including the quality of parenting, the affect of siblings, and the time spent in group day care.

Concern about the association of middle ear disease and development of speech and language was expressed in a recent policy statement of the American Academy of Pediatrics. Although recognizing the validity of criticism of published studies, the Committee on Early Childhood, Adoption, and Dependent Care concluded that "there is growing evidence demonstrating a correlation between middle ear disease with hearing impairment and delays in the development of speech, language, and cognitive skills. . . . When a child has frequently recurring acute otitis media and/or middle ear effusion persisting for longer than three months, hearing should be assessed and the development of communicative skills must be monitored" (American Academy of Pediatrics, 1984). Until definitive answers are available from studies of appropriate design to evaluate the sequelae of otitis media in early infancy, the physician must decide, for each child in his or her care, the optimal management of persistent middle ear effusion. Chapter Eight, on management, provides guidelines for such care.

PERFORATION OF THE TYMPANIC MEMBRANE

Perforation of the tympanic membrane that is secondary to otitis media (and certain related conditions, such as atelectasis of the tympanic membrane) can be classified according to duration, area of the eardrum involved, size, and presence or absence of associated conditions, such as otitis media or cholesteatoma. In addition, perforation may be a complication of a surgical procedure to manage otitis media, such as myringotomy or tympanostomy tube insertion. An acute perforation is most frequently secondary to an episode of acute otitis media; if it persists for more than two months it is considered chronic. Perforations occur in the pars tensa and involve one or more quadrants. The defect may involve almost the entire pars tensa or be so small as to be detectable only when visualized with the otomicroscope or when the electroacoustic impedance bridge measures a volume larger than the expected ear canal volume. Otitis media (with or without discharge) may be present or absent; when chronic otitis media with discharge is present, the condition is called chronic suppurative otitis media, which is described in detail in the next section (page 216). Likewise, a perforation may be associated with some of the other complications and sequelae described in this chapter.

In the past, perforations have been classified into "central" and "marginal" types. Regardless of size, if there is a rim of tympanic membrane remaining at all borders, the perforation has been classified as "central," whereas when any part of the perforation extends to the annulus, it has been termed "marginal."

A defect in the pars flaccida has been commonly called an "attic perforation." The so-called marginal perforation of the pars tensa, which usually occurs in the posterosuperior portion, and the "perforation" are in reality either a deep retraction pocket or a cholesteatoma (Fig. 9–6). For the "attic perforation" and "marginal perforation" there is usually no continuity between the defect in the membrane and the middle ear until late

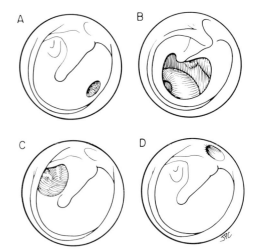

Figure 9–6. Examples of defects in the tympanic membrane. *A,* A small "central" perforation in the anteroinferior portion of the pars tensa of the tympanic membrane. *B,* A "central" perforation that involves approximately half of the pars tensa. *C,* A deep retraction pocket in the posterosuperior portion of the pars tensa that has been incorrectly called a "marginal perforation." *D,* A deep retraction pocket in the pars flaccida that has been inappropriately called an "attic perforation."

in the disease process, when infection destroys the membrane of the pocket or the matrix of the cholesteatoma. Therefore, the terms "marginal perforation" and "attic perforation" are misnomers; they were applied on the basis of observations made prior to the availability of the otomicroscope, modern middle ear surgery, advances in temporal bone histopathological techniques, the use of the electroacoustic impedance bridge, and a better understanding of the pathogenesis of a retraction pocket and cholesteatoma.

Acute Perforation

An acute perforation (not due to trauma) is usually secondary to acute otitis media but may also occur during the course of chronic otitis media with effusion. Since a spontaneous perforation commonly accompanies an episode of acute middle ear infection, it may be considered part of the disease process rather than a complication. Because such a perforation allows purulent material to drain into the external canal and enhances drainage of pus down the eustachian tube (owing to the effects of an opening in the eardrum), a perforation of the eardrum may prevent further spread of infection within the temporal bone or, more importantly, into the intracranial cavity. Infants and children of certain racial groups, such as Alaskan natives (Eskimos) and American Indians, have a high incidence of spontaneous perforation with discharge: the eardrum is perforated spontaneously with almost every episode of acute otitis media. The disease runs a similar course in certain other children not belonging to these high-risk populations.

Pathogenesis

The perforation may occur in high-risk populations because of the presence of a semipatulous eustachian tube (Beery et al., 1980): a eustachian tube with low resistance would permit a larger bolus of bacteria-laden purulent material from the nasopharynx to enter the middle ear, causing a more fulminating infection than would occur if the eustachian tube had either normal or high resistance. An alternative explanation of why some children seem to suffer a perforated eardrum with each episode of acute otitis media while others do not could be that there are differences in the virulence of the bacteria or decreased resistance of the host.

Microbiology

The organisms that are most frequently cultured from an aural discharge when acute otitis media is present are the same as those that have been cultured from acute middle ear effusions when a tympanocentesis has been performed (e.g., *Streptococcus pneumoniae* and *Haemophilus influenzae*). *Streptococcus pyogenes*, when present and untreated, has been associated with acute perforation of the tympanic membrane.

Management

Antimicrobial therapy for children with acutely perforated eardrums should be the same as that recommended for those with acute otitis media when a perforation is not present. However, when an aural discharge is present, it may be desirable to culture the drainage. The antimicrobial regimen can then be adjusted according to the results of the smear, culture, and sensitivity testing. The most effective method to obtain a sample of the discharge is to remove as much as possible of the purulent material from the external canal by suction or cotton-tipped applicator and then to aspirate pus directly at or through the perforation, using a spinal needle attached to a tuberculin syringe or an Alden-Senturia trap (Storz Instrument Co., St. Louis) and suction.

Some experts would argue against use of ototopical medication when a perforation is present because of the potential danger of ototoxicity. However, some children are benefited when otic drops are instilled into the external canal. Ototopical medication will usually be beneficial when infectious eczematoid external otitis complicates the picture. The application of an antibiotic-cortisone otic medication whenever a discharge is present has been advocated by many clinicians despite the possibility of ototoxiciy, since the topical medication may treat or prevent an external canal infection and hasten the resolution of the middle ear infection.

The discharge, especially when profuse, should be prevented from draining onto the pinna and adjacent areas, since this usually results in dermatitis. The parent should be instructed to keep cotton in the external auditory meatus and change it as often as necessary to keep the canal dry. Cotton-tipped applicators should not be used by child or parent.

Healing of the tympanic membrane frequently follows cessation of the suppurative process in the middle ear. The defect usually closes within a week after onset of infection; when persistent discharge lasts longer than the initial 10-day course of antibiotic treatment, the child requires more intensive evaluation and aggressive management. In addition to obtaining a culture of the purulent material from the middle ear and adjusting antimicrobial agents, frequent cleaning of the canal, followed by instillation of ototopical drops, may also be required. The presence of acute mastoiditis with periosteitis or acute mastoid osteitis should be suspected if the child has persistent otalgia, tenderness of the ear to touch, erythema, and swelling in the postauricular area. Roentgenograms of the mastoids may be helpful but are not always diagnostic of mastoid osteitis. Spread of infection outside the middle ear and mastoid may be diagnosed on computerized tomograms. Even if an intratemporal (or intracranial) complication is not readily apparent, if the aural discharge persists two or three weeks after onset of acute otitis media that has been treated with appropriately administered oral antibiotics, the child should be hospitalized. The child should be evaluated again thoroughly in a search for an underlying illness that would interfere with resolution of the infection. The otological assessment should include an examination of the entire external canal and tympanic membrane, using the otomicroscope to determine if another otological condition such as a cholesteatoma or neoplasm, is present. If an adequate examination cannot be performed with the child awake, it should be carried out under general anesthesia, at which time a culture directly from the middle ear can be obtained. If no condition other than the perforation and subacute otitis media is found, parenteral antimicrobial agents should be administered. The selection of both the systemic and topical antimicrobial agents should be based on the results of cultures. Frequently, a gram-negative organism (e.g., *Pseudomonas aeruginosa*) is present at this stage, and management is essentially as recommended in the section on chronic suppurative otitis media (page 216).

With this method of management, the infection will usually subside; however, if the discharge persists, an exploratory tympanotomy and complete simple mastoidectomy is indicated, even if there are no signs and symptoms of mastoid osteitis present and the roentgenograms fail to show osteitis (i.e., "coalescence"). During surgery on the middle ear and mastoid, a thorough search for another cause of the persistent infection must be made. On occasion, a cholesteatoma that could not be visualized through the otomicroscope will be found. Resolution of infection in the middle ear and mastoid will invariably follow the surgery, since mastoid osteitis is the usual cause of this complication of acute otitis media.

Fortunately, nowadays, the occurrence of such cases is uncommon and the perforation usually heals rapidly; however, not infrequently, the defect will remain open without evidence of otitis media (with or without discharge). If the perforation remains free of infection, it will frequently close in a few months. At this stage, no attempt at surgical closure of an uncomplicated perforation is indicated. If there is no sign of progressive healing after three or more months, management should be as described below for a chronic perforation of the tympanic membrane.

Chronic Perforation

A perforation of the tympanic membrane may remain open after an episode of acute otitis media or following spontaneous extrusion (or removal) of a tympanostomy tube. When the perforation is present with no signs of healing and there are no signs of otitis media for several months, the perforation is considered to be chronic and possibly "permanent." If chronic suppurative otitis media is present, the perforation may close spontaneously following appropriate treatment. The healing of the perforation is most likely being prevented by the presence of squamous epithelium at the edges of the perforation. The effect on hearing of a small chronic perforation, regardless of its location, and in the absence of other middle ear abnormalities, is not significant. However, a large perforation can be associated with an appreciable conductive hearing loss (e.g., 20 to 30 dB).

The incidence of chronic perforation in the pediatric population has not been formally studied, but chronic perforation is a frequent reason for referral to an otolaryngologist. The incidence of tympanoplasties performed in children would not accurately reflect the true incidence of chronic perforation, since many physicians elect to withhold surgery until later in the child's life. However, next to myringotomy, with or without tympanostomy tube insertion, tympanoplasty is the most common ear operation performed in children (Avery et al., 1976).

Chronic perforations, as complications of otitis media, are more prevalent in racial groups that also have a high prevalence and incidence of perforations associated with acute middle ear infection. In 1970, new cases of chronic peforation (with or without chronic suppurative otitis media), were reported in 8 percent of the native population of Alaska, although this rate appears to be dropping (Wiet et al., 1980). Similar rates have been reported in American Indian populations. Zonis (1968) reported that of 207 Apache Indian children examined in Canyon Day, Arizona, 17 (8 percent) had chronic perforations as their only sign of otitis media, whereas 16 years later, Todd (1985) returned to the same village in 1983, examined 145 Indian children living there at the time, and found only one child who had a perforation of the tympanic membrane but 12 (8 percent) children who had other evidence of otitis media. Of 1062 ears of children who received tympanostomy tubes in one study reported from West Germany, 26 ears (2.5 percent) had a persistent perforation (Muenker, 1980). However, this figure is dependent on the site of the tube placement and the type of tube used (see section on tympanostomy tubes, page 175).

Management

The management of so-called dry chronic perforations in children is both difficult and controversial. The perforation provides ventilation and drainage of the middle ear, but the physiological protective function of the eustachian tube–middle ear system is impaired. The middle ear and mastoid air cells no longer have an air cushion to prevent nasopharyngeal secretions from entering the ear, which can result in "reflux otitis media" (Figs. 9–7 and 9–8). In addition, the open tympanic membrane can permit contaminated water to enter the middle ear during bathing and swimming. Therefore, the dilemma of when to close such a perforation is comparable to that regarding the most appropriate time to remove a tympanostomy tube: a small, uncomplicated chronic perforation and a tympanostomy tube have similar benefits and risks. Like a tympanostomy tube, a perforation may be beneficial for a child who had had recurrent or chronic otitis media with effusion prior to the development of the perforation, but recurrent acute "reflux otitis media" with discharge may become a problem, making closure of the eardrum defect a consideration. Recurrent acute otitis media that results in otorrhea through a chronic perforation can be effectively treated and even prevented without repair of the tympanic membrane.

When the episodes are infrequent, the treatment of each bout should be the same as recommended for an acute perforation that is associated with acute otitis media. If the episodes of acute infection are frequent and the interval between bouts short, then a prolonged course of a prophylactic antimicrobial agent, e.g., amoxicillin, 20 mg/kg

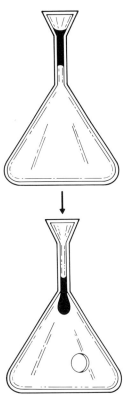

Figure 9–8. Flask model showing how a perforation of the tympanic membrane may result in reflux of nasopharyngeal secretions into the middle ear. The nasopharynx–eustachian tube–middle ear–mastoid air cell system is likened to a flask with a narrow neck. When the system is intact, liquid is prevented from entering the body of the flask, but when the body of the flask is not intact (i.e., a perforation is present), liquid can readily flow through the system.

given in one dose before bedtime, may be considered to prevent recurrent middle ear infection and discharge (see Chapter 8). The selection of the agent should be based on the results of the cultures obtained from previous episodes of discharge. Dosage and duration of treatment should be the same as those recommended for children who have had frequently recurrent acute otitis media without a perforation (see Chapter 8). Children in whom an attack of acute middle ear infection and discharge persists despite adequate medical treatment and in whom the infection is thought to be chronic should be evaluated and managed as described in the section on chronic suppurative otitis media in this chapter (page 216).

Most children who have a defect in the eardrum that is thought to be preventing otitis media can be watched until the risk of recurrence of infection is low enough to consider surgical closure of the perforation.

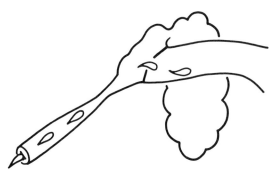

Figure 9–7. The presence of a perforation of the tympanic membrane may promote the reflux of secretions into the middle ear from the nasopharynx, since the middle ear air cushion is not present (see also Fig. 9–8).

Since the perforation, like a tympanostomy tube, may be preventing the development of a retraction pocket and, subsequently, of a cholesteatoma if the function of the eustachian tube is poor, it is desirable to delay such surgery as long as possible in order to prevent such complications. Surgery for a chronic perforation should not necessarily be withheld in children because of recurrent episodes of otitis media and discharge, since the perforation may be causing the middle ear infection (due to reflux from the nasopharynx) rather than preventing disease.

The results of this type of surgery are not as successful in children as they are in adults (Armstrong, 1965; Goodey and Smyth, 1972; Mawson and Ludman, 1979). These findings may be due to the higher incidence of upper respiratory tract infection leading to otitis media in children and the unpredictability of their eustachian tube function. Optimal ages at which to perform tympanoplastic surgery have variously been stated to be from three years to puberty (Bailey, 1976; Glasscock, 1976; Mawson and Ludman, 1979; Storrs, 1976). Lau and Tos (1986) reviewed the outcome of 124 tympanoplasties performed on 116 children who were between the ages of two and 14 years and found a 92 percent success rate of grafts; these authors recommend tympanoplasty in children of all ages, as does Paparella (1977). However, Sheehy and Anderson (1980) do not recommend elective tympanic membrane grafting on children who are younger than seven years of age because of the possibility of postoperative otitis media.

Studying eustachian tube function before the patient with a chronic perforation of the tympanic membrane is operated upon may be helpful in determining the potential results of tympanoplastic surgery. Bluestone, Cantekin, and Douglas (1979), in a study of 45 children with chronic perforation, found that the assessment of eustachian tube function was an aid in preoperative assessment.

Thus, children are uncertain candidates for tympanoplastic surgery, since as a group their eustachian tube function is not as good as that of adults. Improvement may occur in some children, indifferent results in others, and more problems with middle ear infections in a third group. The problem for the clinician is deciding which child should have the perforation repaired. The development of an improved method of testing the eustachian tube, a method that is more indicative of the actual function available for clinical use, could possibly help in this decision-making process.

CHRONIC SUPPURATIVE OTITIS MEDIA

Chronic suppurative otitis media is a stage of ear disease in which there is chronic inflammation of the middle ear and mastoid and in which a nonintact tympanic membrane (perforation or tympanostomy tube) and discharge (otorrhea) are present. Mastoiditis is invariably a part of the pathological process. The condition has been called chronic otitis media, but this term can be confused with chronic otitis media with effusion, in which no perforation is present. It is also called chronic suppurative otitis media and mastoiditis, chronic purulent otitis media, and chronic otomastoiditis. The most descriptive term is "chronic otitis media with perforation, discharge, and mastoiditis" (Senturia et al., 1980a), but this is not common usage. When a cholesteatoma is also present, the term "chronic suppurative otitis media with cholesteatoma" is used; however, because an acquired aural cholesteatoma does not have to be associated with chronic suppurative otitis media, cholesteatoma is not part of the pathological features of the type of ear disease described in this section and is presented as a separate entity in the following section (page 221).

Epidemiology

Most studies that have reported the prevalence of chronic suppurative otitis media in children include children who also have cholesteatoma, so that accurate data on the incidence of chronic suppurative otitis media alone are not available. In a study conducted by the School Health Service in Great Britain, the proportion of children found to have chronic otitis media at the periodic medical inspections was about nine per 1000 (Mawson and Ludman, 1979).

This type of chronic ear disease has a high prevalence in children of certain racial groups. The studies of American Indians (Cambon et al., 1965; DeBlanc, 1975; Wiet et al., 1980; Zonis, 1970), Canadian and Alaskan (Eskimo) natives (Baxter and Ling, 1974; Maynard, 1969), Australian aboriginal children (McCafferty et al., 1977), and the

Maoris of New Zealand have shown an extremely high rate of chronic suppurative otitis media. The prevalence of chronic suppurative otitis media is higher in children in these racial groups than in the Caucasian population living in the same area (Ratnesar, 1977). More recently, Todd (1985) reported a sharp decline in the incidence of chronic draining ears in Apache Indian children living in the southwestern United States. Cholesteatoma is not commonly associated with chronic ear disease found in these populations. In a study of 4193 Alaskan native schoolchildren conducted in 1971, 1274 (30 percent) had perforated tympanic membranes, but in only 144 (3 percent) was a cholesteatoma also diagnosed (Tschopp, 1977). Similar findings were reported for Canadian Eskimos and Indians, but a higher incidence of cholesteatoma was found in the Caucasians living in the same area (Ratnesar, 1977). Similarly, McCafferty and coworkers (1977) studied 3663 Australian aboriginal children and found that 70 percent of their ears were abnormal; 12 percent had chronic otitis media but less than 1 percent had a cholesteatoma. Ear disease has an early onset in these children: Maynard (1969) reported that most Eskimo children had chronic otitis media before the age of two years. Thus, these epidemiological studies describe chronic suppurative otitis media that is *not* associated with cholesteatoma.

Pathogenesis

The pathogenesis of chronic suppurative otitis media is not completely known, but it is considered to be the chronic stage that follows an attack of acute otitis media in which a perforation has developed, followed by continuous discharge. The sequence of events does not have to progress directly from acute to chronic form. A perforation secondary to acute otitis media can become chronic without evidence of middle ear inflammation (i.e., "dry" perforation). Some authors consider this stage to be an "inactive" stage of chronic otitis media, since middle ear (and mastoid) infection with discharge through the perforation may occur at any time. However, some children have a perforation that rarely, if ever, has a discharge after the initial acute episode in which the perforation developed, and the middle ear mucous membrane remains normal. Therefore, only a chronic perforation that is associated with chronic inflammation of the middle ear–mastoid system should be considered to be chronic suppurative otitis media (see section on perforation of the tympanic membrane in this chapter, page 212). However, the pathogenesis may be the same for acute or chronic perforations with or without otitis media.

In addition to perforations that occur as part of the natural history of otitis media, an extremely large number of temporary perforations (tympanostomy tubes) are created by the surgical treatment of otitis media. It has been estimated that over one million tympanostomy tubes are inserted annually for recurrent acute otitis media and otitis media with effusion (Paradise, 1977). Herzon (1980) reported that of 140 patients, 21 percent developed otorrhea one or more times with tubes in place, whereas McLelland (1980) reported that chronic drainage developed in 3.6 percent of patients with tympanostomy tubes. Most likely, the pathogenesis of chronic infection in the middle ear when a tympanostomy tube is in place is similar to that proposed earlier when a perforation is present (Fig. 9–9).

Anatomical differences in bony segment of the eustachian tube were identified in studies of the bony craniofacial structures of Eskimo, American Indian, Caucasian, and Negro individuals (Doyle, 1977). Beery and coworkers (1980) studied 25 White Mountain Apache Indians ranging in age from three to 36 years and found that their eustachian tubes were semipatulous (of low resistance) in comparison to those of a group of Caucasians. In this study, the function of the eustachian tube was assessed directly through chronic perforations of the eardrum, employing the inflation-deflation and forced-response tests. These studies would appear to indicate that

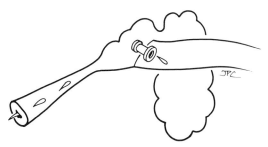

Figure 9–9. This drawing shows a mechanism similar to the one described when a perforation is present (see Fig. 9–7). A patent tympanostomy tube may promote reflux of secretions from the nasopharynx into the middle ear.

these racial groups and the segment of the Caucasian population that have chronic suppurative otitis media have eustachian tubes that permit reflux of nasopharyngeal secretions into the middle ear; reflux acute otitis media develops and the tympanic membrane perforates. In some individuals, the reflux of nasopharyngeal secretions continues after the initial episode, whereas in others the process recurs with each upper respiratory tract infection. The perforation enhances the reflux of the secretions from the nasopharynx, since the middle ear–mastoid air cushion is abolished.

Individuals with a patulous eustachian tube rarely have a cholesteatoma in the posterosuperior quadrant of the pars tensa or in the pars flaccida, and if a cholesteatoma is present, it is usually due to migration of epithelium through the "central" perforation, an uncommon condition. An even more rare and unproven pathogenesis of cholesteatoma is that which is secondary to metaplasia of the middle ear mucous membrane. Since most cholesteatomas are the final step in a sequence of events that begins with negative middle ear pressure, progresses to atelectasis, and then leads to a retraction pocket, the development of a cholesteatoma should be rare when a "central" perforation is present, since the middle ear pressure is ambient. Therefore, even though children who have chronic suppurative otitis media have a morbid process, they appear to be protected from developing an attic or posterosuperior type of cholesteatoma. It is important to keep these facts in mind when considering the surgical management of the perforation after elimination of the chronic middle ear and mastoid infection.

Microbiology

Chronic suppurative otitis media develops from a chronic bacterial infection. However, the bacteria that caused the initial episode of acute otitis media with perforation are usually not those that are isolated from the chronic discharge when there is chronic infection in the middle ear and mastoid. Thus, the antimicrobial therapy recommended for acute otitis media will not be effective for most cases of chronic suppurative otitis media. Kenna, Bluestone, and Reilly (1986) reported that the most common organisms are *P. aeruginosa* and *Staphylococcus aureus* (Table 9–2). Anaerobic bacteria were isolated infre-

Table 9–2. **MICROBIOLOGICAL FINDINGS IN MIDDLE EAR ASPIRATES FROM 36 INFANTS AND CHILDREN (51 EARS) WITH CHRONIC SUPPURATIVE OTITIS MEDIA***

Species	Number of Isolates
Pseudomonas aeruginosa	34
Staphylococcus aureus (7 beta-lactamase–positive strain)	10
Diphtheroids	10
Staphylococcus epidermidis	6
Streptococcus, alpha	4
Streptococcus pneumoniae	3
Escherichia coli	2
Candida albicans	2
Haemophilus influenzae, nontypable	2
Candida parapsilosis	2
Enterococcus species	2
Pseudomonas maltophilia	2
Proteus mirabilis	2
Streptococcus pyogenes	1
Pseudomonas cepacia	1
Eikenella corrodens	1
Moraxella species	1
Alcaligenes odorans	1
Haemophilus influenzae, type b	1
Branhamella catarrhalis	1
Acinetobacter calcoaceticus	1
Citrobacter freundii	1
Streptococcus, nonhemolytic	1
No growth	2
Total	93

*From Kenna, M., Bluestone, C. D., and Reilly, J.: Medical management of chronic suppurative otitis media without cholesteatoma in children. Laryngoscope 96:146–151, 1986.

quently in this study. These organisms are most likely secondary invaders that gain entrance to the middle ear and mastoid from the external auditory canal during an episode of acute otitis media and otorrhea. In contrast, Brook isolated *Bacteroides melaninogenicus* in 40 percent and *Peptococcus* species in 35 percent of middle ear exudates; collection of exudate was performed through the perforation in the tympanic membrane using an 18-gauge needle covered by a plastic cannula (Brook, 1985).

Pathology

It is important to understand the pathological process of chronic otitis media, since the decision for or against surgical intervention may depend on the pathological changes in the middle ear and mastoid. These include edema, submucosal fibrosis, and infiltration with chronic inflammatory cells, which together cause thickening of the mucous membrane (Schuknecht, 1974). Polyps may result from excessive mucosal edema; in the more advanced stage not only polypoid tissue and granulation tissue but also osteitis of the mastoid bone, ossicles, and labyrinth may be present. Adhesive otitis media and sclerosis of bone may occur with healing. Tympanosclerosis may also be present and is commonly associated with this disease in Alaskan (Eskimo) natives (Wiet et al., 1980). If intensive medical treatment is instituted early, these pathological changes may be reversible without surgery. However, when long-standing chronic disease has led to irreversible changes, middle ear and mastoid surgery is usually indicated to eradicate the infection.

Diagnosis

A purulent, mucoid, or serous discharge through a "central" perforation of the tympanic membrane for at least two or three months is evidence of chronic suppurative otitis media. Frequently, a polyp will be seen emerging through the perforation or tympanostomy tube (Fig. 9–10). The size of the perforation has no relation to the duration or severity of the disease, but frequently the defect involves most of the pars tensa. There is no otalgia, mastoid or pinna tenderness, vertigo, or fever. When any of these signs or symptoms is present, the examiner should look for a possible suppurative intratemporal or intracranial complication. A search for the underlying cause of the infection may reveal the presence of paranasal sinusitis, which must be actively treated, since the ear infection may not respond to medical treatment until the sinusitis resolves. An upper respiratory tract allergy or a nasopharyngeal tumor may also contribute to the pathogenesis of chronic otitis media and will need to be managed appropriately.

The discharge should be appropriately examined by a Gram-stained smear and cultured as described in the section on perforation of the tympanic membrane in this chapter (page 213).

One of the most important parts of the evaluation is a complete examination, with the aid of the otomicroscope, of the ear canal, tympanic membrane, and, if the perforation is large enough, the middle ear. If a satisfactory examination cannot be performed with the child awake, then an examination under general anesthesia will be necessary. At this time, the discharge can be aspirated and a culture from the middle ear can be obtained; in addition, a search for a polyp or unsuspected cholesteatoma or neoplasm should be conducted.

A conductive hearing loss usually accompanies chronic otitis media. If a greater than 20- to 30-dB hearing loss is found, the ossicles may be involved; however, the patient may also have a sensorineural component, which is most likely due to a serous labyrinthitis (Paparella et al., 1972). Impedance testing may be helpful if purulent material in the ear canal prevents visualization of the eardrum adequate to identify a possible perforation. If perforation is present, the measured volume of the external canal will be larger than expected; however, the tympanometric pattern may be flat, despite the presence of a perforation, if the volume of air in the middle ear and mastoid is small. When this is suspected, the pressure on the pump-manometer of the impedance bridge can be increased in an attempt to force open the eustachian tube: if the tube can be opened with positive air pressure from the pump-manometer, a perforation must be present.

Roentgenograms of the mastoid should be obtained since cholesteatoma must be ruled out; computerized tomograms, if available, are most informative. In the typical case, the sclerotic or undeveloped mastoid will appear "cloudy." However, if a defect in the bone due to osteitis is present, the area will appear

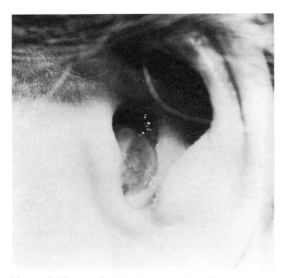

Figure 9–10. Aural polyp in external auditory meatus. The polyp came through a large perforation of an ear with chronic suppurative otitis media.

on the roentgenogram. Discontinuity of the ossicular chain, if present, may be visualized if tomography is used.

Unusual causes of a chronic draining ear, including neoplasms and eosinophilic granuloma, must be considered in the differential diagnosis of chronic suppurative otitis media.

Management

Medical management of chronic otitis media is directed toward eliminating the infection from the middle ear and mastoid. Since the bacteria most frequently cultured are gram-negative, antimicrobial agents should be selected to be effective against these organisms. A suspension containing polymyxin B, neomycin, and hydrocortisone (Cortisporin) or one that has neomycin, polymyxin E, and hydrocortisone (ColyMycin) have been advocated, but owing to the concern over the potential ototoxicity of these agents, caution is advised (Brummett et al., 1976; Meyerhoff et al., 1983). Orally administered antibiotics are usually not effective unless the organisms are highly susceptible.

If topical antibiotic medication is elected, the child should return to the outpatient facility daily so that the discharge can be thoroughly aspirated and ototopical medication can be directly instilled into the middle ear through the perforation or tympanostomy tube, employing the otomicroscope. Frequently, the discharge will rapidly improve with this type of treatment within a week, after which the ear drops may be administered at home until there is complete resolution of the middle ear–mastoid inflammation.

Because of concern over toxicity of the ototopical agents, parents should be informed of this potential danger if such medications are used. As an alternative, we hospitalize our patients and administer a parenteral beta-lactam antipseudomonal drug such as ticarcillin, azlocillin, piperacillin and ceftazidime. The regimen can be altered when results of culture and susceptibility tests are available. The middle ear is aspirated daily. In almost all children the middle ear will be free of discharge and the signs of otitis media will be greatly improved or absent within several days. If resolution does occur, the child should be discharged and followed on an ambulatory basis at periodic intervals to watch for signs of spontaneous

closure of the perforation, which frequently happens after the middle ear and mastoid are no longer infected. If the perforation (or tympanostomy tube) and middle ear are not infected, and it is desirable to maintain middle ear ventilation through a nonintact eardrum, recurrent episodes of otorrhea can usually be prevented with antimicrobial prophylaxis. The agent selected should be effective against the usual organisms that cause acute otitis media, e.g., pneumococci, *H. influenzae* (see Chapter 8).

If the perforation persists or another abnormality requiring surgery is present, such as an ossicular chain disarticulation, tympanoplastic surgery should be considered. When a chronic ("dry") perforation is present, the indications for repair of the tympanic membrane would be similar to those outlined in the previous section. Frequent episodes of acute and chronic infection would be a possible indication to explore the middle ear (and possibly the mastoid) and perform tympanoplasty. Routine mastoidectomy is not necessary if the perforation is not associated with another abnormality that would warrant an exploration of the mastoid. In most children who have had complete resolution of the infection in the middle ear and mastoid but who have a persistent, chronic ("dry") perforation and in whom a tympanoplasty is performed, the addition of a mastoidectomy is of limited value for either diagnosis or management. In such cases, the mastoid is likely to be converted to a more normal state if the discharge is absent for several months.

When the discharge fails to respond to intensive medical therapy, surgery on the middle ear and mastoid is indicated. Kenna, Bluestone, and Reilly (1986) conducted a study in 36 pediatric patients with chronic suppurative otitis media in which all received parenteral antimicrobial therapy and daily aural toilet. Thirty-two patients (89 percent) had resolution of their infection with medical therapy alone; four children required tympanomastoidectomy.

A child who has a chronic suppurative aural discharge and who develops one or more of the intratemporal suppurative complications, such as acute mastoid osteitis, labyrinthitis, facial paralysis, or an intracranial suppurative complication, will require immediate surgical intevention. It is not uncommon that a cholesteatoma is present when an ear with chronic suppurative otitis media fails to respond to intensive medical treatment, even though no preoperative evidence for the presence of cholesteatoma was identified by otomicroscopy or roentgenography. The cholesteatoma usually is found in the middle ear (and mastoid), following migration of the squamous epithelium through the perforation in the tympanic membrane. When a cholesteatoma is found, surgical removal, as outlined in the next section, is indicated.

CHOLESTEATOMA AND RETRACTION POCKET

Keratinizing stratified squamous epithelium and an accumulation of desquamating epithelium of keratin within the middle ear or other pneumatized portions of the temporal bone is called a keratoma or, more commonly, a cholesteatoma. Aural cholesteatomas can be classified into two types: "congenital" and acquired. A "congenital" cholesteatoma is a congenital rest of epithelial tissue and appears as a white, cyst-like structure within the middle ear (intratympanic) or temporal bone. The tympanic membrane is intact and the cholesteatoma is not a sequela of otitis media or eustachian tube dysfunction (Cawthorne and Griffith, 1961; Derlacki and Clemis, 1965). Acquired cholesteatoma may be secondary to implantation or may be a sequela of otitis media or a retraction pocket, or both. Implantation cholesteatoma may develop either from epithelium that has migrated through a traumatic perforation of the tympanic membrane or from epithelium that has been inadvertently overlooked in the middle ear or mastoid during surgery of the ear (iatrogenic) (Brandow, 1977).

The most common cholesteatoma is the acquired type secondary to middle ear disease. In a study of 1024 patients (adults and children) with cholesteatoma, the location was the attic in 42 percent and the posterosuperior quadrant in 31 percent; in 18 percent there was a "total" perforation, in 6 percent there was a "central" perforation, and in 3 percent there was no perforation (Sheehy et al., 1977). It is possible that the patients in whom the cholesteatoma was associated with a "total" perforation originally had involvement of the posterosuperior portion of the pars tensa. In children, the most common defect in the tympanic membrane begins developing in the posterosuperior quadrant of the pars tensa or, somewhat less

commonly, in the pars flaccida. The term "marginal perforation" has been used to describe the defect in the posterosuperior quadrant, and the defect in the pars flaccida has been called an "attic perforation," but in reality, these are not perforations but either retraction pockets or cholesteatomas that appear otoscopically to be perforations (Fig. 9–6). No continuity between the defect and the middle ear occurs until later in the disease process.

Epidemiology

In a study of the general population in Iowa, the overall incidence of cholesteatoma was six per 100,000; in children between zero and nine years of age the incidence was 4.7 per 100,000, whereas, in children 10 to 19 years old, the incidence of 9.2 per 100,000 was the highest for all age groups (Harker and Koontz, 1977). Cholesteatoma is a common sequela in children with cleft palate. Severeid (1977) reviewed the records of 160 children and young adults with cleft palates (70 percent were 10 to 16 years of age), all of whom had had a history of ear disease, and found the incidence of cholesteatoma to be 7.1 percent; the posterosuperior portion of the pars tensa was the most common site. In contrast to this high incidence of cholesteatoma in the cleft palate population is the rare occurrence of cholesteatoma in Alaskan (Eskimo) natives, American Indians (Hinchcliffe, 1977), and Australian aboriginal children (McCafferty et al., 1977), in whom other middle ear disease is very common. This remarkable difference in the incidence of cholesteatoma in children with cleft palates and in certain racial groups, both of which have a high prevalence and incidence of otitis media, is most likely related to differences in the pathogenesis and natural history of the respective middle ear disease processes.

Cholesteatoma in children is considered to be a more aggressive disease than that occurring in adults (Baron, 1969; Derlacki, 1973, Schuknecht, 1974) for two reasons: very extensive disease is found at the time of surgery more frequently in children than in adults, and higher rates of residual (persistent) and recurrent cholesteatoma following surgery have been found in children than have been seen in adults (Abramson et al., 1977). Palva and coworkers (1977) compared 65 children and 65 adults with cholesteatomas; 22 percent of the children had disease that filled the middle ear and mastoid, but only 6 percent of adults had such extensive disease. Despite the finding that cholesteatomas in children tend to be more extensive than those occurring in adults, childhood cholesteatoma may still be confined to the middle ear.

Ritter (1977) compared an epidemiological study in Michigan of 152 cases of cholesteatoma identified during the period from 1965 to 1970 with a similar study from Massachusetts of 303 cases that were identified during 1925 to 1936, a period prior to the use of antimicrobial agents. He found in both series that about 45 percent of cases of cholesteatoma were operated on before the patient was 20 years of age, that in approximately 65 percent of patients the aural discharge had begun by 11 years of age, and that the distribution of sites on the tympanic membrane where the defect was located were about the same. He concluded that antimicrobial agents have not altered the incidence and natural history of cholesteatoma during the 40 years between the two studies.

Prior to the advent of widespread use of antimicrobial agents and modern otological surgery, complications of cholesteatoma were common, and many children died when infection involved the intracranial cavity. Nowadays, serious complications of cholesteatoma in children are uncommon. In a study of 181 children who had cholesteatoma, 8 (4.4 percent) developed a labyrinthine fistula and one suffered facial paralysis, but none had intracranial complications (Sheehy et al., 1977). In the same study, which also included 843 adults, the incidence of both intratemporal and intracranial complications increased the longer the cholesteatoma was present. Because most adults could date the onset of their disease to childhood and because diagnosis of and surgery for cholesteatoma is the best way to prevent serious complications, physicians dealing with ear problems in children should treat suspected cholesteatoma early and aggressively.

The incidence of retraction pockets has not been formally studied, but a retraction pocket is a common sequela of atelectasis of the tympanic membrane with or without otitis media with effusion. The incidence of retraction pockets in children with cleft palates must be greater than that of cholesteatoma (7.1 percent), since a retraction pocket precedes development of a cholesteatoma in this population (Bluestone et al., 1982).

Pathogenesis

Many hypotheses regarding the pathogenesis of cholesteatoma have been proposed; the following are the most popular: (1) metaplasia of the middle ear and attic due to infection (Tumarkin, 1938; Wendt, 1873), (2) invasive hyperplasia of the basal layers of the meatal skin adjoining the upper margin of the tympanic membrane (Hellman, 1925; Lange, 1932; Nager, 1925; Ojala and Saxen, 1952; Ruedi, 1958), (3) invasive hyperkeratosis of the deep external auditory canal (McGuckin, 1961), and (4) retraction or collapse of the tympanic membrane with invagination secondary to eustachian tube dysfunction (Bezold, 1889; Habermann, 1888; Wittmaack, 1933). There are those who consider the condition not to be acquired at all but an embryonic epidermal rest occurring in the attic (Diamant, 1952; McKenzie, 1931; Teed, 1936).

Varying degrees of functional rather than mechanical (anatomical) obstruction of the eustachian tube occurred in 13 children and adults who had a retraction pocket or an acquired cholesteatoma (Bluestone et al., 1977). Subsequently, the findings in 12 children with acquired cholesteatoma, all of whom had functional obstruction of the eustachian tube, were also reported by the same group (Bluestone et al., 1978). Children were specifically studied, since development of an acquired cholesteatoma with its attendant irreversible changes was thought to occur early in life, and function of the eustachian tube might improve with growth and development. In these children, the function of the eustachian tube was assessed by the modified inflation-deflation technique (after Ingelstedt et al., 1963). Another study was undertaken by Bluestone and coworkers (1982) to clarify further the cause of this functional obstruction by employing a new test of eustachian tube function, the forced-response test (Cantekin et al., 1979), and to evaluate a larger group of children who had either a cholesteatoma or a retraction pocket. In addition, children with an apparent "congenital" cholesteatoma were also studied, and the results obtained in both groups were then compared with the results of testing children who had traumatic perforation of the tympanic membrane but who otherwise were considered to be otologically "normal." Another goal of the study was to determine if there were any differences in eustachian tube function among ears that had a posterosuperior or pars flaccida retraction pocket or cholesteatoma, ears with a central perforation and a cholesteatoma, and ears with "congenital" cholesteatoma.

From these studies, the basic problem in children with acquired cholesteatoma is functional obstruction of the eustachian tube due to *constriction* rather than dilatation of the tube during swallowing. (This type of functional obstruction of the eustachian tube was present in subjects with a retraction pocket or cholesteatoma regardless of the site.) Abnormal functioning of the tube then results in impaired ventilation of the middle ear–mastoid air cell system, which in turn causes fluctuating or sustained high negative middle ear pressure. Periodic, rather than regular, ventilation could result in wide variations in middle ear pressures that would produce greater than normal excursions of the tympanic membrane. The membrane would then lose elasticity and become flaccid and, eventually, atelectatic. The most flaccid parts of the tympanic membrane are the posterosuperior and pars flaccida areas (Khanna and Tonndorf, 1972). When the atelectasis becomes severe and localized in these sites, a retraction pocket forms. Inflammation between the medial portion of the retracted or collapsed tympanic membrane could then result in adhesive changes and could fix the pocket to the ossicles or surrounding structures, or both. The next stage in this cascade of events would be discontinuity of the ossicles or cholesteatoma formation, or both. Figures 9–11 and 9–12 show the progression from the stage of a retraction pocket and atelectasis to adhesive otitis and finally to cholesteatoma.

The distinction between a deep retraction pocket and a cholesteatoma in either the posterosuperior quadrant of the pars tensa or the pars flaccida can be difficult even with the aid of the otomicroscope. The transition between the two conditions usually follows a progressive change from a retraction pocket to cholesteatoma; however, the factors involved in this transition remain obscure at present, although infection within the retraction pocket–sac appears to be important in the process.

Children who have a central perforation and cholesteatoma are of particular interest. The cholesteatoma in these cases most likely develops as a result of migration of epithelium from the tympanic membrane through the perforation and into the middle ear. However, it must be stressed that in children this type of acquired cholesteatoma is less common than the posterosuperior or attic types.

It is uncertain that "congenital" cholesteatomas are truly congenital in origin. Children who have an intratympanic cholesteatoma may have had otitis media with effusion; the cholesteatoma is the result of metaplasia secondary to middle ear inflammation and is not "congenital" (Sade, 1977). The fact that children who have "congenital" cholesteatomas tend to be younger than those who present with a retraction pocket or acquired cholesteatoma would support the origin of a cholesteatoma medial to an intact tympanic membrane as being congenital. Most acquired cholesteatomas not due to implantation are secondary to otitis media or a retraction pocket, or both, and some children who have an apparently "congenital" cholesteatoma may have developed the disease in the same way (Sobol et al., 1980).

Cholesteatoma is a common sequela of middle ear disease in patients with cleft palate (Severeid, 1977). It has been shown that all infants with an unrepaired cleft palate have otitis media with effusion (Paradise et al., 1969; Stool and Randall, 1967) and that they have functional obstruction of the eustachian tube due to impairment of the tubal opening mechanism (Bluestone, 1971; Bluestone et al., 1972, 1975). Recent studies of infants, children, and adolescents with cleft palate demonstrated *constriction* of the eustachian tube during the forced-response test (Doyle et al., 1980). The cleft-palate child, therefore, represents an *in vivo* model of the type of functional eustachian tube obstruction that can result in an acquired cholesteatoma. Because this type of dysfunction also occurs commonly in Caucasian children who have recurrent otitis media or atelectasis but who do not have cleft palate (Cantekin et al., 1979), they are also at risk for developing cholesteatoma.

On the other hand, cholesteatoma has rarely been identified in American Indian populations (Wiet et al., 1980). Jaffe (1969) reported that attic "perforations" are rarely found in Navajo children: in over 200 tympanoplasties performed to repair central perforations, no cholesteatoma was found. Wiet (1979), in a study of 600 White Mountain Apache Indians, also reported a low incidence of cholesteatoma; the few cases he

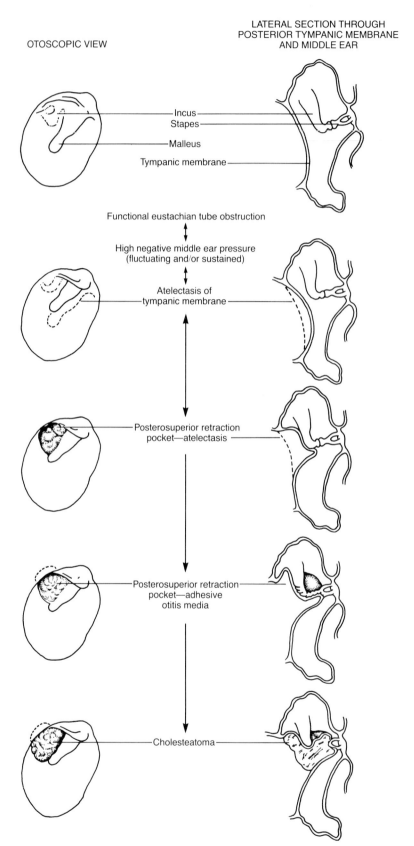

OTOSCOPIC VIEW

LATERAL SECTION THROUGH
POSTERIOR TYMPANIC MEMBRANE
AND MIDDLE EAR

Incus
Stapes
Malleus
Tympanic membrane

Functional eustachian tube obstruction

High negative middle ear pressure
(fluctuating and/or sustained)

Atelectasis of
tympanic membrane

Posterosuperior retraction
pocket—atelectasis

Posterosuperior retraction
pocket—adhesive
otitis media

Cholesteatoma

Figure 9–11. Chain of events in the pathogenesis of acquired aural cholesteatoma in the posterosuperior portion of the pars tensa or the tympanic membrane.

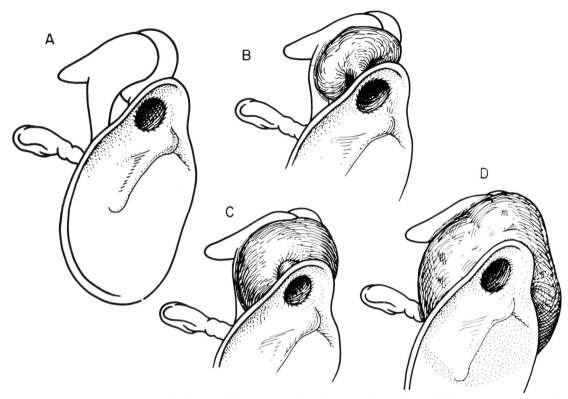

Figure 9–12. Evolution of acquired attic cholesteatoma. *A*, Attic retraction pocket, which appears on otoscopic examination to be a "perforation." *B*, Narrow neck sac developing. *C*, Enlargement of sac with erosion of ossicles. *D*, Large cholesteatoma sac, a portion of which can be seen through the eardrum.

found were mostly of the attic type. In a subsequent study by Beery and coworkers (1980), otoscopic examination of 25 Apache Indians revealed no cholesteatoma. Eustachian tube function was tested in these Indians by employing the inflation-deflation and forced-response tests, which revealed the presence of eustachian tubes that had low resistance to airflow (semipatulous) but had active muscle function. This type of tube would probably preclude the development of high negative middle ear pressure, a retraction pocket, or cholesteatoma. Apache Indians appear to have eustachian tubes that allow for easier passage of gas and liquid than do Caucasians, with or without cleft palate. The middle ear of the Apache individual is very easily ventilated and, consequently, not protected from unwanted secretions from the nasopharynx. It appears that the structure of the eustachian tubes of the Apache Indians of the White Mountain Reservation are conducive to the development of "reflux" otitis media, perforation, and discharge.

Therefore, some American Indian tribes would appear to be *in vivo* models of the semipatulous eustachian tube that actively dilates during swallowing. Cholesteatoma formation is rarely seen in such ears, since the middle ear is aerated either by the eustachian tube or by a central perforation, or both. By studying these *in vivo* models, we can gain a clearer perspective of the whole spectrum of eustachian tube dysfunction.

Microbiology

When a cholesteatoma is infected, the organisms cultured from the discharge are similar to those identified from ears with chronic suppurative otitis media: *P. aeruginosa* and *Proteus* species are the most commonly identified aerobic bacteria, and *Bacteroides* and *Peptococcus-Peptostreptococcus* species are the most commonly seen anaerobic organisms (Table 9–3). Many bacteria were cultured from discharges of over half of 30 patients with cholesteatomas studied by Harker and Koontz (1977). Karma and coworkers (1978) reported that when they cultured 18 infected cholesteatomas, half of the cultures revealed both aerobic and anaerobic bacteria. From the results of the above studies, it seems that

Table 9–3. **BACTERIOLOGICAL FINDINGS IN INFECTED CHOLESTEATOMAS IN 30 CHILDREN AND ADULTS***

Organism	Number of Cases Present
Aerobes	
Pseudomonas aeruginosa	11
Pseudomonas fluorescens	2
Proteus species	4
Escherichia coli	4
Klebsiella, Enterobacter, and Serratia species	4
Streptococcus species	8
Alcaligenes and Achromobacter species	3
Staphylococcus aureus	1
Staphylococcus epidermidis	2
Anaerobes	
Bacteroides species	13
Peptococcus and Peptostreptococcus species	11
Propionibacterium acnes	8
Fusobacterium species	4
Bifidobacterium species	3
Clostridium species	3
Eubacterium species	2

*From Harker, L. A., and Koontz, F. P.: The bacteriology of cholesteatoma. *In* McCabe, B. F., Sade, J., and Abramson, M. (Eds.): *Cholesteatoma: First International Conference.* Birmingham, Alabama, Aesculapius Pub., 1977, pp. 264–267.

the most appropriate ototopical medication and systemic antimicrobial therapy for patients who have an infected cholesteatoma would be agents that are effective against gram-negative organisms and anaerobic bacteria; however, the results of culturing the discharge will aid in selecting the proper antimicrobial therapy. These considerations may be life-saving when an intratemporal or intracranial complication of cholesteatoma is present.

Diagnosis

The signs and symptoms of cholesteatoma are such that the disease may go undetected for many years in all age groups, but in children this is an even greater problem. Most adults have a history of hearing loss, which is usually progressive and associated with recurrent ear discharge. Children rarely complain of hearing loss, especially if the disease is unilateral. Frequently there is no discharge, and otalgia may be absent. Children are usually unaware of or unable to relate the more subtle symptoms associated with the disease, such as fullness in the ear, tinnitus or mild vertigo, and the foul smell of discharge, when present. Fever is not a

sign of cholesteatoma: when it accompanies this disease, and especially when otalgia is also present, a search for an intratemporal or intracranial complication must be made. Other signs and symptoms, such as facial paralysis, severe vertigo, vomiting, and headache, should also alert the physician to the presence of a suppurative complication. In children, the attic type of cholesteatoma appears to be less symptomatic than a cholesteatoma in the posterosuperior quadrant, since the latter type is frequently preceded by symptomatic recurrent or chronic otitis media with effusion and an early onset of ossicular discontinuity with a significant hearing loss. However, in both types, the preceding atelectasis and retraction pocket may not be associated with significant symptoms in children. The intratympanic "congenital" cholesteatoma, which may be secondary to otitis media, is even more obscure, since hearing loss may be a late sequela and discharge is not present.

Examination of the ear with an otoscope or, for greater accuracy, with the otomicroscope, is the most effective way to diagnose cholesteatoma. Usually white, shiny, greasy flakes of debris that may or may not be associated with a foul-smelling discharge will be seen in a defect in the posterosuperior portion of the pars tensa or the attic or through a large perforation. A polyp may be seen coming through the defect, which, like a crust, can prevent adequate visualization of the tympanic membrane. A crust overlying the area of the posterosuperior quadrant or the pars flaccida must be removed, since a retraction pocket or cholesteatoma may be present. The size of the defect in the tympanic membrane may not be indicative of the extent of the cholesteatoma, since a small defect, especially in the attic, may be associated with extensive cholesteatoma. On the other hand, the cholesteatoma may be confined only to the attic or middle ear despite the presence of a large defect. If an adequate examination of the child's ear is not possible with the child awake, then an examination under anesthesia is indicated. Every child who must be given a general anesthetic for myringotomy (with or without the insertion of typanostomy tube) should have an examination of the entire tympanic membrane in order to identify a possible cholesteatoma or its precursor, a retraction pocket. In addition, an intratympanic cholesteatoma may be visualized through the tympanic membrane or through the incision following a myringotomy.

It is not always possible to determine if the defect is a retraction pocket or a cholesteatoma without discharge; however, even though this distinction cannot be made, the management of the defect will usually be the same.

There is no tympanometric pattern that is diagnostic of a cholesteatoma. An abnormal tympanogram should alert the clinician to the presence of middle ear disease, but the result of the tympanogram may be normal even when a cholesteatoma is present. Impedance testing may reveal a perforation of the tympanic membrane, but in children this occurs less commonly than in adults. Likewise, audiometric testing may reveal a conductive hearing impairment, or possibly a mixed conductive and sensorineural deficit, but a cholesteatoma may be present without a loss of hearing. A sensorineural hearing loss is presumably due to serous labyrinthitis (Paparella et al., 1972) or possibly to a labyrinthine fistula.

Roentgenograms of the temporal bone should be obtained when a cholesteatoma is suspected; computerized tomography is even more helpful. The roentgenograms should be studied carefully to identify the extent of the cholesteatoma, possible ossicular involvement, and any complication that might be present, such as a labyrinthine fistula. The radiographs should be restudied preoperatively when the surgical procedure is planned.

When aural discharge accompanying cholesteatoma is profuse, microbiological assessment of the discharge is indicated so that the infection can be controlled preoperatively by administering one or more of the most appropriate antimicrobial agents. If possible, purulent material within the cholesteatoma sac should be aspirated with the aid of the operating microscope.

Prevention and Management

Rational management of children with cholesteatoma and conditions that may be causally related to this disease should be based upon an understanding of its pathogenesis. The presence of a deep retraction pocket in the posterosuperior or pars flaccida area of the tympanic membrane, if persistent, must be managed promptly by insertion of a tympanostomy tube in an effort to return the tympanic membrane to the neutral position and prevent formation of adhesions between the tympanic membrane and middle ear structures (Fig. 9–13, *upper panel*). If the retraction pocket persists after the middle ear has been ventilated by a tympanostomy tube that has been in place for several weeks or months (Fig. 9–13, *lower panel*), then the physician should consider performing tympanoplasty to prevent ossicular discontinuity or the development of a cholesteatoma, or both.

When a cholesteatoma is present, surgical intervention is indicated. The surgical procedures that are currently employed to eradicate a cholesteatoma are briefly described below. These procedures may also be performed for other conditions described in this monograph, but for detailed descriptions of the surgical techniques the reader is referred to current texts and atlases.

The procedures can be divided into those that provide exposure and removal of disease from the middle ear and mastoid and those that are designed to reconstruct the middle ear to preserve or restore hearing.

Tympanotomy is a surgical procedure that opens the middle ear space.

RETRACTION POCKET—ATELECTASIS

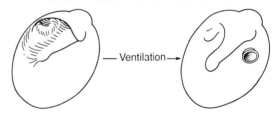

RETRACTION POCKET—ADHESIVE OTITIS

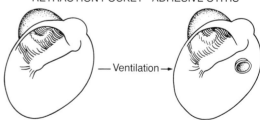

Figure 9–13. When a retraction pocket is in the posterosuperior portion of the pars tensa of the tympanic membrane and adhesive otitis media is not present between the eardrum and ossicles, the insertion of a tympanostomy tube may return the tympanic membrane to the neutral position. However, if adhesive otitis media is present, the retraction pocket will persist in spite of the presence of a tympanostomy tube and middle ear ventilation.

Exploratory tympanotomy is indicated when it is suspected that there is an abnormality, such as an intratympanic cholesteatoma or ossicular chain abnormality; it can also be a planned second-stage procedure after tympanoplasty, with or without mastoidectomy.

Myringoplasty is the surgical repair of a defect in the tympanic membrane, with no attempt made to explore the middle ear. A perforation (or retraction pocket) is commonly repaired by utilizing autogenous connective tissue graft (temporalis fascia, compressed adipose from the earlobe) as a lattice onto which epithelial cells can migrate from the edges of the existing perforation. The procedure is employed to manage a simple uncomplicated tympanic membrane perforation without cholesteatoma.

Tympanoplasty is the surgical reconstruction of the tympanic membrane–transformer mechanism. If a perforation is present, it is repaired with a connective tissue graft but, unlike the case in myringoplasty, the middle ear is explored. Ossicles can be repositioned (ossiculoplasty) to restore ossicular chain continuity. Traditionally, tympanoplastic operations are characterized according to the degree to which the reconstructed ossicular chain approximates the anatomical juxtaposition of ossicles in the normal middle ear.

Mastoidectomy involves the surgical exposure and removal of mastoid air cells. There are several types of mastoidectomy (Fig. 9–14). In a *complete simple "cortical" mastoidectomy* (Fig. 9–14A) the mastoid air cell system is exenterated, including the epitympanum, but the canal wall is left intact. The operation is performed when acute or chronic mastoid osteitis is present, and it is frequently part of the surgical procedure advocated by some surgeons for cholesteatoma. A *posterior tympanotomy* or *facial recess tympanotomy* (Fig. 9–14B) involves exenteration of mastoid air cells, followed by formation of an opening between the mastoid and middle ear that is created in the posterior wall of the middle ear lateral to the facial nerve and medial to the chorda tympani. This procedure is an extension of the complete simple mastoidectomy and allows better visualization of the facial recess without removing the canal wall; it is primarily advocated for ears in which a cholesteatoma is present. A *modified radical mastoidectomy* (Fig. 9–14C) is an operation in which a portion of the posterior ear canal wall is removed and a permanent mastoidectomy cavity is created, but the tympanic membrane and some or all of the ossicles are left. The procedure is usually performed when a cholesteatoma cannot be removed without removing the canal wall; some function may be preserved. *Radical mastoidectomy* (Fig. 9–14D) involves exenteration of all mastoid air cells, opening of the epitympanum, and

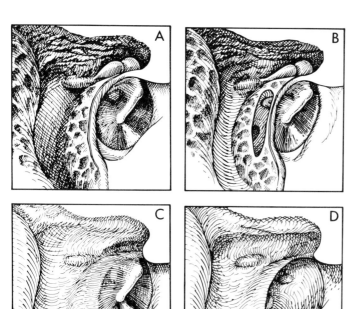

Figure 9–14. Examples of four types of mastoid surgery. *A,* Complete simple ("cortical") mastoidectomy in which the canal wall has been left intact. However, the exposure of the epitympanum is an important part of the surgical procedure. *B,* A posterior tympanotomy–facial recess access to the middle ear has been added to the complete simple mastoidectomy. *C,* Modified radical mastoidectomy. *D,* Radical mastoidectomy.

removal of the posterior ear canal wall along with the tympanic membrane, the malleus, and the incus. Only the stapes, or the footplate of the stapes, remains. No attempt is made to preserve or improve function. With removal of the posterior ear canal wall, the exenterated mastoid cellular area, middle ear, and external auditory canal communicate, forming a common single cavity. The procedure is indicated when there is extensive cholesteatoma present in the middle ear and mastoid that cannot be removed by a less radical procedure. In addition, the operation may be indicated when a suppurative complication of otitis media is present.

When a tympanoplastic operation is done in conjunction with mastoidectomy, the combined procedure is termed "mastoidectomy-tympanoplasty." Mastoidectomy operations that leave the posterior ear canal wall intact are termed "closed cavity," "canal wall up," or "intact canal wall" procedures, whereas those in which the posterior canal is partially removed are called "open cavity" or "canal wall down" procedures.

The type of surgery chosen to manage these conditions in children should be selected on the basis not only of the site and extent of the cholesteatoma but also on the basis of other factors such as patient age, presence or absence of otitis media, eustachian tube function, and availability of health care. The operation must be tailored for each child. Prevention of the pathological conditions that predispose to this type of cholesteatoma is the most effective method of management.

ADHESIVE OTITIS MEDIA

Adhesive otitis media is a result of healing following chronic inflammation of the middle ear and mastoid. The mucous membrane is thickened by proliferation of fibrous tissue, which frequently impairs movement of the ossicles, resulting in conductive hearing loss.

The pathological process is a proliferation of fibrous tissue within the middle ear and mastoid termed fibrous sclerosis (Schuknecht, 1974). When there are cystic spaces present it is called fibrocystic sclerosis, and when there is new bone growth in the mastoid it is termed fibro-osseous sclerosis.

There are no data available on the prevalence of adhesive otitis media in children, but the condition is common in those who have had recurrent acute or chronic otitis media with effusion or atelectasis of the tympanic membrane—middle ear region, or both. We also have no data for establishing the probability with which a child who has a middle ear effusion or atelectasis might develop adhesive otitis media. The possibility of adhesive changes occurring when inflammation is present in the middle ear and mastoid must be considered when the most appropriate medical or surgical treatment is selected for children who have recurrent acute and chronic otitis media with effusion or atelectasis. In addition to fixation of the ossicles, adhesive otitis media may result in ossicular discontinuity and conductive hearing loss due to rarefying ossicular osteitis, especially of the long process of the incus. When there is severe localized atelectasis (a retraction pocket) in the posterosuperior portion of the pars tensa of the tympanic membrane, adhesive changes may bind the eardrum to the incus, stapes, and other surrounding middle ear structures and cause resorption of the ossicles. Once adhesive changes bind the tympanic membrane in this area, the development of a cholesteatoma is also possible (Fig. 9–15). Timely ventilation of the middle ear and mastoid prior to adhesive changes may return the tympanic membrane to normal position, thus preventing ossicular damage. If middle ear effusion is also present, a course of antimicrobial agent may be useful, but if medical treatment fails, then myringotomy should be performed and a tympanostomy tube should be inserted to reverse the potentially progressive disorder. However, if the tympanic membrane is still attached to the ossicles in spite of tympanostomy tube insertion, then adhesive otitis media is present, and, in children, tympanoplasty should be considered to prevent further structural damage, since the process may progress due to persistent eustachian tube obstruction.

When ossicular discontinuity or fixation has occurred, reconstruction of the ossicles may be tried to restore function, but this procedure is not always successful. When the middle ear and mastoid are bound by adhesive otitis media, the results of ossiculoplasty frequently are not permanent owing to recurrence of the adhesive process. The best method for management of adhesive otitis media is prevention, which involves treating of its precursor, acute otitis media and chronic otitis media with effusion and atelectasis.

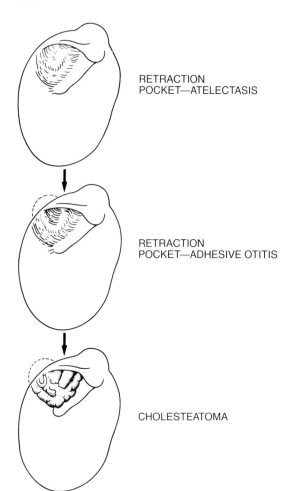

RETRACTION
POCKET—ATELECTASIS

RETRACTION
POCKET—ADHESIVE OTITIS

CHOLESTEATOMA

Figure 9–15. Sequence of events leading from a localized area of atelectasis (retraction pocket) in the posterosuperior portion of the pars tensa of the tympanic membrane to a cholesteatoma and ossicular discontinuity. Adhesive otitis media in this area is shown as the stage between atelectasis and the development of a cholesteatoma.

TYMPANOSCLEROSIS

Tympanosclerosis may be a sequela of chronic middle ear inflammation or the result of trauma. It is characterized by the presence of whitish plaques in the tympanic membrane and nodular deposits in the submucosal layers of the middle ear (Igarashi et al., 1970). The pathological process in the tympanic membrane occurs in the lamina propria, whereas within the middle ear the basement membrane is affected; in both sites, there is hyalinization followed by deposition of calcium and phosphate crystals. Conductive hearing loss may occur if the ossicles become embedded in the deposits.

The condition was first described by von Troltsch (1869), who called it sclerosis, but it was Zollner (1956) who called the disorder tympanosclerosis and differentiated it from otosclerosis. Schuknecht (1974) prefers the term "hyalinization" rather than "tympano-

sclerosis," since the histopathological features are those of hyalin degeneration, which is the result of a healing reaction characterized by fibroblastic invasion of the submucosa, followed by thickening and fusion of collagenous fibers into a homogeneous mass. The hyalinized collagen may extend around the ossicles.

Pathogenesis

Tympanosclerosis of the tympanic membrane is a common sequela in children who have or have had recurrent or chronic otitis media with effusion. It is common in the site of a healed, spontaneous perforation or following myringotomy, especially if a tympanostomy tube has been inserted. The chalky patch seen in the tympanic membrane may be due to inflammation or trauma, or both. Even though the condition is commonly seen affecting the tympanic membranes of children, the condition is not common within the middle ear. Ossicular involvement is rare in very young children. Of 311 cases of tympanosclerosis studied by Kinney (1978), only 20 percent occurred in individuals 30 years of age or younger. This would imply that the condition in the middle ear may take many years to develop. However, Schiff and co-workers (1980) hypothesize that tympanosclerosis has an immune component that occurs in the middle ear following an insult or mucosal disruption and that there is also a genetic component, which would explain the low incidence of the condition in children who have a high prevalence and incidence of otitis media.

The genetic hypothesis may be the explanation for the relatively high rate of tympanosclerosis among children who are Alaskan natives (Eskimos) and American Indians (DeBlanc, 1975; Jaffe, 1969; Wiet, 1979). Other factors may predispose these children to the disease, such as differences in eustachian tube function. Wiet and coworkers (1980) reported that tympanosclerosis affected a higher percentage of Alaskan native children than children of a similar age in New Hampshire: tympanosclerosis of the tympanic membrane or the ossicles, or both, was found in 78 (68 percent) of 114 Alaskan native children who had tympanoplastic surgery, whereas only seven such cases were diagnosed in 377 consecutive tympanoplasties performed on children in Wieder's New Hampshire practice. Far advanced tympanosclerosis that resulted in fixation of the ossicular chain occurred at an early age in the Alaskan native children but not in children in the private practice.

Management

No surgical correction, such as tympanoplasty, is indicated when tympanosclerosis of the tympanic membrane, even though extensive, is the only abnormality of the middle ear. If a middle ear effusion is present and myringotomy, with or without tympanostomy tube insertion, is indicated, the incision should be placed, if possible, in an area without involvement, leaving the affected area untouched. Removal of large tympanosclerotic plaques may result in a permanent perforation of the tympanic membrane. When an incision must be made in an area of tympanosclerosis, then only that amount necessary to perform the procedure should be removed. When tympanosclerosis is the cause of ossicular fixation and a tympanoplasty procedure is elected, removal of the plaques and ossiculoplasty are appropriate for the rare child with this advanced stage of tympanosclerosis (Shambaugh and Glasscock, 1980). Refixation of the ossicles is common even after apparently adequate surgical removal of plaques and ossiculoplasty. If surgery is not performed or is not successful in restoring hearing loss, a hearing aid should be considered.

Even though the pathogenesis of tympanosclerosis is not understood, it seems most likely that appropriate management of recurrent and chronic middle ear inflammation in infants and children is the best method of prevention. The disorder also occurs following trauma to the tympanic membrane. Myringotomy with tube placement can result in tympanosclerosis of the drum, i.e., myringosclerosis. Tympanosclerosis that involves the tympanic membrane does not appreciably affect function, although when the ossicles are involved, the patient may have a significant conductive hearing loss. Tympanostomy tubes may, on the one hand, increase the incidence of tympanosclerosis of the tympanic membrane, but on the other hand, their placement may decrease the frequency of ossicular fixation due to this disease later in life.

OSSICULAR DISCONTINUITY AND FIXATION

Ossicular interruption is the result of rarefying osteitis secondary to chronic middle ear inflammation. A retraction pocket or cholesteatoma may also cause resorption of ossicles. The long process of the incus is most commonly involved, which results in incudostapedial disarticulation. The commonly accepted reason given for erosion of this portion of the incus is its poor blood supply; however, since the tympanic membrane frequently becomes attached to this part of the incus when a posterosuperior retraction pocket is present, adhesive otitis media may be the cause of the osteitis and subsequent erosion. Also, cholesteatoma is commonly found in the same area (Bluestone et al., 1977). The stapes, or more specifically its crural arches, is the second most commonly involved ossicle. The cause of stapes fixation is more likely to be associated with presence of a retraction pocket or cholesteatoma rather than with decreased vascular supply. Less commonly, the body of the incus and manubrium of the malleus may also be eroded. The ossicles may become fixed by fibrous tissue secondary to adhesive otitis media or, more rarely in children, secondary to tympanosclerosis. Neither the incidence of ossicular discontinuity and fixation nor the natural history of pathological conditions that precede these abnormalities has been formally studied in chidren; however, ossicular discontinuity is commonly associated with a deep retraction pocket or cholesteatoma in the posterosuperior portion of the tympanic membrane. Disarticulation or fixation of the ossicles may also occur when there is a central perforation of the tympanic membrane with or without the presence of chronic suppurative otitis media and, more rarely, when the tympanic membrane is intact.

The hearing loss is conductive when the ossicular chain is affected, and the degree is dependent upon the site and degree of involvement of the ossicles as well as upon the presence or absence of associated conditions such as a perforation of the tympanic membrane. When there is a discontinuity of the incudostapedial joint and the tympanic membrane is intact, a maximum conductive hearing loss may be present (i.e., 50 to 60 dB). However, when the same ossicular disorder is present in addition to a perforation, the hearing loss may be less severe. Erosion of the manubrium of the malleus is usually associated with a perforation of the tympanic membrane but does not contribute to the hearing loss.

Diagnosis

The diagnosis of ossicular chain abnormalities that are secondary to otitis media and its related conditions can frequently be made by visualization of the defect through the otoscope or, more accurately, with the otomicroscope. Erosion of the long process of the incus can usually be seen when a deep posterosuperior retraction pocket is present. The occurrence of a significant conductive hearing loss (e.g., greater than 30 dB) when a perforation of the tympanic membrane is present would be presumptive evidence of ossicular involvement. When the tympanic membrane is normal, a significant conductive loss may be due to inflammatory ossicular

involvement that has occurred in the past; congenital ossicular abnormalities and otosclerosis must be considered. In addition to the history, otoscopic examination, and conventional audiometric testing, impedance audiometry may aid in the diagnosis. A tympanogram showing high compliance would be presumptive evidence of ossicular chain discontinuity when there is a significant conductive hearing loss. If the compliance is low, ossicular fixation would be more likely. However, the accuracy with which tympanometry can differentiate between ossicular discontinuity and fixation is not high, since several other parameters in the middle ear, such as mobility of the tympanic membrane, affect the shape of the tympanogram. Computerized tomography may also aid in identifying ossicular discontinuity but usually is only of diagnostic benefit when a large defect is present. The most accurate way to diagnose these defects is exploration of the middle ear, either during exploratory tympanotomy, when the tympanic membrane is intact, or inspection of the entire ossicular chain when middle ear and mastoid surgery (e.g., tympanoplasty) is indicated.

Management

Management of ossicular deformities in children is similar to that described for adults, except for some notable exceptions. Most adults who have ossicular discontinuity or fixation no longer are at risk of developing otitis media with effusion or high negative pressure within the middle ear due to eustachian tube dysfunction, but many children still have or will have these conditions, which could interfere with the success of reconstructive middle ear surgery in general and ossiculoplasty in specific. Therefore, the indications for the timing and the type of middle ear surgery may be different for children. When an ossicular deformity is suspected and the tympanic membrane is intact, without evidence of otitis media or any other of its complications or sequelae (e.g., retraction pocket or cholesteatoma), then the decision to perform an exploratory tympanotomy to diagnose and possibly repair the ossicular deformity would depend on several considerations. First, and most important, is the child still at risk of developing a middle ear effusion or atelectasis (retraction pocket), or both? As a general rule, if neither condition has occurred in either ear for a year or longer, the risk is low; however, the younger the child, the higher the risk. If further middle ear disease may still occur, the operation should be delayed. The second consideration is the degree of hearing loss and whether or not the defect is unilateral or bilateral. A child who has a maximum conductive hearing loss in both ears would be a very likely candidate for surgical intervention, whereas the child who has only a unilateral mild conductive loss should not be operated upon. Another important consideration is the need for a general anesthetic to perform the surgery in all children. The benefit of surgery must be weighed against the risk of a general anesthetic. For the child who has a bilateral maximum conductive hearing loss, the benefit of hearing improvement may outweigh the risk of general anesthesia, whereas the risk of an anesthetic may not override the potential chance of improving the hearing in a child with only a unilateral loss of hearing. Withholding reconstructive surgery until the child is able to tolerate a local anesthetic (adolescence) is a preferred option when the hearing loss is unilateral and especially when it is only mild to moderate in degree. Whenever the decision to operate is delayed until the child is older, a hearing aid should be considered, even when the hearing loss is unilateral.

When middle ear surgery is indicated owing to the presence of a perforation of the tympanic membrane with or without chronic suppurative otitis media, a cholesteatoma, or a retraction pocket, the fact that the patient is a child still affects the decision as to whether or not ossiculoplasty is performed. This is because children are at increased risk of suffering future episodes of otitis media and of developing atelectasis or adhesive otitis media. When these conditions are a possibility, the surgeon should consider staging the surgery and performing the ossiculoplasty when the child is older.

MASTOIDITIS

The proximity of the mastoid to the middle ear cleft suggests that most cases of suppurative otitis media are associated with inflammation of the mastoid air cells. The incidence of clinically significant mastoiditis, however, has been low since the introduction of antimicrobial agents. Nevertheless, acute and chronic disease still occur and may be responsible for significant morbidity and life-threatening disease.

At birth, the mastoid consists of a single cell, the antrum, connected to the middle ear by a small channel, the aditus ad antrum. Pneumatization of the mastoid bone takes place soon after birth and is usually extensive by two years of age. The process may continue throughout life. The clinical importance of the mastoid is related to contiguous structures, including the posterior cranial fossa, the middle cranial fossa, the sigmoid and lateral sinuses, the canal of the facial nerve, the semicircular canals, and the petrous tip of the temporal bone. The mastoid air cells are lined with modified respiratory mucosa, and all are interconnected with the antrum.

Infection in the mastoid proceeds after middle ear infection through the following stages: (1) hyperemia and edema of the mucosal lining of the pneumatized cells; (2) accumulation of serous and then purulent exudates in the cells; (3) demineralization of the cellular walls and necrosis of bone due to pressure of the purulent exudate on the thin bony septa and ischemia of the septa, caused by decrease in blood flow; (4) formation of abscess cavities due to coalescence of adjacent cells following destruction of cell walls; and (5) escape of pus into contiguous areas.

This process may halt at any stage with subsequent resolution. When infection persists for more than a week or 10 days, however, inflammatory granulation tissue forms in the pneumatic cavity. A hypertrophic osteitis develops that results in thickening and sclerosis of cellular walls and reduction in size of cellular space. There may be repeated cycles of absorption and deposition of bone. If the infection remains chronic but low grade, there is thickening of the mucosa caused by a fibrinous exudate, which may become organized and lead to permanent adhesions. Columnar metaplasia with new gland formation may result in extensive production of mucus in the former cells.

Mastoiditis can be classified into acute and chronic types. Acute mastoiditis is further subdivided according to the pathological stage present, which has clinical significance because management is dependent upon the stage of the disease. Unfortunately, because of failure to appreciate the natural history and pathological features of acute mastoiditis, there is confusion in the minds of clinicians, as well as in the current literature, regarding the most appropriate management of each stage.

Acute Mastoiditis

In almost every child who has acute otitis media, the mastoid air cells are also inflamed; thus, acute mastoiditis is a natural extension and part of the pathological process of acute middle ear infection. No specific signs or symptoms of mastoid infection are present in this most common stage of mastoiditis. The hearing loss, otalgia, and fever are due primarily to acute infection within the middle ear. Roentgenograms of the mastoid area are usually read as "cloudy mastoids," which is, in reality, indicative of inflammation. No mastoid osteitis is evident on computerized tomography (Fig. 9–16). The process is usually reversible, as the middle ear–mastoid effusion resolves, either as a natural process or as a result of treatment of the acute infection. If resolution of the infection does not occur at this stage, one or more of the following conditions can develop: (1) acute mastoiditis with periosteitis, (2) acute mastoid osteitis (with or without subperiosteal abscess), or (3) chronic mastoiditis.

A condition has been described called

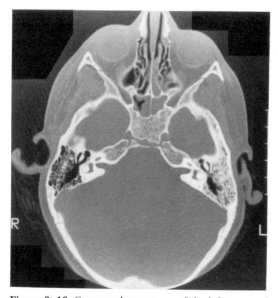

Figure 9–16. Computed tomogram of the left temporal bone of a child with acute otitis media in which the mastoid air cells show signs of inflammation without osteitis. The diagnosis was acute mastoiditis, which is usually present during episodes of acute middle ear infection and is most frequently self-limited.

masked mastoiditis, for which a complete simple mastoidectomy has been advocated (Mawson and Ludman, 1979). The disease appears to be a subacute stage of otitis media and mastoiditis (without osteitis) that is characterized by the same signs and symptoms as acute otitis media (such as persistent fever and ear pain), except that they are persistent and less severe. The progression to this stage is attributed to failure of the intitial antimicrobial agent to resolve the middle ear infection within a short period. Persistent otalgia and fever in a patient receiving an antimicrobial agent is an indication for tympanocentesis and myringotomy in order to identify the causative organism and to promote drainage. In selected children, especially those patients who have had frequently recurrent episodes of acute otitis in the past, the insertion of a tympanostomy tube (in addition to the appropriate antimicrobial therapy) will resolve the problem. Mastoid surgery is not indicated unless mastoid osteitis is present.

Acute Mastoiditis with Periosteitis

At this stage, the infection within the mastoid air cells spreads to the periosteum covering the mastoid process, causing periosteitis. The route of infection from the mastoid cells to the periosteum is by venous channels, usually the mastoid emissary vein. The condition should not be confused with the presence of a subperiosteal abscess, since management of the latter condition requires incision and drainage of the abscess and a complete simple (cortical) mastoidectomy, whereas the former usually responds to immediate but less aggressive surgical intervention.

Children with acute mastoiditis with periosteitis have fever, otalgia, and postauricular erythema, tenderness, and slight swelling. The pinna may be displaced inferiorly and anteriorly, with loss of the postauricular crease. When acute mastoiditis with periosteitis occurs in the absence of roentgenographic evidence of osteitis of the mastoid, management should consist of hospitalization, immediate tympanocentesis (for aspiration and microbiological assessment of the middle ear–mastoid effusion), and myringotomy for drainage of the system. The insertion of a tympanostomy tube is desirable and will enhance drainage over a longer period of time than myringotomy alone. Parenteral antimicrobial agents should be administered as described under acute mastoid osteitis.

Resolution of the periosteal involvement should occur with 24 to 48 hours after the tympanic membrane has been opened for drainage and adequate and appropriate antimicrobial therapy has been begun. Surgical drainage of the mastoid (i.e., complete simple mastoidectomy) should be performed if the symptoms of the acute infection, such as fever and otalgia, persist, if the postauricular involvement does not progressively improve, or if a subperiosteal abscess develops.

Failure to institute immediate treatment at this stage may result in the development of acute mastoid osteitis, with or without a subperiosteal abscess, or, more dangerous to the child, a suppurative intratemporal or intracranial complication such as lateral sinus thrombosis, extradural abscess, or meningitis. Immediate surgical intervention is indicated when acute mastoid infection develops in a child with a chronic suppurative otitis media or cholesteatoma, or both.

Acute Mastoid Osteitis (Acute "Coalescent" Mastoiditis, Acute Surgical Mastoiditis)

If the infection within the mastoid progresses, rarefying osteitis can cause destruc-

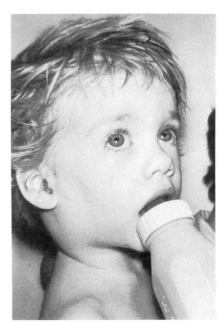

Figure 9–18. An abscess in the neck (Bezold's abscess) can be seen in this child who has a draining ear owing to acute otitis media. The pus has extended from acute mastoid osteitis and empyema into the neck.

tion of the bony trabeculae that separate the mastoid cells so that there is a "coalescence" of the cells. At this stage, a mastoid empyema is present. The pus may spread in one or more of the following directions: (1) anterior to the middle ear through the aditus ad antrum, in which case spontaneous resolution usually occurs; (2) lateral to the surface of the mastoid process, resulting in a subperiosteal abscess (Fig. 9–17); (3) anterior, burrowing beneath the skin to form a soft tissue abscess below the pinna or behind the attachment of the sternocleidomastoid muscle in the neck, which is known as a Bezold abscess (Fig. 9–18); (4) medial to the petrous air cells, resulting in petrositis; or (5) posterior to the occipital bone, which can result in osteomyelitis of the calvarium or a Citelli abscess. Infection may also spread to the labyrinth and facial nerve or into the intracranial cavity, causing one or more suppurative complications such as an extradural abscess or meningitis.

Clinically, the major signs of mastoid osteitis are a reflection of the underlying inflammatory process and include swelling, redness, and tenderness to touch over the mastoid bone. The pinna is displaced outward and downward (Fig. 9–19), and swelling or sagging of the posterosuperior canal wall may also be present. A purulent discharge may issue through a perforation in the tympanic

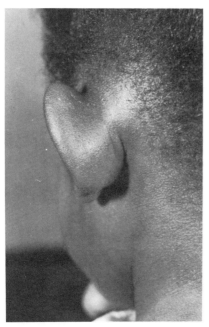

Figure 9–17. An example of a subperiosteal abscess in a child who had acute mastoid osteitis. Note that the pinna is displaced inferiorly and anteriorly, with obliteration of the postauricular crease due to the abscess.

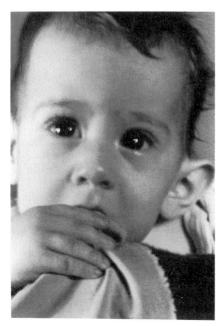

Figure 9–19. Acute mastoid osteitis in an infant, showing the outward displacement of the pinna.

membrane. Ear drainage may be persistent, with the ear canal filled with pus and debris, or there may be a nipple-like protrusion at the site of the perforation of the tympanic membrane. A fluctuant subperiosteal abscess or even a draining fistula from the mastoid to the postauricular area may be present (Fig. 9–20). The patient may have toxic symptoms and be febrile with systemic signs of acute illness. In the subacute disease, fever may be prolonged and low grade with occasional temperature spikes.

Conversely, the tympanic membrane and middle ear may appear almost normal when mastoid osteitis is present. In such cases, the acute middle ear effusion drains through the eustachian tube, in which case there is resolution of the otitis media, but if an obstruction between the middle ear and mastoid is present, then infection in the mastoid becomes trapped and can cause osteitis. The obstruction is usually due to the presence of mucosal swelling or granulation tissue at the aditus ad antrum, the "bottle neck" of the middle ear–mastoid system. In these cases, the condition of the tympanic membrane and middle ear may not be a reliable indication of mastoid infection. When no external stigmata of extension of pus from the mastoid, such as a subperiosteal abscess, is evident, roentgenograms of the mastoids must be obtained to rule out presence of an acute mastoid osteitis when otitis media is not obvious.

Children with fever of unknown origin may have, as part of the search for cause of the fever, radiographs taken of the mastoids to rule out acute mastoid osteitis (without otitis media).

Epidemiology

Before antimicrobial agents were widely used; acute mastoid osteitis was the most common suppurative complication of acute otitis media and frequently resulted in death. The frequency of mastoidectomy for acute mastoiditis in 1938 was 20 percent, whereas it was 2.8 percent in 1948, with an almost 90 percent reduction in the mortality rate during that period (Sorensen, 1977). A more recent study from Finland found that 29 cases of acute mastoiditis were reported during the period from 1956 to 1971 (Juselius and Kaltiokallio, 1972). It would appear that the frequency of this complication has significantly dropped, but it is still present.

Microbiology

Acute mastoiditis may be caused by the same organisms responsible for acute otitis media, *S. pneumoniae* and *H. influenzae*. In subacute or chronic cases, *S. aureus* and gram-negative enteric bacilli, including *E. coli, Pro-*

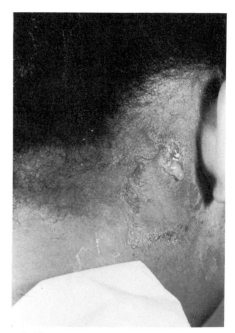

Figure 9–20. An example of a postauricular fistula with purulent discharge in a child who had acute mastoid osteitis.

teus species, and *P. aeruginosa*, may be present and are responsible for a persistent and indolent discharge.

Diagnosis

The diagnosis should be suspected on the basis of clinical signs. Computed tomograms of the mastoid area may show one or more of the following:

1. Haziness, distortion, or destruction of the mastoid outline.

2. Loss of sharpness of the shadows of cellular walls due to demineralization, atrophy, and ischemia of the bony septa (Fig. 9–21).

3. Decrease in density and cloudiness of the areas of pneumatization due to inflammatory swelling of the air cells.

4. In long-standing cases, there is a chronic osteoblastic inflammatory reaction that may obliterate the cellular structure. Small abscess cavities in sclerotic bone may be confused with pneumatic cells.

Cultures for bacteria from ear drainage must be taken with care and concern for discriminating fresh drainage from debris in the external canal. The canal must be initially cleaned, and if fresh pus is exuding through a perforation in the tympanic membrane, the discharge is cultured at the point of exit from the tympanic membrane, with a cotton-tipped, wire swab or, preferably, a needle

and syringe under direct view. A Gram stain of the pus provides immediate information about the responsible organisms.

Management

Antimicrobial agents are the mainstay of treatment of acute disease. If the case is otherwise uncomplicated (i.e., there was no prior infection) it is likely that *S. pneumoniae* or *H. influenzae* is responsible, and ampicillin in a dosage schedule for severe disease is suitable. If the disease has persisted for weeks or longer, coverage for *S. aureus* and gram-negative organisms must be provided. It is of the utmost importance to obtain cultures from the site of infection to guide therapy, but initial treatment may begin with a penicillinase-resistant penicillin (nafcillin, oxacillin, or methicillin) and an aminoglycoside (gentamicin, tobramycin or amikacin). This regimen may be altered by the findings from a Gram stain of purulent material or the results of cultures and sensitivity tests.

A complete simple ("cortical") mastoidectomy must be performed when there is evidence of acute mastoid osteitis, especially when the mastoid empyema has extended outside the mastoid bone. The procedure should be considered an emergency, but the timing of the operation must be dependent upon the status of the child. Ideally, sepsis should be under control, and the patient must be able to tolerate a general anesthetic. The principle is to clean out the mastoid infection, to drain the mastoid air cell system into the middle ear by eliminating any obstruction that is caused by edema or granulation tissue in the aditus ad antrum, and to provide external drainage. If a suppurative intratemporal or intracranial complication is also present, surgical intervention for these conditions may also be required.

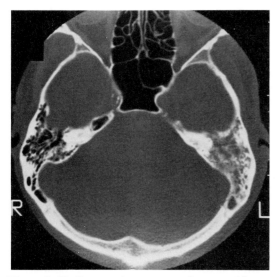

Figure 9–21. Computed tomogram of temporal bones showing left acute osteitis with loss of septa between the mastoid air cells, which has been termed acute "coalescent" mastoiditis; right mastoid is normal. Mastoid surgery was performed in this case.

Chronic Mastoiditis

Chronic mastoiditis is invariably associated with chronic suppurative otitis media. The mastoid may be poorly pneumatized or sclerotic. The chronic infection at this stage may be brought under control by medical treatment, but when there are extensive amounts of granulation tissue and osteitis in the mastoid, mastoidectomy is usually necessary to eliminate the chronic mastoid osteitis, especially if a cholesteatoma is present. When signs and symptoms of acute mastoiditis, such as periosteitis, develop in a child with chronic suppurative otitis media, immediate surgical intervention is almost always required to prevent a more serious intratemporal or intracranial suppurative complication.

PETROSITIS

Petrositis is a rare suppurative complication that is secondary to an extension of infection from the middle ear and mastoid into the petrous portion of the temporal bone. All the inflammatory and cellular changes described as occurring in the mastoid can also occur in the pneumatized petrous pyramid. Only about 30 percent of individuals have well-pneumatized petrous bones (Ranier, 1938). Petrositis may be more frequent than appreciated by clinical and roentgenographic signs, since there is commuication of the petrosal air cells with the mastoid–middle ear system. Pneumatization usually does not occur before three years of age.

Petrositis may be either acute or chronic. In the acute form, there is extension of acute otitis media and mastoiditis into the pneumatized petrous air cells. The condition, like acute mastoiditis, usually is self-limited with resolution of the acute middle ear and mastoid infection, but on occasion the infection in the petrous portion of the temporal bone does not drain owing to mucosal swelling or because granulation is obstructing the passage from the petrous air cells to the mastoid and middle ear, which results in acute petrous osteomyelitis. The widespread use of antimicrobial agents has made this an extremely rare complication. However, chronic petrous osteomyelitis can be a complication of chronic suppurative otitis media or cholesteatoma, or both, and it is much more common than the acute type. Pneumatization of the petrous portion of the temporal bone does not have to be present, since the infection can invade the area by thrombophlebitis, osteitis, or along fascial planes (Allam and Schuknecht, 1968). The infection may persist for months or years, with mild and intermittent signs and symptoms, or may spread to the intracranial cavity and result in one or more of the suppurative complications of ear disease, such as an extradural abscess or meningitis.

Microbiology

The organisms that cause acute petrositits are the same as those that cause acute mastoid osteitis: *S. pneumoniae, H. influenzae,* and beta-hemolytic streptococci. However, chronic petrous osteomyelitis may be caused by the bacteria found in association with chronic suppurative otitis media and cholesteatoma, such as *P. aeruginosa* or *Proteus* species.

Diagnosis

The disease is characterized by pain behind the eye, deep ear pain, persistent ear discharge, and sixth nerve palsy. Eye pain is due to irritation of the ophthalmic branch of the fifth cranial nerve. On occasion, the maxillary and mandibular divisions of the fifth nerve will be involved, and pain will occur in the teeth and jaw. A discharge from the ear is common with acute petrositis but may not be present with chronic disease. Paralysis of the sixth cranial nerve leading to diplopia is a late complication (Glasscock, 1972). Acute petrous osteomyelitis should be suspected when persistent purulent discharge follows a complete simple mastoidectomy for mastoid osteitis. The triad of pain behind the eye, aural discharge, and sixth nerve palsy is known as Gradenigo syndrome.

The diagnosis of acute petrous osteomyelitis is suggested by the unique clinical signs. Standard roetgenograms of the temporal bones may show clouding with loss of trabeculation of the petrous bone. The visualization is uncertain, however, because of normal variation in pneumatization (including asymmetry) and the obscuring of the petrous pyramids by superimposed shadows of other portions of the skull. However, computed tomograms of the temporal bones can lead to diagnosis, and should be obtained if there might be the possibility of an extension of infection into the cranial cavity.

Management

Management of acute petrositis is similar to that described for acute mastoiditis, since at this stage it can be considered as further spread of infection within the pneumatized petrous portion of the temporal bone. However, when acute petrous osteomyelitis and acute mastoid osteitis are present together, a more aggressive surgical approach to management will be required than needed when only the mastoid is involved.

LABYRINTHITIS

This complication of otitis media occurs when infection spreads into the cochlear and vestibular apparatus. The usual portal of entry is the round window, and, less commonly, the oval window, but invasion may take place from an infectious focus in an adjacent area, such as the mastoid antrum, the petrous bone, and the meninges, or as a result of bacteremia. Schuknecht (1974) has classified labyrinthitis into four types: (1) acute serous (toxic) labyrinthitis, in which there may be bacterial toxins or biochemical involvement, but no bacteria are present; (2) acute suppurative (purulent) labyrinthitis, in which bacteria have invaded the otic capsule; (3) chronic labyrinthitis, which is secondary to soft tissue invasion, usually by cholesteatoma and granulation tissue or fibrous tissue; and (4) labyrinthine sclerosis, in which there is replacement of the normal labyrinthine structures by fibrous tissue and bone. Labyrinthitis has also been classified into localized (circumscribed) and generalized types.

Acute Serous (Toxic) Labyrinthitis (With or Without Perilymphatic Fistula)

The acute serous type of labyrinthitis is considered to be one of the most common complications of otitis media. Paparella and coworkers (1972) described the histopathological evidence of serous labyrinthitis in most of the temporal bone specimens from patients who had otitis media. They hypothesized that bacterial toxins from infection in the middle ear enter the inner ear, primarily through an intact round window, or through a congenital defect. The portal of entry may also be through an acquired defect of the labyrinth, such as from head trauma or previous middle ear or mastoid surgery. Biochemical changes within the labyrinth have also been found. The cochlea is usually more severely involved than the vestibular system. Paparella, Goycoolea, and Meyerhoff (1980) reviewed the audiograms of 232 patients who had surgery for chronic otitis media and found a significant degree of bone conduction loss in the younger age groups. In addition, there was a marked difference in the presence and degree of sensorineural loss in the affected ear, compared with the normal ear, in patients of all age groups who had

unilateral disease. They postulated that the high-frequency sensorineural hearing loss that frequently accompanies this disease is due to a pathological insult to the basal turn of the cochlea. Fluctuating sensorineural hearing loss has been described in patients with otitis media and has been thought to be due to either endolymphatic hydrops (Paparella et al., 1979) or a perilymphatic fistula (Grundfast and Bluestone, 1978; Supance and Bluestone, 1983).

The signs and symptoms of serous labyrinthitis (especially when a perilymphatic fistula is present) are a sudden, progressive, or fluctuating sensorineural hearing loss or vertigo, or both, in association with otitis media or one or more of its complications or sequelae, such as mastoid osteitis. The loss of hearing is usually mixed (i.e., there are both conductive and sensorineural components) when serous labyrinthitis is a complication of otitis media. However, in some children who have recurrent middle ear infection, hearing may be normal between episodes, whereas in other children only a mild or moderate sensorineural hearing loss will be present at all times. The presence of vertigo may not be obvious in children, especially infants. Older children may describe a feeling of spinning or turning, whereas younger children may not be able to talk about the symptoms but may manifest disequilibrium by falling, stumbling, or "clumsiness." The vertigo may be mild and momentary, and it may tend to recur over months or years. Spontaneous nystagmus may also be present, but the signs and symptoms of acute suppurative labyrinthitis, such as nausea, vomiting, and deep-seated pain, are usually absent. Fever, if present, is usually due to a concurrent upper respiratory tract infection or acute otitis media.

The presence of a labyrinthine fistula may be identified by performing a fistula test employing a Siegle pneumatic otoscope or by applying positive and negative external canal pressure using the pump-manometer system of an impedance bridge. Results of the fistula test are considered positive if nystagmus or vertigo is produced by the application of the pressures. Electronystagmography is an objective way of documenting the presence or absence of the nystagmus, but the findings of the fistula test may be misleading, since there can be false-positive and false-negative results. The test can be done in the presence of a perforation of the tympanic membrane or tympanostomy tube. Fistulas are frequently associated with congenital or acquired defects in the temporal bone, such as the Mondini malformation. Computerized tomography may be helpful in identifying such defects.

When otitis media with effusion is present, tympanocentesis and myringotomy should be performed to determine the microorganisms present in the middle ear effusion and drainage. If possible, a tympanostomy tube should also be inserted for more prolonged drainage and an attempt to ventilate the middle ear. Antimicrobial agents with efficacy against *S. pneumoniae* and *H. influenzae*, such as ampicillin, should be administered. Following resolution of the otitis media with effusion, the signs and symptoms of the labyrinthitis should rapidly disappear; however, sensorineural hearing loss may persist. If the diagnostic assessment is indicative of a possible congenital or acquired defect of the labyrinth, an exploratory tympanotomy should be performed as soon as the middle ear is free of infection. If a perilymphatic fistula is found, it should be repaired employing muscle. Even when no defect of the oval or round window is identified but a fistula is still suspected, the stapes footplate and round window should be covered with muscle, since a leak may not be present at the time of the tympanotomy but may recur (Supance and Bluestone, 1983). A tympanostomy tube should be reinserted if recurrent otitis media persists.

When acute mastoid osteitis, chronic suppurative otitis media, or cholesteatoma is present, definitive medical and surgical management of these conditions is essential in eliminating the labyrinthine involvement. A careful search for a labyrinthine fistula must be performed when mastoid surgery is indicated. However, a labyrinthectomy is not indicated for serous labyrinthitis.

Any child with sensorineural hearing loss (with or without vertigo) who also has recurrent acute otitis media or chronic otitis media with effusion should be carefully evaluated for the possible existence of serous labyrinthitis, which can be secondary to a perilymphatic fistula. This combination appears to be common, and failure to identify this complication can result in irreversible severe to profound hearing loss, making early diagnosis and prevention imperative. Since prevention of sensorineural hearing loss due to other causes (e.g., congenital, viral) is not yet

possible, our goal should be to prevent this loss of function in those children in whom it can be prevented. In addition, serous labyrinthitis may develop into acute suppurative labyrinthitis.

Acute Suppurative Labyrinthitis

Suppurative (purulent) labyrinthitis may develop as a complication of otitis media or may be one of its complications and sequelae when bacteria migrate from the middle ear into the perilymphatic fluid through the oval or round window, or through a pre-existing temporal bone fracture or an area where bone has been eroded by cholesteatoma or chronic infection, or a congenital defect. (The most common way that bacteria enter the labyrinth is from the meninges, rather than as a complication of otitis media.)

Suppurative labyrinthitis as a complication of otitis media is rare subsequent to the widespread use of antibiotics. In a series of 96 cases of suppurative intratemporal and intracranial complications of acute and chronic otitis media treated during the period from 1956 to 1971, there were only five cases of suppurative labyrinthitis, all of which were secondary to cholesteatoma that had caused a labyrinthine fistula (Juselius and Kaltiokallio, 1972).

The sudden onset of vertigo, disequilibrium, deep-seated pain, nausea and vomiting, and sensorineural hearing loss during an episode of acute otitis media or an exacerbation of chronic suppurative otitis media indicates that labyrinthitis has developed. The hearing loss is severe, and there is loss of the child's ability to repeat words shouted in the affected ear when sound in the opposite ear is masked. Often, spontaneous nystagmus and past-pointing can be observed. Initially, the quick component of the nystagmus is toward the involved ear and there is a tendency to fall toward the opposite side. However, when there is complete loss of vestibular function, the quick component will be toward the normal ear. Laboratory and radiographic studies are not of much diagnostic value. In the absence of associated meningitis, the cerebrospinal fluid pressure and cell count are normal.

Frequently, the onset of suppurative labyrinthitis may be followed by facial paralysis, meningitis, or both. In later stages, cerebellar abscess can develop. Thus, suppurative labyrinthitis is a serious complication of otitis media. The development of purulent labyrinthitis means that infection has spread to the inner ear fluid, and infection can then spread to the subarachnoid space through the cochlear aqueduct, the vestibular aqueduct, or the internal auditory canal.

The treatment of suppurative labyrinthitis in the absence of meningitis consists of otological surgery combined with intensive antimicrobial therapy. If this complication is due to acute otitis media, immediate tympanocentesis and myringotomy with tympanostomy tube insertion is indicated, as described when serous labyrinthitis is present. If acute mastoid osteitis is present, a complete simple mastoidectomy should be performed; however, because this complication is usually secondary to cholesteatoma, a radical mastoidectomy is required. A radical or modified radical mastoidectomy is also appropriate when chronic suppurative otitis media is present without cholesteatoma. If meningitis has also occurred in association with suppurative labyrinthitis, then otological surgery other than a diagnostic and therapeutic tympanocentesis and myringotomy should be delayed until the meningitis is under control. A labyrinthectomy should be performed only if there is complete loss of labyrinthine function or if the infection spreads to the meninges in spite of adequate antimicrobial therapy. Initially, parenteral antimicrobial agents appropriate to manage the primary middle ear and mastoid disease present should be administered, but since cholesteatoma and chronic suppurative otitis media are the most frequent causes of suppurative labyrinthitis, antimicrobials effective for the gram-negative organisms (*P. aeruginosa* and *Proteus* species) are frequently required. However, the results of cultures of middle ear effusion, purulent discharge, or cerebrospinal fluid may alter the selection of antibiotics.

Chronic Labyrinthitis

The most common cause of chronic labyrinthitis as a complication of middle ear disease is a cholesteatoma that has eroded the labyrinth, resulting in a fistula. Osteitis may also cause bone erosion of the otic capsule. The fistula most commonly occurs in the lateral semicircular canal, and it is filled by squamous epithelium of a cholesteatoma, granulation tissue, or fibrous tissue entering

the labyrinth. The middle ear and mastoid are usually separated at the site of the fistula from the inner ear by the soft tissue, but when there is continuity, acute suppurative labyrinthitis may develop.

The signs and symptoms of chronic labyrinthitis are similar to those of the acute forms of the disease (e.g., sensorineural hearing loss, vertigo) except that they are of more subtle rather than of more sudden onset. The disease is characterized by slowly progressive loss of cochlear and vestibular function over a prolonged period of time. The fistula test may be helpful in making the diagnosis of a labyrinthine fistula, and computerized tomography may reveal a defect. When there is complete loss of function, no signs or symptoms of labyrinthine dysfunction may be present.

Since a cholesteatoma is the most common cause of this type of labyrinthitis, middle ear and mastoid surgery must be performed. For children with a labyrinthine fistula due to a cholesteatoma, a modified radical or radical mastoidectomy is the procedure of choice. When labyrinthine function is still present, the cholesteatoma matrix overlying the fistula should be left undisturbed, since removal can result in total loss of function.

Failure to make the diagnosis of this complication and perform the surgery as soon as possible may result in complete loss of cochlear and vestibular function, with possible development of labyrinthine sclerosis or acute suppurative labyrinthitis, which can cause a life-threatening intracranial complication such as meningitis.

FACIAL PARALYSIS

Facial paralysis may occur during an episode of acute otitis media because of exposure of the facial nerve from a congenital bony dehiscence within the middle ear (Figs. 9–22 and 9–23). Facial paralysis is a relatively frequent complication of acute otitis media in infants and children, and when it occurs as an isolated complication, tympanocentesis and myringotomy should be performed and parenteral antibiotics effective for *S. pneumoniae* and *H. influenzae* should be administered. The paralysis will usually improve rapidly without requiring further surgery (i.e., facial nerve decompression). Mastoidectomy is not indicated unless acute mastoid osteitis (acute "coalescent" mastoiditis) is present.

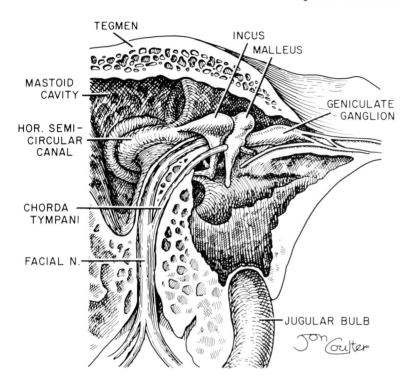

Figure 9–22. The course of the facial nerve in the middle ear and mastoid. The nerve can be involved by infection in these areas and can result in facial paralysis.

However, if there is complete loss of facial function and electrophysiological testing indicates the presence of degeneration or progressive deterioration of the nerve, then facial nerve decompression may be necessary to achieve complete return of function.

During the period from 1960 to 1980, there were 35 cases of facial paralysis associated with acute otitis media at the Children's Hospital of Pittsburgh and The Eye and Ear Hospital of Pittsburgh. The paralysis was partial in 22 (63 percent) and complete in 13 (37 percent). In most instances, initial treatment consisted of antimicrobial therapy and myringotomy. However, of these 35 individuals, seven (20 percent) had further surgery: five underwent facial nerve decompression, and two had simple mastoidectomies (all seven of these children had complete facial paralysis) (Bluestone, C. D., unpublished data).

When a facial paralysis develops in a child who has chronic suppurative otitis media with or without cholesteatoma, immediate surgical intervention is indicated.

CHOLESTEROL GRANULOMA

Cholesterol granuloma is a sequela of chronic otitis media with effusion. It has been described as "idiopathic hemotympanum," since the tympanic membrane appears to be dark blue: a so-called blue eardrum. Unfortunately, this term is a misnomer. There is no evidence that bleeding within the middle ear is related to the cause of this disease; in addition, neither fresh blood nor a microscopic amount of old blood is present (Sade et al., 1980). The condition is rare in all age groups but does occur in children, and it is most likely due to long-standing changes associated with chronic otitis media with effu-

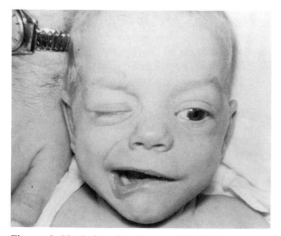

Figure 9–23. Infant in whom a left facial paralysis developed a day after the onset of acute otitis media.

sion (Paparella and Lim, 1967; Sheehy et al., 1969). The blue color of the tympanic membrane as visualized through the otoscope is probably caused by the reflection of light from the thick liquid (granuloma) within the middle ear. The condition must be differentiated from an uncovered, high jugular bulb and a glomus tumor, either tympanicus or jugulare (Valvassori and Buckingham, 1974), and, more commonly, chronic otitis media with effusion or barotitis.

The tissue has been described as being composed of chronic granulations, with foreign body giant cells and foam cells within the middle ear or mastoid, or both. Cholesterol crystals are usually present. The condition is similar to a chronic middle ear effusion except that a soft brownish material that contains shining golden-yellow specks is present. The pathological features of cholesterol granuloma should not be confused with that of a cholesteatoma (Schuknecht, 1974). Similar granulomas have been described in other parts of the body: atheromatous and dermoid cysts, periapical and follicular cysts of the jaw, old infarcts, and hematomas (Korthals Altes, 1966). When the granulomas are stained, prominent iron deposits or hemosiderin may be found (Bak-Pederson and Tos, 1972; Nager and Vanderveen, 1976) but not in sufficient quantities to account for the otoscopic appearance of the blue tympanic membrane.

Cholesterol granulomas occur when the eustachian tube is obstructed by a muscle pedicle flap (Linthicum, 1971) or by a tumor (Sheehy et al., 1969). In addition to occurring as an isolated pathological entity, cholesterol granuloma can be associated with chronic suppurative otitis media with or without cholesteatoma or any inflammation that may obstruct portions of the middle ear or mastoid, or both.

The condition will not respond to medical treatment, middle ear inflation, or myringotomy with tympanostomy tube insertion. However, when a child is observed to have a tympanic membrane that has a dark blue appearance and is unresponsive to nonsurgical management, a myringotomy under general anesthesia should be performed, since, on occasion, chronic otitis media with effusion may also be associated with a blue tympanic membrane (again, probably as the result of the way light from the otoscope is reflected from the middle ear effusion). However, if a thick brown liquid is found at the procedure, successful aspiration of the

material will not be possible, and if a tympanostomy tube is inserted, it will become occluded immediately. The treatment of choice for a cholesterol granuloma is middle ear and mastoid surgery. The granuloma in the mastoid can be removed by performing a complete simple mastoidectomy, and the middle ear portion can be removed by using a tympanomeatal approach. There is no reason to remove the canal wall unless a cholesteatoma is present. A tympanostomy tube should be inserted into the tympanic membrane at the time of the procedure and reinserted as often as needed (i.e., until the middle ear remains normally aerated following spontaneous extubation).

INFECTIOUS ECZEMATOID DERMATITIS

Otitis media with perforation (also a patent tympanostomy tube) can be associated with an infection of the external auditory canal (i.e., external otitis), or occur secondary to a discharge from the middle ear and mastoid. An infection in the mastoid may also erode the bone of the ear canal or the postauricular area, resulting in a dermatitis (Fig. 9–1A). The ear canal skin is erythematous, edematous, and filled with purulent drainage, and yellow-crusted plaques may be present. The organisms involved are usually the same as those found in the middle ear–mastoid infection, but the flora of the external canal may contribute to the infectious process. *Pseudomonas* and *Proteus* species are frequently present. Fungi may also be present in chronic cases; most commonly *Aspergillus niger* or *A. alba* are found. A culture of the external auditory canal should be obtained and the results compared with those of a needle aspiration of the middle ear discharge through the tympanic membrane perforation or the tympanostomy tube; this will aid in determining the offending organisms. Antimicrobial therapy can then be selected by the results of the culture and sensitivity testing. The infection may spread to the auricle, periauricular area, or other parts of the body, possibly as a result of direct implantation of the organisms or, possibly, as an autosensitivity phenomenon. *S. aureus* is the most frequently involved bacterium (Senturia et al., 1980b).

Severe inflammatory stenosis of the external auditory meatus is uncommon and there-

Table 9–4. **OTOTOPICAL AGENTS AVAILABLE TO TREAT OTITIS MEDIA WITH PERFORATION, DISCHARGE, AND SECONDARY ECZEMATOID EXTERNAL OTITIS***

Generic Name	Product Name
Chloramphenicol	Chloromycetin Otic
Colistin sulfate; neomycin sulfate; thonzonium bromide; hydrocortisone acetate	Coly-Mycin S Otic
Polymyxin B; neomycin sulfate; gramicidin; hydrocortisone	Cortisporin Cream and Cortisporin Ointment
Polymyxin B; neomycin sulfate; hydrocortisone	Cortisporin Otic Suspension
Polymyxin B; hydrocortisone	Pyocidin–Otic Solution

*These drugs should be used with care in cases of nonintact eardrum because of the possibility of ototoxicity.

fore can be differentiated from the extreme tenderness and pain that is so commonly present in acute, diffuse external otitis. Also included in the differential diagnosis would be impetigo, secondary infection, and seborrheic dermatitis. Management should be directed toward resolving the middle ear–mastoid infection, which may require medical treatment or surgery, or both. If the skin of the ear canal is the only area of involvement, then a combination of a topical antibiotic with or without hydrocortisone otic drops is usually sufficient to reduce the inflammation (Table 9–4). Polymyxin B, neomycin sulfate with hydrocortisone (Cortisporin Otic Suspension), or colistin sulfate, neomycin sulfate, and thonzonium bromide (Coly-Mycin S Otic) are the most commonly employed medications; however, the ototopical agents may be ototoxic to the cochlea if they penetrate the middle ear and therefore should be used with caution. If a fungal infection is present, *m*-cresyl acetate ear drops (Cresylate) may need to be prescribed. Irrigation of the ear canal with 2 percent acetic acid or frequent suctioning of the ear canal may also hasten the resolution of the external canal infection.

If the adjacent skin around the auricle or other parts of the body is involved, the skin should be cleansed with saline solution or aluminum acetate and treated with a local antibiotic corticosteroid cream (see Table 9–4). The child should be cautioned about spread of the infection from the ear canal to other parts of the body and should refrain from putting his or her finger in the ear or scratching the infected skin. Cotton in the external ear canal can be helpful if profuse drainage is present, but it should be changed as frequently as necessary.

References

Abramson, M., Lachenbruch, P. A., Press, B. H. J., and McCabe, B. F.: Results of conservative surgery for middle ear cholesteatoma. Laryngoscope 87:1281–1287, 1977.

Allam, A. F., and Schuknecht, H. F.: Pathology of petrositis. Laryngoscope 78:1813–1832, 1968.

American Academy of Pediatrics. Committee on Early Childhood, Adoption and Dependent Care. News and Comment 35(9):9, 1984.

Armstrong, B. W.: Tympanoplasty in children. Laryngoscope 75:1062–1069, 1965.

Avery, A. D., Lelah, T., Solomon, N. E., Harris, L. J., Brook, R. H., Greenfield, S., Ware, J. E., Jr., and Avery, C. H.: *Quality of Medical Care Assessment Using Outcome Measures: Eight Disease-Specific Applications.* Prepared for the Health Resources Administration, Department of Health, Education and Welfare by the Rand Corporation, Santa Monica, California, 1976.

Bailey, T. H.: Absolute and relative contraindications to tympanoplasty. Laryngoscope 86:67–69, 1976.

Bak-Pederson, K., and Tos, M.: The pathogenesis of idiopathic haemotympanum. J. Laryngol. Otol. 86:473, 1972.

Baron, S. H.: Management of aural cholesteatoma in children. Otolaryngol. Clin. North Am. 2:71–88, 1969.

Baxter, J. D., and Ling, D.: Ear disease and hearing loss among the Eskimo population of the Baffin zone. Can. J. Otolaryngol. 3:110, 1974.

Beery, Q. C., Doyle, W. J., Cantekin, E. I., Bluestone, C. D., and Wiet, R. J: Eustachian tube function in an American Indian population. Ann. Otol. Rhinol. Laryngol. 89(68):28–33, 1980.

Berko-Gleason, J.: Otitis media and language development (Workshop on Effects of Otitis Media on the Child). Pediatrics 71:639–652, 1983.

Bess, F. H., and Tharpe, A. M.: Unilateral hearing impairment in children. Pediatrics 74:206–216, 1984.

Bezold, F.: Cholesteatom, Perforation der Membrana Flaccida Shrapnelli und Tubenverschluss, eine Atiologische Studie. Ztschrf. Ohrenheilk. 20:5–28, 1889.

Bluestone, C. D.: Eustachian tube obstruction in the infant with cleft palate. Ann. Otol. Rhinol. Laryngol. 80(2):1–30, 1971.

Bluestone, C. D., Wittel, R. A., and Paradise, J. L.: Roentgenographic evaluation of the eustachian tube function in infants with cleft and normal palates. Cleft Palate J. 9:93–100, 1972.

Bluestone, C. D., Beery, Q. C., and Paradise, J. L.: Audiometry and tympanometry in relation to middle ear effusions in children. Laryngoscope 83:594–604, 1973.

Bluestone, C. D., Beery, Q. C., Cantekin, E. I., and Paradise, J. L.: Eustachian tube ventilatory function in relation to cleft palate. Ann. Otol. Rhinol. Laryngol. 84:333–338, 1975.

Bluestone, C. D., Cantekin, E. I., Beery, Q. C., Douglas, G. S., Stool, S. E., and Doyle, W. J.: Functional eustachian tube obstruction in acquired cholesteatoma and related conditions. *In* McCabe, B. F., Sade, J., and Abramson, M. (Eds.): *Cholesteatoma: First International Conference.* Birmingham, Alabama, Aesculapius Pub. Co., 1977, pp. 325–335.

Bluestone, C. D., Cantekin, E. I., Beery, Q. C., and Stool, S. E.: Function of the eustachian tube related to surgical management of acquired aural cholesteatoma in children. Laryngoscope 88:1155–1163, 1978.

Bluestone, C. D., Cantekin, E. I., and Douglas, G. S.: Eustachian tube function related to the outcome of tympanoplasty in children. Laryngoscope 89:450, 1979.

Bluestone, C. D., Casselbrant, M. L., and Cantekin, E. I.: Functional obstruction of the eustachian tube in the pathogenesis of aural cholesteatoma in children. *In* Sade, J. (Ed.): *Cholesteatoma and Mastoid Surgery. Proceedings of the Second International Conference on Cholesteatoma and Mastoid Surgery.* Amsterdam, Kugler, 1982, pp. 211–224.

Bluestone, C. D., and Stool, S. E. (Eds): *Pediatric Otolaryngology.* Philadelphia, W. B. Saunders Co., 1983.

Brandow, E. C., Jr.: Implant cholesteatoma in the mastoid. *In* McCabe, B. F., Sade, J., and Abramson, M. (Eds.): *Cholesteatoma: First International Conference.* Birmingham, Alabama, Aesculapius Pub., 1977, pp. 253–256.

Brook, I.: Prevalence of β-lactamase-producing bacteria in chronic suppurative otitis media. Am. J. Dis. Child. 139:280–283, 1985.

Brown, D. T., Marsh, R. R., and Potsic, W. P.: Hearing loss induced by viscous fluids in the middle ear. Int. J. Pediatr. Otorhinolaryngol. 5:39–46, 1983.

Brummet, R. E., Harris, R. F., and Lindgren, J. A.: Detection of ototoxicity from drugs applied topically to the middle ear space. Laryngoscope 86:1177–1187, 1976.

Cambon, K., Galbreath, J. D., and Kong, G.: Middle ear disease in Indians on the Mount Currie Reservation, British Columbia. Can. Med. Assoc. J. 93:1301–1305, 1965.

Cantekin, E. I., Saez, C. A., Bluestone, C. D., and Bern, S. A.: Airflow through the eustachian tube. Ann. Otol. Rhinol. Laryngol. 88:603–612, 1979.

Cawthorne, T., and Griffith, A.: Primary cholesteatoma of the temporal bone. Arch. Otolaryngol. 73:252–261, 1961.

DeBlanc, G. B.: Otologic problems in Navajo Indians of the southwestern United States. Hear. Instr. 26:15, 1975.

Derlacki, E. L.: Congenital cholesteatoma of the middle ear and mastoid. A third report. Arch. Otolaryngol. 97:177–182, 1973.

Derlacki, E. L., and Clemis, J. D.: Congenital cholesteatoma of the middle ear and mastoid. Ann. Otol. Rhinol. Laryngol. 74:706–727, 1965.

Diamant, M.: *Chronic Otitis. A Critical Analysis.* New York, S. Karger, 1952.

Downs, M. P.: Audiologist's overview of sequelae of early otitis media. Pediatrics 71:643–644, 1983.

Doyle, W. J.: A functiono-anatomic description of eustachian tube vector relations in four ethnic populations: An osteologic study. Microfilm, Ann Arbor, University of Michigan, 1977.

Doyle, W. J., Cantekin, E. I., and Bluestone, C. D.: Eustachian tube function in cleft palate children. Ann. Otol. Rhinol. Laryngol. 89(68):34–40, 1980.

Fischler, R. S., Todd, N. W., and Feldman, C. M.: Otitis media and language performance in a cohort of Apache Indian children. Am. J. Dis. Child. 139:355–360, 1985.

Fisher, B.: The social and emotional adjustment of children with impaired hearing attending ordinary classes. Br. J. Educ. Psychol. 36:319–321, 1966.

Fria, T. J., Cantekin, E. I., and Eichler, J. A.: Hearing acuity of children with otitis media with effusion. Arch. Otolaryngol. 111:10–16, 1985.

Friel-Patti, S., Finitzo-Hieber, T., Conti, G., and Brown, K. C.: Language delay in infants associated with middle ear disease and mild fluctuating hearing impairment. Pediatr. Inf. Dis. 1:104–109, 1982.

Glasscock, M. E.: Chronic petrositis: Diagnosis and treatment. Ann. Otol. Rhinol. Laryngol. 81:677–685, 1972.

Glasscock, M. E.: An exercise in clinical judgment. Laryngoscope 86:70–76, 1976.

Goetzinger, D. P., Harrison, C., and Baer, C. J.: Small perceptive hearing loss: Its effect in school age-children. Volta Rev. 66:124–132, 1964.

Goodey, R. J., and Smyth, G. D.: Combined approach tympanoplasty in children. Laryngoscope 82:166–171, 1972.

Gray, S. W.: Cognitive development in relation to otitis media. Pediatrics 71:645–646, 1983.

Grundfast, K. M., and Bluestone, C. D.: Sudden or fluctuating hearing loss and vertigo in children due to perilymph fistula. Ann. Otol. Rhinol. Laryngol. 87:761–771, 1978.

Habermann, J.: Zur Entstehung des Cholesteatoms des Mittelohrs (Cysten in der Schleimhaut der Paukenhohle, Atrophie der Nerven in der Schnecke). Arch. Ohrenh. (Leipz.) 27:42–50, 1888.

Harker, L. A., and Koontz, F. P.: The bacteriology of cholesteatoma. *In* McCabe, B. F., Sade, J., and Abramson, M. (Eds.): *Cholesteatoma: First International Conference.* Birmingham, Alabama, Aesculapius Pub., 1977, pp. 264–267.

Hellman, K.: Studien uber das Sekundare Cholesteatoma des Felsenbeins. Z. Hals Nas Ohrenheilk. 11:406, 1925.

Herzon, F. S.: Tympanostomy tubes: Infectious complications. Arch. Otolaryngol. 106:645–647, 1980.

Hignett, W.: Effect of otitis media on speech, language, and behavior. Ann. Otol. Rhinol. Laryngol. 92(Suppl. 107):47–48, 1983.

Hinchcliffe, R.: Cholesteatoma: Epidemiological and quantitative aspects. *In* McCabe, B. F., Sade, J., and Abramson, M. (Eds.): *Cholesteatoma: First International Conference.* Birmingham, Alabama, Aesculapius Pub., 1977, pp. 277–286.

Holm, V. A., and Kunze, L. H.: Effects of chronic otitis media on language and speech development. Pediatrics 43:833–839, 1969.

Hubbard, T. W., Paradise, J. L., McWilliams, B. J., Elster, B. A., and Taylor, F. H.: Consequences of unremitting middle ear disease in early life: Otologic, audiologic and developmental findings in children with cleft palate. N. Engl. J. Med. 312:1529–1534, 1985.

Igarashi, M., Konishi, S., Alford, B., and Guilford, F.: The pathology of tympanosclerosis. Laryngoscope 80:233, 1970.

Ingelstedt, S., Flisberg, K., and Ortegren, U.: On the function of middle ear and eustachian tube. Acta Otolaryngol. (Stockh.) Suppl. 182, 1963.

Jaffe, B. R.: The incidence of ear disease in the Navajo Indians. Laryngoscope 79:2126–2134, 1969.

Juselius, H., and Kaltiokallio, K.: Complications of acute and chronic otitis media in the antibiotic era. Acta Otolaryngol. (Stockh.) 74:445–450, 1972.

Kaplan, G. J., Fleshman, J. K., Bender, T. R., Baum, C., and Clark, P. S.: Long-term effects of otitis media: A ten-year cohort study of Alaskan Eskimo children. Pediatrics 52:577–585, 1973.

Karma, P., Jokipii, L., Ojala, K., and Jokipii, A. M. M.:

Bacteriology of the chronically discharging middle ear. Acta Otolaryngol. (Stockh.) 86:110–114, 1978.

Kenna, M., Bluestone, C. D., and Reilly, J.: Medical management of chronic suppurative otitis media without cholesteatoma in children. Laryngoscope 96:146–151, 1986.

Khanna, S. M., and Tonndorf, J.: Tympanic membrane vibrations in cats studied by time-averaged holography. J. Acoust. Soc. Am. 51:1904–1920, 1972.

Kinney, S. E.: Postinflammatory ossicular fixation in tympanoplasty. Laryngoscope 88:821–838, 1978.

Klein, J. O., Teele, D. W., Menyuk, P., Chase, C., Rosner, B., and Greater Boston Otitis Media Study Group: Otitis media and development of speech, language and cognitive abilities. In preparation.

Kodman, F.: Educational status of hard of hearing children in the classroom. J. Speech Hear. Res. 28:297–299, 1963.

Kokko, E.: Chronic secretory otitis media in children. Acta Otolaryngol. (Stockh.) 327:7–44, 1974.

Korthals Altes, A. J.: Cholesterol granuloma in the tympanic cavity. J. Laryngol. Otol. 80:691–698, 1966.

Lange, W.: Tief Eingezogene Membrana Flaccida und Cholesteatom. Z. Hals. Nas. Ohrenheilk. 30:575–582, 1932.

Lau, T., and Tos, M.: Tympanoplasty in children. An analysis of late results. Am. J. Otol. 7:51–59, 1986.

Leviton, A., and Bellinger, D.: Consequences of unremitting middle ear infection in early life. N. Engl. J. Med. 313:1352, 1985.

Lewis, N.: Otitis media and linguistic incompetence. Arch. Otolaryngol. 102:387–390, 1976.

Linthicum, F. H., Jr.: Cholesterol granuloma (iatrogenic), further evidence of etiology, a case report. Ann. Otol. Rhinol. Laryngol. 80:207–210, 1971.

Lowe, J. F., Bamforth, J. S., and Pracy, R.: Acute otitis media: one year in a general practice. Lancet 2:1129–1132, 1963.

Lous, J., and Fiellau-Nikolajsen, M.: A 5-year prospective case-control study of the influence of early otitis media with effusion on reading achievement. Int. J. Pediatr. Otorhinolaryngol. 8:19–30, 1984.

Mawson, S. R., and Ludman, H.: *Diseases of Ear: A Textbook of Otology.* Chicago, Yearbook Medical Publ., 1979, pp. 378–380.

Maynard, J.: Otitis media in Alaskan Eskimo children, an epidemiological review with observation/s on control. Alaska Med., Sept.:93, 1969.

McCafferty, G. J., Coman, W. B., Shaw, E., and Lewis, N.: Cholesteatoma in Australian aboriginal children. *In* McCabe, B., Sade, J., and Abramson, M. (Eds.): *Cholesteatoma: First International Conference.* Birmingham, Alabama, Aesculapius Pub. Co., 1977, pp. 293–301.

McLelland, C. A.: Incidence of complications from use of tympanostomy tubes. Arch. Otolaryngol. 106:97–99, 1980.

McGuckin, F.: Concerning the pathogenesis of destructive ear disease. J. Laryngol. Otol. 75:949–961, 1961.

McKenzie, D.: The pathogeny of aural cholesteatoma. J. Laryngol. Otol. 46:163–190, 1931.

Menyuk, P.: Effects of hearing loss on language acquisition in the babbling stage. *In* Jaffee, B. F. (Ed.): *Hearing Loss in Children.* Baltimore, University Park Press, 1977, pp. 621–629.

Meyerhoff, W. L., Morizono, T., Shaddock, L. C., Wright, C. G., Shea, D. A., and Sikora, M. A.: Tympanostomy tubes and otic drops. Laryngoscope 93:1022–1027, 1983.

Morizono, T., Giebink, G. S., Paparella, M. M., Sikora, M. A., and Shea, D.: Sensorineural hearing loss in experimental purulent otitis media due to *Streptococcus pneumoniae.* Arch. Otolaryngol. 111:794–798, 1985.

Muenker, G.: Results after treatment of otitis media with effusion. Ann. Otol. Rhinol. Laryngol. 89:308–311, 1980.

Nager, F.: The cholesteatoma of the middle ear. Ann. Otol. Rhinol. Laryngol. 34:1249–1258, 1925.

Nager, G. T., and Vanderveen, T. S.: Cholesterol granuloma involving the temporal bone. Ann. Otol. Rhinol. Laryngol. 85:204, 1976.

Needleman, H.: Effects of hearing loss from early recurrent otitis media on speech and language development. *In* Jaffe, B. F. (Ed.): *Hearing Loss in Children.* Baltimore, University Park Press, 1977, pp. 640–649.

Neil, J. F., Harrison, S. H., Morbey, R. D., Robinson, G. A., Tate, G. M., and Tate, H. T.: Deafness in acute otitis media. Br. Med. J. 1:75–77, 1966.

Ojala, L., and Saxen, A.: Pathogenesis of middle ear cholesteatoma arising from Shrapnell's membrane (attic cholesteatoma). Acta Otolaryngol. (Stockh.) Suppl. 100:33–54, 1952.

Olmstead, R. W., Alvarez, M. C., Moroney, J. D., and Eversden, M.: The pattern of hearing following acute otitis media. J. Pediatr. 65:252–255, 1964.

Palva, A., Karma, P., and Karja, J.: Cholesteatoma in children. Arch. Otolaryngol. 103:74–77, 1977.

Paparella, M. M.: Otologic surgery in children. Otolaryngol. Clin. North Am. 10:145–151, 1977.

Paparella, M. M., and Lim, D. J.: Pathogenesis and pathology of the "idiopathic" blue drum. Arch. Otolaryngol. 85:249, 1967.

Paparella, M. M., Oda, M., Hiraida, F., and Brady, D.: Pathology of sensorineural hearing loss in otitis media. Ann. Otol. Rhinol. Laryngol. 81:632–647, 1972.

Paparella, M. M., Goycoolea, M. V., Shea, D., and Meyerhoff, W. L.: Endolymphatic hydrops in otitis media. Laryngoscope 89:43–54, 1979.

Paparella, M. M., Goycoolea, M. V., and Meyerhoff, W. L.: Inner ear pathology and otitis media: A review. Ann. Otol. Rhinol. Laryngol. 89(68):249–253, 1980.

Paradise, J. L.: On tympanostomy tubes: Rationale, results, reservations, and recommendations. Pediatrics 60:86–90, 1977.

Paradise, J. L.: Long-term effects of short-term hearing loss—menace or myth? Pediatrics 71:647–648, 1983.

Paradise, J. L., Bluestone, C. D., and Felder, H.: The universality of otitis media in fifty infants with cleft palate. Pediatrics 44:35–42, 1969.

Paradise, J. L., and Rogers, K. D.: On otitis media, child development, and tympanostomy tubes: New answers or old questions. Pediatrics 77:88–92, 1986.

Peckham, C. S., Sheridan, M., and Butler, N. R.: School attainment of seven-year-old children with hearing difficulties. Dev. Med. Child. Neurol. 14:592–602, 1972.

Ranier, A.: Development and construction of the pyramidal cells. Arch. Ohren.-Nasen-U., Kehlkopfh. 145:3, 1938.

Rapin, I.: Conductive hearing loss effects on children's language and scholastic skills: A review of the literature. Ann. Otol. Rhinol. Laryngol. 88(60):3–12, 1979.

Ratnesar, P.: Aeration: A factor in the sequelae of chronic ear disease among the Labrador and northern Newfoundland coast. *In* McCabe, B., Sade, J., and Abramson, M. (Eds.): *Cholesteatoma: First International Conference.* Birmingham, Alabama, Aesculapius Pub., 1977.

Reed, D., Struve, S., and Maynard, J. E.: Otitis media and hearing deficiency among Eskimo children. A cohort study. Am. J. Publ. Health 57:1657–1662, 1967.

Ritter, F. N.: Complications of cholesteatoma. In McCabe, B. F., Sade, J., and Abramson, M. (Eds.): *Cholesteatoma: First International Conference.* Birmingham, Alabama, Aesculapius Pub., 1977, pp. 430–437.

Ruedi, L.: Cholesteatosis of the attic. J. Laryngol. Otol. 72:593–609, 1958.

Sade, J.: Pathogenesis of attic cholesteatoma: The metaplasia theory. In McCabe, B. F., Sade, J., and Abramson, M. (Eds.): *Cholesteatoma: First International Conference.* Birmingham, Alabama, Aesculapius Pub., 1977, pp. 212–232.

Sade, J., Halevy, A., Klajman, A., and Mualem, T.: Cholesterol granuloma. Acta Otolaryngol. (Stockh.) 89:233–239, 1980.

Sak, R. J., and Ruben, R. J.: Recurrent middle ear effusion in childhood: Implications of temporary auditory deprivation for language and learning. Ann. Otol. Rhinol. Laryngol. 90:546–551, 1982.

Schiff, M., Poliquin, J. F., Catanzaro, A., and Ryan, A. F.: Tympanosclerosis: A theory of pathogenesis. Ann. Otol. Rhinol. Laryngol. 89(70):1–16, 1980.

Schlieper, A., Kisilevsky, H., Mattingly, H., and Yorke, L.: Mild conductive hearing loss and language development: A one year follow-up study. Dev. Behav. Pediatr. 6:65–68, 1985.

Schuknecht, H. F.: *Pathology of the Ear.* Cambridge, Harvard University Press, 1974, pp. 227, 228–233.

Senturia, B. H., Bluestone, C. D., Lim, D. J., and Klein, J. O.: Recent advances in otitis media with effusion. Ann. Otol. Rhinol. Laryngol. 89(68):1–362, 1980a.

Senturia, B. H., Marcus, M. D., and Lucente, F. E.: *Diseases of the External Ear: An Otologic-Dermatologic Manual.* 2nd ed. New York, Grune & Stratton, 1980b.

Severeid, L. R.: Development of cholesteatoma in children with cleft palate: A longitudinal study. In McCabe, B. F., Sade, J., and Abramson, M. (Eds.): *Cholesteatoma: First International Conference.* Birmingham, Alabama, Aesculapius Pub., 1977, pp. 287–292.

Shambaugh, G. E., and Glasscock, M. E.: *Surgery of the Ear.* 3rd ed. Philadelphia, W. B. Saunders Co., 1980, pp. 432–436.

Sheehy, J. L., Linthicum, F. H., Jr., and Greenfield, E. C.: Chronic serous mastoiditis, idiopathic hemotympanum and cholesterol granuloma of the mastoid. Laryngoscope 79:1189–1217, 1969.

Sheehy, J. L., Brachman, D. E., and Graham, M. D.: Complications of cholesteatoma: A report on 1024 cases. In McCabe, B. F., Sade, J., and Abramson, M. (Eds.): *Cholesteatoma: First International Conference.* Birmingham, Alabama, Aesculapius Pub., 1977, pp. 420–429.

Sheehy, J. L., and Anderson, R. G.: Myringoplasty: A review of 472 cases. Ann. Otol. Rhinol. Laryngol. 89(68):331–334, 1980.

Skinner, M. W.: The hearing of speech during language acquisition. Otolaryngol. Clin. North Am. 11:631–650, 1978.

Sobol, S. M., Reichert, T. J., Faw, K. D., Stroud, M. H., Spector, G. J., and Ogura, J. H.: Intramembranous and mesotympanic cholesteatomas associated with an intact tympanic membrane in children. Ann. Otol. Rhinol. Laryngol. 89:312–317, 1980.

Sorensen, H.: Antibiotics in suppurative otitis media. Otolaryngol. Clin. North Am. 10:45–50, 1977.

Stool, S. E., and Randall, P.: Unexpected ear disease in infants with cleft palate. Cleft Palate J. 4:99–106, 1967.

Storrs, L. A.: Contraindications to tympanoplasty. Laryngoscope 86:79–81, 1976.

Supance, J. S., and Bluestone, C. D.: Perilymph fistulas in infants and children. Otolaryngol. Head Neck Surg. 91:663–671, 1983.

Teed, R. W.: Cholesteatoma verum tympani. Its relationship to first epibranchial placode. Arch. Otolaryngol. 24:455–474, 1936.

Teele, D. W., Klein, J. O., Rosner, B. A., and the Greater Boston Otitis Media Study Group: Otitis media with effusion during the first three years of life and development of speech and language. Pediatrics 74: 282–287, 1984.

Todd, W. N.: Otitis media at Canyon Day, Arizona: A 16-year follow-up in Apache Indians. Arch. Otolaryngol. 111:606–698, 1985.

Tschopp, C. H.: Chronic otitis media and cholesteatoma in Alaskan native children. In MCabe, B., Sade, J., and Abramson, M. (Eds.): *Cholesteatoma: First International Conference.* Birmingham, Alabama, Aesculapius Pub., 1977, pp. 290–292.

Tumarkin, A.: A contribution to the study of middle ear suppuration with special reference to the pathogeny and treatment of cholesteatoma. J. Laryngol. Otol. 53:685–710, 1938.

Valvassori, G. E., and Buckingham, R. A.: Middle ear masses mimicking glomus tumors: Radiographic and otoscopic recognition. Ann. Otol. Rhinol. Laryngol. 83:606–612, 1974.

Ventry, I. M.: Research design issues in studies of effects of middle ear effusion. Pediatrics 71:644–645, 1983.

vonTroltsch, A. F.: *Handbuch der Ohrenheilkunde.* Leipzig, 1869.

Watanabe, H., Shin, T., Fukaura, J., Nakaaki, K., and Tsuda, T.: Total actual speaking time in infants and children with otitis media with effusion. Int. J. Pediatr. Otorhinolaryngol. 10:171–180, 1985.

Webster, D. B.: Conductive loss affects auditory neural soma size only during a sensitive postnatal period. In Lim, D. J., Bluestone, C. D., Klein, J. O., and Nelson, J. D. (Eds.): *Recent Advances in Otitis Media with Effusion.* Burlington, Ontario, B. C. Decker Inc., 1983, pp. 344–346.

Wendt, H.: Desquamative Entzundung des Mittelohrs (Cholesteatom des Felsenbeins). Arch. Ohrenheilk. (Leipzig) 14:428, 1873.

Weiderhold, M. L., Zajtchuk, J. T., Vap, J. G., and Paggi, R. E.: Hearing loss in relation to physical properties of middle ear effusions. Ann. Otol. Rhinol. Laryngol. 89:185–189, 1980.

Wiet, R. J.: Patterns of ear disease in the southwestern American Indian. Arch. Otolaryngol. 105:381–385, 1979.

Wiet, R. J., DeBlanc, G. B., Stewart, J., and Weider, D. J.: Natural history of otitis media in the American native. Ann. Otol. Rhinol. Laryngol. 89(68):14–19, 1980.

Wittmaack, K.: Wie ensteht ein genuines Cholesteatom? Arch. Ohren-Nasen-U. Kehlkopfh. 137:306–332, 1933.

Young, C., and McConnell, F.: Retardation of vocabulary development in hard of hearing children. Except. Child Ann. 1957, pp. 368–370.

Zollner, F.: Tympanosclerosis. J. Laryngol. Otol. 70:77–85, 1956.

Zonis, R. D.: Chronic otitis media in the southwestern American Indians: Prevalence. Arch. Otolaryngol. 88:360–365, 1968.

Zonis, R. D.: Chronic otitis media in the Arizona Indian. Ariz. Med. 27:1–6. 1970.

Complications and Sequelae: Intracranial

10

There has been an overall decline in the incidence of suppurative intracranial complications of otitis media since the advent of antimicrobial agents. Today, these complications occur more often in association with chronic suppurative otitis media and mastoiditis, with or without cholesteatoma, than in association with acute otitis media (Juselius and Kaltiokallio, 1972).

The middle ear and mastoid air cells are adjacent to important structures, including the dura of the posterior and middle cranial fossa, the sigmoid venous sinus of the brain, and the inner ear. Suppuration in the middle ear or mastoid, or both, may spread to these structures, producing the following suppurative intracranial complications: meningitis, extradural abscess, subdural empyema, focal encephalitis, brain abscess, lateral (sigmoid) sinus thrombosis, and otitic hydrocephalus (Fig. 10–1).

Multiple complications are frequently dependent on the route of infection. Thus, a patient may have meningitis, lateral sinus thrombosis, and cerebellar abscess or other combinations of suppurative disease involving adjacent areas.

Any child who has acute or chronic otitis media who develops one or more of the following signs or symptoms, especially while receiving medical treatment, should be suspected of having a suppurative intracranial complication: persistent headache, lethargy, malaise, irritability, severe otalgia, onset of fever, nausea, and vomiting. The following would be signs and symptoms demanding an intensive search for an intracranial complication: stiff neck, focal seizures, ataxia, blurred vision, papilledema, diplopia, hemiplegia, aphasia, dysdiadochokinesia, intention tremor, dysmetria, and hemianopsia. Conversely, children with intracranial infection such as meningitis or brain abscess must have middle ear–mastoid disease ruled out as the origin of or concomitant with the central nervous system disease.

In children who have acute or chronic suppurative otitis media, the presence of headache, even though a nonspecific symptom, should indicate a potential complication. Irritability, lethargy, or other changes in personality may be secondary to intracranial spread of the infection. Fever is common when acute infection of the ear is present, but persistent or recurrent fever, particularly after apparently appropriate antimicrobial therapy, may be a potentially dangerous sign of spread. Fever is rarely present in children with chronic suppurative otitis media and, when present, may be a hallmark of an impending intracranial complication.

The diagnosis of intracranial complications has been greatly improved since the advent of computerized tomography, but when not

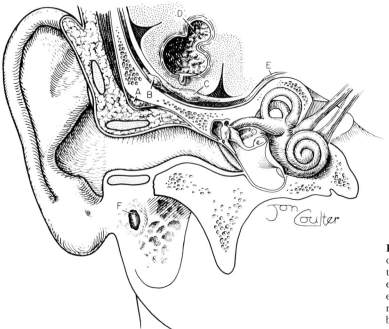

Figure 10–1. Suppurative complications of otitis media and mastoiditis. *A*, Subperiosteal abscess; *B*, extradural abscess; *C*, subdural empyema; *D*, brain abscess; *E*, meningitis; *F*, lateral sinus thrombosis.

available, arteriography should be used. For lesions above the tentorium, electroencephalography and radionuclide brain scanning may be of value as diagnostic procedures. When the lesions are below the tentorium, these methods are not as helpful (du Boulay, 1979).

Intracranial extension of infection may take place because of:

1. Progressive thrombophlebitis permitting the inflammatory process to spread through the intact bone (osteothrombophlebitis),

2. Erosion of the bony walls of the middle ear or mastoid (osteitis), and

3. Extension along preformed pathways—round window, dehiscent sutures, skull fracture, or congenital or surgically acquired bony dehiscenses (mastoidectomy with dura exposure).

In this chapter the incidence, pathogenesis, etiology, diagnosis, management, and outcome for each of these complications as they relate to children will be presented.

INCIDENCE

Prior to the introduction of antimicrobial agents, 2.3 percent of all patients with acute and chronic suppurative otitis media developed intracranial complications, and two thirds of the cases were due to chronic middle ear disease (Turner and Reynolds, 1931). In the antibiotic era, intracranial complications are uncommon, but approximately two thirds are still caused by chronic ear disease (Jeanes, 1962). However, Dawes (1979) reported that most intracranial complications in children were secondary to acute otitis media. Ritter (1977) reviewed 152 cases of cholesteatoma, about half of which were present in patients younger than 20 years of age. The study, which represented cases seen between 1965 and 1970, included four cases with suppurative intracranial complications: two patients with sigmoid sinus thrombosis and one patient each with extradural abscess and brain abscess. In a review by Sheehy, Brackmann, and Graham (1977), of 1024 operations for cholesteatoma performed during the years 1965 through 1974 in 949 patients, 17.7 percent of whom were 15 years of age or younger, only one patient had meningitis and in only two patients was an extradural abscess present; however, neither of these complications occurred in children. The relative incidence of suppurative intracranial complications of acute and chronic otitis media is indicated in a report of 29 consecutive patients treated at a medical center in Finland during the years 1956 through 1971 (Table 10–1). Meningitis was the most common of these complications. This has also been the

Table 10–1. **SUPPURATIVE INTRACRANIAL COMPLICATIONS OF ACUTE OR CHRONIC OTITIS MEDIA IN 29 CHILDREN AND ADULTS—VASA, FINLAND 1956–1971***

	Acute Otitis Media	Chronic Otitis Media	Total
Meningitis	9	5	14
Extradural or perisinuous abscess	3	5	8
Lateral sinus thrombosis	2	3	5
Temporal lobe abscess	0	2	2
Total	14	15	29

*Adapted from Juselius, H., and Kaltiokallio, K.: Complications of acute and chronic otitis media in the antibiotic era. Acta Otolaryngol. (Stockh.) 74:445–450, 1972.

case in other reports in the antibiotic era (Krajina, 1956; Proctor, 1966).

MENINGITIS

Meningitis may be associated with infections of the middle ear in three circumstances:

1. Direct invasion—a suppurative focus in the middle ear or mastoid spreads through the dura and extends to the pia-arachnoid, causing generalized meningitis.

2. Inflammation in an adjacent area—the meninges may become inflamed if there is suppuration in an adjacent area such as a subdural abscess, brain abscess, or lateral sinus thrombophlebitis.

3. Concurrent infection—otitis media arises by contiguous spread from an infectious focus in the upper respiratory tract, and meningitis results from invasion of the blood from the upper respiratory focus. The infections are simultaneous, but meningitis does not arise from the middle ear infection.

The most common route is the third one, concurrent infection with simultaneous bacteremia. Less common is direct extension through congenital preformed pathways or by thrombophlebitis, which usually extends to the middle cranial fossa through the petrosquamous suture or to the posterior cranial fossa through the subarcuate fossa (i.e., the first route). In the preantibiotic era, Lindsay (1938) examined the histopathological features of temporal bones of patients who had had acute otitis media and meningitis

and found that most of the specimens had evidence of direct spread of infection through the petrous apex. However, since the widespread use of antimicrobial agents, extension of infection has been thought to be along preformed pathways or by direct extension through the dura. Spread of infection from the middle ear and mastoid through the inner ear to the meninges is another pathway but is thought to be rare in comparison with the other pathogenic mechanisms. More recently, Eavey and coworkers (1985) examined 16 temporal bones from eight children who had died of meningitis and found otitis media in 14 bones but could not find any evidence that the middle ear infection had spread to the meninges.

The symptoms of meningitis caused by any one of the three mechanisms include fever, headache, neck stiffness, and altered consciousness. Examination of cerebrospinal fluid reveals pleocytosis and elevation of protein concentration in all, but depression of sugar is common in only the first and third types. Polymorphonuclear leukocytes are the predominant cell type in the early phase of meningitis caused by the first and third mechanisms. When infection occurs by the second mechanism, it is likely to be chronic; lymphocytes usually predominate in the cerebrospinal fluid. Organisms are usually isolated from the spinal fluid when meningitis is caused by the first and third mechanisms but not from the second. Thus, meningitis from the second mechanism may be defined as an aseptic meningitis (clinical signs of meningitis associated with cells in the cerebrospinal fluid but without bacteria isolated by usual laboratory techniques).

The organisms associated with meningitis arising from acute otitis media are the common agents of meningitis, *Streptococcus pneumoniae* and *Haemophilus influenzae* type b. About 20 percent of all cases of acute otitis media are due to *H. influenzae*, but less than 10 percent of these are type b. Some of the children with otitis media due to *H. influenzae* show very toxic symptoms, and up to one quarter have concomitant bacteremia or meningitis (Feigin, 1981; Harding et al., 1973).

Initial management of meningitis involves the administration of high doses of appropriate antimicrobial agents. If the causative agent is unknown, ampicillin and chloramphenicol are started. The regimen may be modified after results of cultures are known. If cultures are negative and there is concern that a suppurative focus may be producing the aseptic process, diagnostic tests should be performed to identify the focus, to obtain material for culture, and to clear, usually by incision and drainage, the local infection. If an acute or chronic otitis media with effusion is present, then tympanocentesis, for identification of the causative organism within the middle ear, and myringotomy, for drainage, should be performed immediately. If an acute mastoiditis with osteitis is present, a complete simple mastoidectomy is indicated as soon as the child is able to tolerate a general anesthetic. If chronic suppurative otitis media with or without cholesteatoma is present, then a radical mastoidectomy is frequently required and should be performed when the patient is stable. Appropriate management of any of the suppurative intratemporal (petrositis, labyrinthitis) or intracranial complications (extradural abscess) will also require surgical management.

Occasionally, after trauma to the temporal bone, an acute otitis media develops that is complicated by meningitis. Tympanocentesis and myringotomy should be performed immediately for culture and drainage or culture of the otorrhea, if present. However, exploration of the middle ear and mastoid may be necessary later to search for and repair possible defects in the dura, especially if otorrhea of cerebrospinal fluid is present.

Appropriate management of both the meningitis and the suppurative focus within the temporal bone should result in a favorable outcome, although many studies still report a considerable mortality associated with otitic meningitis. Kessler, Dietzmann, and Krish (1970) reported a mortality rate of 33 percent in their series of 51 patients with otitic meningitis.

EXTRADURAL ABSCESS

Extradural (epidural) abscess usually results from the destruction of bone adjacent to dura by cholesteatoma or infection, or both. This occurs when granulation tissue and purulent material collect between the lateral aspect of the dura and the adjacent temporal bone. Dural granulation tissue within a bony defect is much more common than an actual accumulation of pus. When an abscess is present, a dural sinus thrombosis or, less commonly, a subdural or brain abscess may also be present. If extensive bone

destruction has occurred when acute mastoid osteitis is present, an extradural abscess may develop in the area of the sigmoid dural sinus.

Symptoms can include severe earache, low-grade fever, and headache in the temporal region with deep local throbbing pain, but the more common extradural abscess encountered today may produce no signs or symptoms. Frequently, an asymptomatic extradural abscess is found in patients undergoing elective mastoidectomy for cholesteatoma.

When otorrhea accompanies an extradural abscess, it is characteristically profuse, creamy, and pulsatile. Compression of the ipsilateral jugular vein may increase the rate of discharge and the degree of pulsation. Usually fever is absent, malaise and anorexia are present, but there are no specific neurological signs. Cerebrospinal fluid cell count and pressure are normal unless meningitis is also present. Computerized tomography may demonstrate a sizeable extradural abscess (Fig. 10–2).

Although identification of the infecting organism and appropriate antimicrobial therapy can help prevent the development of an intradural complication from an extradural abscess, the treatment of the extradural abscess consists of surgical drainage. A mastoidectomy is indicated.

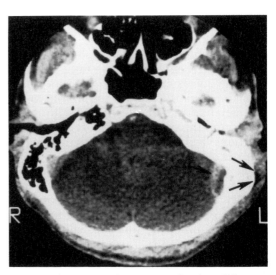

Figure 10–2. Computed tomogram showing a left extradural abscess (*arrow*) as a complication of acute mastoiditis with osteitis and a subperiosteal abscess (*double arrows*).

SUBDURAL EMPYEMA

A subdural empyema is a collection of purulent material within the potential space between the dura externally and the arachnoid membrane internally. Since the pus collects in a preformed space, it is correctly termed empyema rather than abscess. Subdural empyema may develop as a direct extension or, more rarely, by thrombophlebitis through venous channels. It is a rare complication of otitis media.

Children with subdural empyema are febrile and extremely toxic. There are usually signs and symptoms of a locally expanding intracranial mass. Severe headache in the temporoparietal area is often present. Central nervous system findings may include seizures, hemiplegia, dysmetria, belligerent behavior, somnolence, stupor, deviation of the eyes, dysphagia, sensory deficits, stiff neck, and a positive Kernig sign. Hemiplegia and recurrent seizures in a child with suppurative disease of the middle ear and mastoid are indicative of a subdural empyema. Results of computerized tomography often lead to diagnosis. The peripheral white blood cell count is high. The cerebrospinal fluid pressure is high, pleocytosis is present with increased numbers of polymorphonuclear leukocytes, the glucose concentration is normal, and no microorganisms are seen on smear or culture.

Treatment of subdural empyema includes intensive intravenous antimicrobial therapy and neurosurgical drainage of the empyema through burr holes or craniectomy. Mastoid surgery to locate and drain the source of infection is usually delayed until after neurosurgical intervention has yielded some improvement in neurological status. The condition still has a high mortality rate, and more than half of those children who recover will have some neurological deficit.

FOCAL OTITIC ENCEPHALITIS

Focal areas of the brain may become edematous and inflamed as a complication of acute or chronic otitis media or of one or more of the suppurative complications of these disorders, such as an extradural abscess or dural sinus thrombophlebitis. This localized inflammation is called focal otitic encephalitis, and its signs and symptoms may be similar to those that are characteristic of a brain abscess, except that suppuration within the brain is absent. Ataxia, nystagmus, vomiting, and giddiness would indicate a possible focus within the cerebellum, whereas drowsiness, disorientation, restlessness, seizures, and coma may indicate a cerebral focus. In both sites, headache may be present. However, since these signs and symptoms are also commonly associated with a brain abscess or subdural empyema, needle aspiration may be necessary to rule out the presence of an abscess. Computerized tomography is helpful in making this distinction. If an abscess is not thought to be present, then focal encephalitis should be treated by administering antimicrobial agents and by an appropriate otological surgical procedure to remove the infection from within the temporal bone. Failure to control the source of infection may result in development of a brain abscess. Anticonvulsive medication is given when there is cerebral involvement.

BRAIN ABSCESS

Of all age groups, infants and children have the highest incidence of brain abscess (Brewer et al., 1975). However, the incidence of brain abscess has decreased significantly in the antibiotic era. From 1930 to 1960 there were 89 cases of otogenic brain abscess at the Otolaryngological Hospital of the University of Helsinki, whereas between 1961 and 1969 there were only three cases (Tarkkanen and Kohonen, 1970). Several studies have reported that infection of the middle ear and mastoid was the predominant source of infection when abscess in the brain occurred in children (Beller et al., 1973; Liske and Weikers, 1964; Morgan et al., 1973). However, Jadavji and coworkers (1985) reviewed 74 cases of brain abscess diagnosed at Toronto Hospital for Sick Children between 1960 and 1984 and found cyanotic congenital heart disease (24 percent) was the most common cause; 10 children (14 percent) had chronic otitis media with or without mastoiditis. Chronic suppurative otitis media with cholesteatoma is thought to be more commonly the cause when brain abscess is present, but Browning (1984) reviewed 26 consecutive patients with brain abscess and found that 10 of them had chronic ear disease without cholesteatoma.

Otogenic abscess of the brain may follow directly from acute or chronic middle ear and mastoid infection or may follow the development of an adjacent infection, such as lateral sinus thrombophlebitis, petrositis, or meningitis. The dura overlying the infected mastoid is invaded either along vascular pathways or by adherence of the dura to underlying infected bone. Chronic otitis media or mastoiditis with or without cholesteatoma may lead to erosion of the tegmen tympani by pressure necrosis and perforation of the bone, with resultant inflammation of the dura and invasion by pathogenic organisms. An extradural abscess occurs with subsequent infiltration of the dura and spreads to the subdural space. A localized subdural abscess or leptomeningitis ensues. Invasion of brain tissue follows, and the various stages of abscess formation take place: inflammatory reaction, suppuration, necrosis and liquefaction, and development of a fibrinous capsule. If delimitation of the abscess does not occur, infection may extend to the meninges or may rupture into the ventricles.

The site of the abscess is the area closest to the primary source of infection. Thus, temporal lobe abscesses occur after invasion through the tegmen tympani or petrous bone. Cerebellar abscesses occur when the infectious focus is the posterior surface of the petrous bone or thrombophlebitis of the lateral sinus. An abscess in the temporal lobe occurs more commonly than does one in the cerebellum, and multiple abscesses are frequent.

The natural history of brain abscesses includes resorption and healing through gliosis and calcification, spontaneous rupture through a fistulous tract, or spillage into the ventricles or subarachnoid space, producing encephalitis or meningitis.

The bacterial pathogens responsible for brain abscesses include the virulent invasive strains associated with acute disease or the more indolent strains associated with chronic disease (Brewer et al., 1975):

1. Gram-positive cocci—*S. pyogenes, S. pneumoniae, S. viridans,* and *Staphylococcus aureus.*

2. Gram-negative coccobacilli—*H. influenzae* and *H. aphrophilus.*

3. Gram-negative enteric bacilli—*Escherichia coli, Proteus* species, *Enterobacter aerogenes, Enterobacter cloacae,* and *Pseudomonas aeruginosa.*

4. Anaerobic bacteria—*Eubacterium* species, *Bacteroides* species, *Peptostreptococcus* spe-

cies, and *Propionibacterium acnes* (Heineman and Braude, 1963).

Signs of invasion of the central nervous system usually occur about a month after an episode of acute otitis media or an acute exacerbation of chronic otitis media. Systemic signs, including fever and chills, are variable and may be absent. Signs of a generalized central nervous system infection that may occur include severe headache, vomiting, drowsiness, seizures, irritability, personality changes, altered levels of consciousness, anorexia and weight loss, and meningismus. In addition to these signs of an expanding intracranial lesion, there may be specific signs of involvement of the temporal or cerebellar lobes, including signs involving the cranial nerves, such as vertigo, focal seizures, visual field defects, and nystagmus. Temporal lobe abscesses may be silent. There may be persistent purulent ear drainage, suggesting the primary site of infection. Terminal signs include coma, papilledema, or cardiovascular changes.

Diagnosis is based on the development of clinical signs, the results of electroencephalography, and roentgenographic evidence. Computerized tomography is an invaluable aid in diagnosis (Fig. 10–3). Results of radionuclide brain scans can be abnormal when focal encephalitis or a brain abscess is present. Of particular concern is the sudden appearance of signs of acute disease—fever

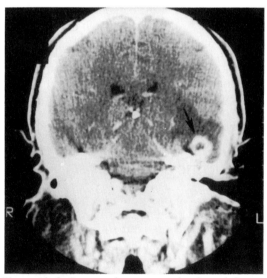

Figure 10–3. Computed tomogram showing a left temporal lobe abscess (*arrow*) as a complication of chronic suppurative otitis media with cholesteatoma.

and headache—in a patient with chronic middle ear disease.

The cerebrospinal fluid may appear normal if the abscess is deep in the tissue and does not produce inflammation of the meninges; if the abscess does produce meningeal inflammation, there may be pleocytosis, initially seen as a predominance of polymorphonuclear leukocytes and then lymphocytes. The concentration of protein may be high, but the sugar level is not usually reduced unless there is bacterial invasion of the meninges. Cultures of spinal fluid are usually negative in the absence of suppurative meningitis. Lumbar puncture should be withheld if there are signs of increased intracranial pressure.

Treatment includes use of antimicrobial agents, drainage or resection of the brain abscess, or both, as well as surgical débridement of the primary focus, the mastoid, or adjacent infected tissues such as is seen in thrombophlebitis of the lateral sinus. The choice of antimicrobial regimen is difficult because of the varied bacteriological characteristics of otogenic brain abscess. Aspiration of the abscess to define its origin is most helpful (Garfield, 1979). Initial therapy should include administration of a penicillin for gram-positive cocci, an aminoglycoside for gram-negative enteric pathogens, and chloramphenicol to combat gram-negative organisms and, more importantly, anaerobic bacteria (see Table 9–4). Even with the administration of antimicrobial agents, the mortality caused by brain abscess has been approximately 30 percent (McGreal, 1962; Morgan et al., 1973). The best results, a mortality rate of zero, were reported in brain abscesses in children treated by catheter drainage (Selker, 1975). More recently, reports have described successful medical treatment of brain abscess without neurosurgical intervention (Berg et al., 1978; Keven and Tyrell, 1984; Rennels et al., 1983).

LATERAL SINUS THROMBOSIS

Lateral and sigmoid sinus thrombosis or thrombophlebitis arises from inflammation in the adjacent mastoid. The superior and petrosal dural sinuses also are intimately associated with the temporal bone, but they are rarely affected. The mastoid infection in contact with the sinus walls produces inflammation of the adventitia, followed by penetration of the venous wall. Formation of a thrombus occurs after the infection has spread to the intima. The mural thrombus may become infected and may propagate, occluding the lumen. Embolization of septic thrombi or extension of infection into the tributary vessels may produce further disease.

This complication is still common in children. Of 13 patients who had otogenic lateral sinus disease at the Groote Schuur Hospital in South Africa during the period from 1967 to 1970, nine were younger than 20 years of age; three children had acute and six had chronic ear infection (Seid and Sellars, 1973).

The clinical signs of lateral sinus thrombosis may be grouped as follows:

1. Systemic—fever, headache, and malaise. With formation of the infectious mural thrombus, the patient may have spiking fever and chills.

2. Signs of increased intracranial pressure—altered states of consciousness, headache, papilledema, and seizures.

3. Signs of intracranial complications—meningitis, cavernous sinus thrombosis, and brain abscess.

4. Signs of disease resulting from metastases of infected thrombi—pneumonia and empyema, bone and joint infection, and, less commonly, thyroiditis, endocarditis, ophthalmitis, and abscess of the kidney (Rosenwasser, 1945).

5. Spread to overlying soft tissue and skin may produce cellulitis or abscess.

Bacteremia is frequent. In Rosenwasser's series of 100 patients published in 1945 (the specific years of the cases are not mentioned but only 19 patients received sulfonamides, so presumably most were evaluated prior to 1935), 80 had presurgery cultures of blood that were positive, and cultures of eight of 17 patients that were negative preoperatively were positive postoperatively. Bacteremia persisted after the operation in 36 cases, for a median of four to five days (range, one to 24 days). The predominant organisms were beta-hemolytic streptococci (68 patients); *S. pneumoniae* type III (three patients), *Bacillus proteus* (*Proteus* species) (two patients), *S. aureus* (one patient), and *Bacillus pyocyaneus* (*P. aeruginosa*) (one patient).

Computerized tomography is an invaluable aid in making the diagnosis and should precede a lumbar puncture whenever lateral sinus thrombosis is suspected. Variations in cerebrospinal fluid pressure occur and can be demonstrated by the Queckenstedt test, which measures changes in cerebrospinal fluid pressure with compression and release of the jugular vein. If the sinus is occluded, there is no rise in pressure when the jugular vein of the affected side is compressed, whereas compression of the contralateral jugular vein results in a brisk rise and fall in pressure. However, if the intracranial pressure is increased, the brain may herniate. In addition to this potential danger, the Queckenstedt test may give falsely negative or inconclusive results (Juselius and Kaltiokallio, 1972). There are usually no other abnormalities in the cerebrospinal fluid, although in some cases leakage of red cells and subsequent xanthochromia may occur (Greer and Berk, 1963).

Management includes use of appropriate antimicrobial agents. The administration of anticoagulant medication has also been advocated. The sinus should be uncovered and any perisinuous abscess drained. The lateral sinus should be opened and the thrombus removed. On rare occasions, the internal jugular vein may have to be ligated. For a complete description of the surgical technique, see the discussion by Shambaugh and Glasscock (1980).

The mortality in the Rosenwasser series (before 1945) was 27 percent, with an increased risk in patients over age 30 years. The mortality rate is still high and has been reported in a large series of cases to be between 10 and 40 percent. Not much has changed with regard to mortality of this intracranial complication 40 years after the introduction of antimicrobial agents.

OTITIC HYDROCEPHALUS

The term "otitic hydrocephalus" was introduced by Symonds in 1931 to describe a syndrome of increased intracranial pressure without abnormalities of cerebrospinal fluid complicating acute otitis media. The pathogenesis of the syndrome is unknown, but since the ventricles are not dilated, the term "benign intracranial hypertension" also seems appropriate. The disease is usually associated with lateral sinus thrombosis.

Symptoms include headache (often intractable), blurring of vision, nausea, vomiting, and diplopia. Signs include a draining ear, abducens paralysis of one or both lateral rectus muscles, and papilledema.

If the diagnosis is suspected, lumbar puncture should be performed after computerized tomography, with a neurosurgeon in attendance. The cerebrospinal fluid pressure is high, sometimes above 300 mm H_2O, but protein, cells, and sugar concentrations are normal and the ventricles are of normal or small size. Although thought of as benign, otitic hydrocephalus in some cases has proceeded to loss of vision secondary to optic atrophy.

Treatment includes use of antimicrobial agents and mastoidectomy. An aggressive surgical approach is warranted because of the possibility of optic atrophy.

PREVENTION

The life-threatening complications of middle ear disease in children are relatively uncommon. Our goal should be to reduce the incidence of these complications still further by effective management of acute and chronic otitis media with effusion and prevention of chronic suppurative otitis media and cholesteatoma. Multiple factors may influence the extension of infection from the middle ear and mastoid to the intracranial cavity; these include virulence of the bacteria, defects in anatomy, or altered host immunity. An impending complication may be prevented from developing into a life-threatening condition if tympanocentesis and myringotomy are performed to identify the causative organism and provide adequate drainage when children with acute otitis media have persistent or recurrent fever, otalgia, or other signs and symptoms of toxicity and are not responding to medical management. In such cases, the results of culture of the middle ear effusion should guide the clinician in the selection of the appropriate antimicrobial agent. If persistent or recurrent discharge through a perforation is present, then a culture should be obtained by aspiration of the purulent material within the middle ear cavity. The antimicrobial agent chosen should be administered in a high dosage schedule that is adequate to prevent a suppurative complication.

In children who have had an episode of meningitis as a complication of acute otitis media, presence of a perilymphatic fistula (i.e., cerebrospinal fluid fistula) must be ruled out, especially if more than one episode of meningitis has occurred. The fistula may be in the area of the oval or round window, or both, and may be of congenital origin or due to an acquired defect (Grundfast and Bluestone, 1978). Suppurative labyrinthitis is usually present, and the fistula must be repaired to prevent recurrence of the intracranial complication. Acute mastoid osteitis and petrositis are other possible intratemporal complications of acute otitis media in which the infection may spread to the intracranial cavity. Early diagnosis and appropriate management of these conditions can prevent intracranial complications.

A suppurative complication should be suspected in children who have the signs and symptoms of acute infection when pre-existing chronic suppurative otitis media is present, with or without a cholesteatoma. An acute exacerbation in a chronically infected ear may destroy bone and permit bacteria to enter the intracranial cavity. A persistent aural discharge may indicate the presence of this type of disease.

In children who have chronic suppurative otitis media and in whom the discharge from the ear is persistent in spite of medical treatment (such as ototopical medication and orally administered antimicrobial agents), hospitalization may be required to provide more aggressive therapy. A parenterally administered antimicrobial agent may be necessary, depending upon the results of culture of the discharge, and direct instillation of appropriate ototopical medication through the tympanic membrane perforation after thorough aspiration of the middle ear may be warranted. This procedure is best performed using the otomicroscope. If the suppurative process continues in spite of this type of medical management, then surgical intervention is indicated. Frequently found in the middle ear and, possibly, the mastoid is a cholesteatoma that could not be identified by inspection of the tympanic membrane even when visualized with the aid of the otomicroscope. Nevertheless, if a cholesteatoma is not present, middle ear and mastoid surgery is still indicated in such cases in order to drain the ear and decrease the possibility of further complications. Tympanoplastic surgery, which may be performed at the time of the initial procedure or as a second-stage operation, may be required to prevent subsequent episodes of discharge (see Chapter 9).

When a cholesteatoma is present, the diagnosis should be made as soon as possible, and surgery is indicated, since structural damage to the middle ear and mastoid is usually progressive and suppurative complications are an ever-present danger. The most important goals of surgery on such ears are complete eradication of the cholesteatoma (or its exteriorization), elimination of the infection, and prevention of potential intratemporal or intracranial complications. If these goals are met, the ear is "safe." Prolonged follow-up of children who have had cholesteatoma is mandatory, since recurrence is common. In patients who have had middle ear and mastoid surgery performed and in whom infection in the middle ear or mastoid cavity, or both, persists in spite of medical management, surgical intervention may again be necessary. In cases in which a radical mastoidectomy has been performed, the middle ear–mastoid discharge may be the result of reflux of nasopharyngeal secretions through a patent eustachian tube into the middle ear. Surgical closure of the eustachian tube at the middle ear end may be required to eliminate the reflux and chronic infection. Likewise, identification of an extradural abscess can prevent spread of the infection further into the intracranial cavity. During surgery, a thorough examination of the tegmen tympani should be performed, since such an abscess may be present as a result of cholesteatoma or infection, or both, in the area. If the cholesteatoma is in the region of the lateral semicircular canal, the possibility of a labyrinthine fistula must be ruled out. Juselius and Kaltiokallio (1972) reported that of 42 patients with labyrinthine fistula, five had suppurative labyrinthitis and meningitis.

Antimicrobial agents have greatly reduced the incidence of intracranial complications of infections of the middle ear and mastoid, but the physician must remain alert to the possibility of an unusual event. In underdeveloped areas of the world, where availability of medical facilities is still limited, complications occur with significant morbidity and mortality (Raikundalia, 1975).

References

Beller, A. J., Sahar, A., and Praiss, I.: Brain abscess: Review of 89 cases over a period of 30 years. J. Neurol. Neurosurg. Psych. 36:757–768, 1973.

Berg, B., Franklin, G., Cuneo, R., Boldrey, E., and Strimling, B.: Nonsurgical care of brain abscess: Early diagnosis and follow-up with computerized tomography. Ann. Neurol. 3:474–478, 1978.

Brewer, N. S., MacCarty, C. S., and Wellman, W. E.:

Brain abscess: A review of recent experience. Ann. Intern. Med. 82:571–576, 1975.

Browning, G. G.: The unsafeness of "safe" ears. J. Laryngol. Otol. 98:23–26, 1984.

Dawes, J. D. K.: Complications of infections of the middle ear. *In* Ballantyne, J., and Groves, J. (Eds.): *Scott-Brown's Diseases of the Ear, Nose, and Throat.* 4th ed., Vol. 2. London, Butterworth and Co., 1979, pp. 305–384.

du Boulay, G. H.: Current practice in neurosurgical radiology. *In* Symon, L. (Ed.): *Neurosurgery.* London, Butterworth and Co., 1979, pp. 13–45.

Eavey, R. D., Gao, Y. Z., Schuknecht, H. F., and Gonzalez-Pineda, M.: Otologic features of bacterial meningitis of childhood. J. Pediatr. 106:402–407, 1985.

Feigin, R. D.: Bacterial meningitis beyond the neonatal period. *In* Feigin, R. D., and Cherry, J. D. (Eds.): *Textbook of Pediatric Infectious Diseases,* Vol. I. Philadelphia, W. B. Saunders Co., 1981, pp. 293–308.

Garfield, J.: Intracranial abscess. *In* Symon, R. (Ed.): *Neurosurgery.* London, Butterworth and Co., 1979, p. 335.

Greer, M., and Berk, M. S.: Lateral sinus obstruction and mastoiditis. Pediatrics 31:840–844, 1963.

Grundfast, K. M., and Bluestone, C. D.: Sudden or fluctuating hearing loss and vertigo in children due to perilymph fistula. Ann. Otol. Rhinol. Laryngol. 87:761–771, 1978.

Harding, A. L., Anderson, P., Howie, V. M., Ploussard, J. H., and Smith, D. H.: *Hemophilus influenzae* isolated from children with otitis media. *In* Sell, S. H., and Karzon, D. T. (Eds.): *Hemophilus influenzae.* Nashville, Vanderbilt University Press, 1973, pp. 21–28.

Heineman, H. S., and Braude, A. I.: Anaerobic infection of the brain: Observations on eighteen consecutive cases of brain abscess. Am. J. Med. 35:682–697, 1963.

Jadavji, T., Humphreys, R. P., and Prober, C. G.: Brain abscess in infants and children. Pediatr. Infect. Dis. 4:394–398, 1985.

Jeanes, A.: Otogenic intracranial suppuration. J. Laryngol. Otol. 76:388–402, 1962.

Juselius, H., and Kaltiokallio, K.: Complications of acute and chronic otitis media in the antibiotic era. Acta Otolaryngol. (Stockh.) 74:445–450, 1972.

Kessler, L., Dietzmann, K., and Krish, A.: Beitrag zur otogenen Meningitis. Z. Laryng. Rhinol. Otol. 49:93–100, 1970.

Keven, G., and Tyrell, L. J.: Nonsurgical treatment of brain abscess: Report of two cases. Pediatr. Infect. Dis. 3:331–334, 1984.

Krajina, Z.: Observations on endocranial complications of the ear and sinuses in the era of antibiotics. Pract. Oto-rhino-laryng. (Basel) 18:1–22, 1956.

Lindsay, J. R.: Suppuration in the petrous pyramid. Ann. Otol. Rhinol. Laryngol. 47:3–36, 1938.

Liske, E., and Weikers, N. J.: Changing aspects of brain abscesses: Review of cases in Wisconsin 1940 through 1962. Neurology 14:294–300, 1964.

McGreal, D. A.: Brain abscess in children. Can. Med. Assoc. J. 86:261–268, 1962.

Morgan, H., Wood, M. W., and Murphey, F.: Experience with 88 consecutive cases of brain abscess. J. Neurosurg. 38:698–704, 1973.

Proctor, C. A.: Intracranial complications of otitic origin. Laryngoscope 76:288–308, 1966.

Raikundalia, K. B.: Analysis of suppurative otitis media in children: Aetiology of non-suppurative otitis media. Med. J. Aust. 1:749–750, 1975.

Rennels, M. B., Woodward, C. L., Robinson, W. L., Gumbinas, M. T., and Brenner, J. T.: Medical cure of apparent brain abscesses. Pediatrics 72:220–224, 1983.

Ritter, F. N.: Complications of cholesteatoma. *In* McCabe, B. F., Sade, J., and Abramson, M. (Eds.): *Cholesteatoma: First International Conference.* Birmingham, Alabama, Aesculapius Pub. Co., 1977, pp. 430–437.

Rosenwasser, H.: Thrombophlebitis of the lateral sinus. Arch. Otolaryngol. 41:117–132, 1945.

Seid, A. B., and Sellars, S. L.: The management of otogenic lateral sinus disease at Groote Schuur Hospital. Laryngoscope 83:397–403, 1973.

Selker, R. G.: Intracranial abscess: Treatment by continuous catheter drainage. Childs Brain 1:368–375, 1975.

Shambaugh, G. E., and Glasscock, M. E.: *Surgery of the Ear.* 3rd ed. Philadelphia, W. B. Saunders Co., 1980, pp. 302–312.

Sheehy, J. L., Brackmann, D. E., Graham, M. D.: Complications of cholesteatoma: A report on 1024 cases. *In* McCabe, B. F., Sade, J., and Abramson, M. (Eds.): *Cholesteatoma: First International Conference.* Birmingham, Alabama, Aesculapius Pub. Co., 1977, pp. 420–429.

Symonds, C. P.: Otitic hydrocephalus. Brain 54:55–71, 1931.

Tarkkanen, J., and Kohonen, A.: Otogenic brain abscess. Arch. Otolaryngol. 91:91–92, 1970.

Turner, A. L., and Reynolds, E. E.: *Intracranial Pyogenic Diseases.* Edinburgh, Oliver and Boyd, 1931.

Index

Note: Page numbers in *italics* indicate illustrations; those followed by t indicate tables.